ADVANCES IN CANCER MANAGEMENT

Edited by **Ravinder Mohan**

Advances in Cancer Management
Edited by Ravinder Mohan

Published by InTech
Janeza Trdine 9, 51000 Rijeka, Croatia

Publishing Process Manager Masa Vidovic

Technical Editor Teodora Smiljanic

Cover Designer InTech Design Team

Additional hard copies can be obtained from orders@intechopen.com

Advances in Cancer Management, Edited by Ravinder Mohan
p. cm.
ISBN 978-953-307-870-0

For EU product safety concerns:
IN TECH d.o.o., Prolaz Marije Krucifikse Kozulić 3, 51000 Rijeka, Croatia, info@intechopen.com or visit our website at intechopen.com.

Meet the editor

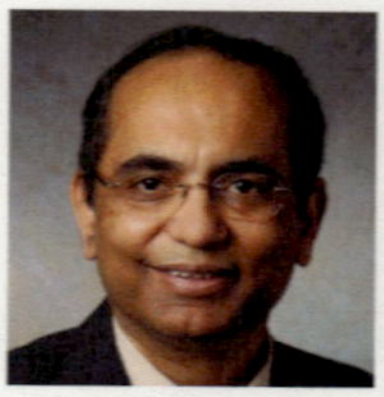

Dr Ravinder Mohan, MD, PhD teaches and practices family medicine in Virginia and also works as a hospitalist physician. He became interested in research on health-related quality of life in Belgium, where he followed clinical outcomes in heart surgery patients. He later used similar methods in Virginia, to evaluate the quality of life of patients who had knee arthritis, and subsequently of patients before and after treatment of localized prostate cancer. Dr. Mohan's research has been published in over 35 high-impact factor peer-reviewed journals and he has also contributed to chapters in five books.

Contents

Preface

Cancer strikes individuals and families both unexpectedly and devastatingly. In the U.S., one in two men and one in three women will be diagnosed with a non-skin cancer. According to a 2008 report by the World Health Organization's International Agency for Research in Cancer, by 2010 cancer would have overtaken heart disease to be the number one cause of death globally with a disproportionate increase in middle- and lower income countries. Accordingly, the war on cancer is being fought on a global scale both in the laboratory and in clinical settings.

This book presents advances in a wide variety of approaches to manage cancer. Some of these include the evolving understanding of how Vitamin D and cancer are related, how psychological factors contribute in the development of cancer, and present newer clinical approaches in the management of cancers of the breast, prostate, rectum, and brain. Other chapters describe novel cell surface markers to help in the diagnosis and prognosis of cancers, the use of proteomics to find newer anti-cancer targets for monoclonal antibodies, newer techniques to expand the use of MALDI mass spectrometry in cancer diagnosis and treatment, and newer computational tools to find anti-cancer drugs. Finally, an author discusses how we can contain the rising cost of cancer treatments and make them more affordable to patients all over the world.

Assoc. Prof. Dr. Ravinder Mohan
Full-time Clinical Faculty,
Department of Family and Community Medicine,
Eastern Virginia Medical School, Norfolk, Virginia,
USA

1

Vitamin D and Cancer

Khanh vinh quốc Lương and Lan Thị Hòang Nguyễn
Vietnamese American Medical Research Foundation,
United States

1. Introduction

Vitamin D has been known as a regulator of bone and mineral metabolism by regulation of calcium absorption in the gut and reabsorption by the kidney, which is mediated by the vitamin D receptor (*VDR*). The expression of *VDR* in a variety of cell lines coupled with increased evidence of *VDR* involvement in cell differentiation and inhibition of cellular proliferation suggests that vitamin D plays a role in many diseases. A meta-analysis of randomized controlled trials demonstrated that intake of vitamin D supplements was associated with a significant 7% reduction in mortality from any causes (Autier & Gandini, 2007). A serum 25-hydroxyvitamin D_3 (25OHD_3) concentration of 25 nmol/l was associated with a 17% reduction in incidence of cancer, a 29% reduction in total cancer mortality, and a 45% reduction in digestive system cancer mortality (Giovannucci et al., 2006). A low serum 25OHD_3 was prospectively associated with an increased risk of fatal cancer in patients referred to coronary angiography (Pilz et al., 2008).

Alphacalcidol, a vitamin D analogue, has been demonstrated significant antitumor activity in patients with low-grade non-Hodgkin's lymphoma of the follicular, small-cleaved cell type (Raina et al., 1991). In patient with parathyroid cancer, vitamin D has been shown to avert or delay the progression of recurrence (Palmieri-Sevier et al., 1993). In locally advanced or cutaneous metastatic breast cancer, topical calcipotriol treatment reduced in the diameter of treated lesions that contained *VDR* (Bower et al., 1991). In a clinical trial, high-dose calcitriol decreased Prostatic-specific antigen (PSA) levels by 50% and reduced thrombosis in prostate cancer patients (Beer et al., 2003 & 2006). In hepatocellular carcinoma, calcitriol and its analogs have been reported to reduce tumor volume, increase apoptosis of hepatocarcinoma cells by 21.4%, and transient stabilization of the serum alpha-fetoprotein levels (Dalhoff et al., 2003; Luo et al., 2004; Morris et al., 2002).

Calcitriol additively or synergistically potentiates the antitumor of other types of chemotherapeutic agents. Calcitriol enhances cellular sensitivity of human colon cancer cells to 5-fluorouracil (Liu et al., 2010). Combination of calcitriol and cytarabine prolonged remission in elderly patients with acute myeloid leukemia (AML) and myelodysplastic syndrome (MDS) (Slapak et al., 1992; Ferrero, et al., 2004). In a prospective study, a combination of active vitamin D and α- interferon has shown to be effective in patients with metastatic renal cell carcinoma (Obara et al., 2008). Calcitriol promotes the anti-proliferative effects of gemcitabine and cisplatin in human bladder cancer models (Ma et al., 2010), and also potentiates antitumor activity of paclitaxel and docetaxel (Hershberger et al., 2001; Ting et al. 2007). A phase II study showed that high-dose calcitriol with docetaxel may increase time to progression in patients with incurable pancreatic cancer when compared with docetaxel monotherapy (Blanke, 2009).

2. Risk factors for the development of both vitamin D deficiency and cancer

It has been noted that vitamin D and cancer share many of the same risk factors, including both environmental (air pollution, geographic and seasonal) and genetic risk factors.

2.1 Environmental factors

Changes in the environment, such as those caused by air pollution, geographic and seasonal factors, may cause diseases that contribute to the development of both vitamin D deficiency and cancer.

2.1.1 Air pollution factors

Atmospheric pollution has been suggested to be a cause of reduced vitamin D synthesis in the skin. In Australia, some authors demonstrated a large difference in vitamin D synthesis between an urban canyon (urbanized environment with tall building) and a typical suburban area (~2.5 km away from urban area) (Kinley et al., 2010). Increased atmospheric pollution may be related to haze from industrial and vehicle sources and lead to decrease in absorption of ultraviolet-B (UVB) photons, thereby reducing the cutaneous vitamin D synthesis (Mimms, 1996; Hollick, 1995). In another study, some reported that the higher atmospheric pollution, the lower the amount of UVB light reaching ground level (Agarwal et al., 2002). They also showed that children living in areas of high atmospheric pollution are at risk of developing vitamin D deficiency rickets. In a study Belgian postmenopausal women who participated in outdoor activities during the summer, urban inhabitants were reported to have an increased prevalence of vitamin D deficiency compared with rural inhabitants (Manicourt & Devogelaer, 2008). In a cross sectional study, living in a polluted area plays a significant independent role in vitamin D deficiency (Hosseinpanah et al., 2010). Similarly, cancer mortality rates (esophagus, stomach, colon-rectum, liver, lung, breast, and bladder) in 263 counties in all Provinces of China were inversely associated with solar UVB exposure by using the National Central Cancer Registries (NCCR) of China, satellite measurements of cloud-adjusted ambient UVB intensity that were obtained from the NASA Goddard Space Flight Center Data Archive Center database, and the Geographic Information System (GIS) methods (Chen et al., 2010). Cancer incidence rates (esophagus, stomach, colon-rectum, and cervix) in 30 counties were inversely correlated with ambient UVB exposure. Lung cancer mortality has been shown the strongest inverse correlation with an estimated 12% fall per 10 mW/(nm m^2) increase in UVB irradiance even adjusted for smoking. These associations were similar to those observed in a number of populations of European origin.

2.1.2 Geographic factors

The relationship between the geographical variation of colon cancer mortality rates and vitamin D related to UVB was first proposed in 1980 (Garland & Garland, 1980). The authors showed that the colon mortality rates are highest in the Northeast and lowest in the Southwest of the United States from 1950 - 1969 and was correlated to the annual hours of sunshine. It has been observed that with each 10 degrees distance from equator, there is a progressive decrease in UVB radiation exposure (Diffey, 1991). Solar UVB is the primary source of vitamin D for most people living on Earth. Nuclear submarine crewmen who were not exposed to UVB for 3 months showed a decrease in an already low circulating $25OHD_3$ level from 13.7 to 7.9 ng/ml (Garland & Garland, 1980). Grant determined that 14 types of cancer (bladder, breast, colon, endometrial, esophageal, gallbladder, gastric, ovarian, pancreatic, rectal, renal and vulvar cancer and both Hodgkin's and non-Hodgkin's lymphoma) had mortality rates inversely correlated with solar UVB levels (Grant, 2009). During the cold weather, latitude was found to determine levels of vitamin D-producing UV radiation. As latitude increase, vitamin D producing UV radiation decreases dramatically and may inhibit vitamin D synthesis in humans (Kimlin et al., 2007).

2.1.3 Seasonal factors

Seasonal variations of $25OHD_3$ were reported either in southern and northern latitudes (Oliveri et al., 1993; Stryd et al., 1979). Another study confirmed and quantified the relatively large seasonal fluctuations in circulating $25OHD_3$ levels in association with summer sun exposure among outdoor workers. Their median serum $25OHD_3$ levels decreased from 122 nmol/L in late summer to 74 nmol/L in late winter (Barger-Lux & Heany, 2002). Similarly, a seasonal pattern has been noticed in many cancers with the highest in the winter and springs – including lung cancer, brain tumors, parathyroid tumor, non-Hodgkin's lymphoma, Hodgkin's lymphoma, childhood leukemia/lymphoma, monocytic leukemia, breast cancer, thyroid cancer, bladder carcinoma, and cervical cancer. In the summer and autumn season, certain cancers (breast, colon, prostate, Hodgkin's lymphoma, and lung) have a better survival rates than during other seasons (Luong & Nguyen, 2010).

2.2 Genetic factors

Genetic studies provide an excellent opportunity to link molecular variations with epidemiological data. *DNA* sequences variations such as polymorphisms have modest and subtle biological effects. Receptors play a crucial role in the regulation of cellular function, and small changes in their structure can influence intracellular signal transduction pathways.

The *VDR* is expressed and regulated in mammary gland during the reproductive cycle (Zinser & Welsh, 2004). *VDR* ablation is associated with ductal ectasia of the primary ducts, loss of secondary and tertiary ductal branches and atrophy of the mammary fat pad (Welsh et al., 2011). *VDR* has also been demonstrated to be lowered in human colorectal adenocarcinoma biopsies (34.5%) than in adjacent normal mucosa (82.5%) (Meggouh et al., 1990). In this colorectal adenocarcinoma, the incidence decreased from right colon (64.7%) to left colon (27.7%), and rectum (15%). Certain allelic variations in the *VDR* may also be genetic risk factors for developing tumors. There are five important common polymorphisms within the *VDR* gene region that are likely to exert functional effects on *VDR* expression. *Cdx2*, located in the promoter region of exon 1, affects the binding ability of *VDR* and subsequent *VDR* transcription activity; *Fok*1 located in translation start of the exon 2; and three other variants (*Bsm*1, *Apa*1 and *Taq*1) located at the 3′ end of *VDR*s that may influence *VDR* expression by altering the *mRNA* stability. In a review of the literature, an association of *VDR* polymorphisms and cancer prognosis are reported to be strongest for prostate cancer (*Fok*1 and *Taq*1), breast cancer (*Bsm*1, *Taq*1 and *Apa*1), malignant melanoma

(*Bsm*1, *Fok*1 and *Taq*1), renal cell carcinoma (*Taq*1), colorectal cancer (*Apa*1, *Fok*1, *Bsm*1, and *Taq*1), epithelial ovarian cancer (*Fok*1), lung cancer (*Taq*1), and oral squamous cell carcinoma (*Taq*1) (Köstner et al., 2009; Mahmoudi et al., 2010; Slattery et al., 2001; Slattery et al., 2006; Taylor et al., 1996; Lundin et al., 1999; Hutchinson et al., 2000; Tamez et al., 2009; Dogan et al., 2009; Bektas-Kayhan et al., 2010). However, other reports are conflicting and the role of *VDR* polymorphisms remains obscure. Their studies revealed no relationship between prostate and breast cancers and *VDR* variants (Ntais et al., 2003; Császá & Abel, 2001; Newcomb et al., 2002; Buyru et al., 2003).

There are numerous potential gene products that are transcriptionally activated by *p53* and are involved in cell cycle arrest or apoptosis (Ko & Prives, 1996). Some authors demonstrated a trend toward lower risk of a *p53* mutation with increased hours of sunshine exposure (Slattery et al., 2010). They also reported specific point mutations of the *p53* gene were associated with the *Fok*1 and *Cdx2 VDR* genotypes. The *p53* is one of the more commonly mutated genes in rectal and pancreatic tumors (Slattery et al., 2009; Slebos et al., 2000). The mutated *p53* gene increases the nuclear accumulation of *VDR*, even in the absence of added vitamin D, and converts vitamin D into an anti-apoptotic agent (Stambolsky et al., 2010).

The cytochrome P_{450} (*CYP*) is responsible for the oxidation, peroxidation, and/or reduction of vitamins, steroids, xenobiotics, and metabolism of drugs. The *CYP27B*1 (25-hydroxyvitamin D_3-1α-hydroxylase) enzyme catalyzes the 1α-hydroxylation of the 25OHD$_3$ to 1,25OHD$_3$, the most active form of vitamin D_3 metabolite. 1α-hydroxylase is down-regulated early in the neoplastic process of prostatic cancer cells (Chen et al., 2003; Hsu et at., 2001). In another study, the common genotypic variation in *CYP27B*1, however, has little or no effect on overall prostate cancer risk (Holt et al., 2009). The *CYP27B1 mRNA* in malignant breast tumors was reported to decrease in comparison with normal mammary tissue (McCarthy et al., 2009). 1α-hydroxylation levels were found elevated in malignant pancreatic cells and their proliferation is inhibited by prohormone 25OHD$_3$ (Schwartz et al., 2004). Calcitriol significantly increased the 24-hydroxylase *mRNA* in the human cervical adenocarcinoma and the human ovarian adenocarcinoma cell lines (Kloss et al., 2010). The *CYP24A1* encodes for the catabolic enzyme 24-hydroxylase and is responsible for inactivating vitamin D metabolites. The *CYP24A1 gene* was found to be amplified in breast cancer (Albertson et al., 2000). In prostate cancer mortality, significantly altered risks of recurrence/progression were observed in relation to genotype for two *tagSNPs* (single-nucleotide polymorphisms) of *VDR*, *CYP24A1*, and one *CYP27B*1 (Holt et al., 2010); *CYP24A1* expression is inversely correlated with promoter *DNA* methylation in prostate cancer cell lines (Luo et al., 2010), and its overexpression was also observed to be associated with poorer survival in patients with lung adenocarcinoma (Chen et al., 2011). The gene encoding for *CYP24A1* and *CYP27B*1 have been observed to be expressed in colon cancer cells (Anderson et al., 2006; Tangpricha et al., 2001). Variants of *CYP24A1* and *CYP27B*1 have also been reported to be associated with risk of distal colon cancer (Dong et al., 2009). There is a deregulation of the vitamin D signaling and metabolic pathways in breast cancer (Lopes et al., 2010). The *VDR* was strongly associated with the estrogen receptor positivity in breast carcinomas. *CYP27B1* expression is slightly lower in invasive carcinomas (44.6%) than in benign lesions (55.8%). In contrast, *CYP24A1* expression was augmented in carcinomas (56% in *in situ* and 53.7% in invasive carcinomas) when compared with that in benign lesions (19%). In another study, however, it has found no difference in the expression of the *VDR*,

CYP27B1, and *CYP24A1 mRNA* in breast cancer and non-neoplastic mammary tissue (de Lyra et al., 2006).

Vitamin D binding protein (DBP) is the main transporter of vitamin D in the bloodstream. DBP-macrophage activating factor (DBP-maf) is considered to be deglycosylated DBP in cancer patients causing inability to activate macrophages and a strong inhibitory activity on prostate tumor cells (Rehder et al., 2009; Gregory et al., 2010). DBP-maf acts as a potent anti-angiogenic factor and inhibits tumor growth *in vivo* (Kalkunte et al., 2005). These authors also reported that DBP-maf also inhibited the vascular endothelial growth factor (VEGF) signaling.

3. Role of vitamin D and its analog in cancer

Calcitriol acts mainly via its high affinity receptor *VDR* through a complex network of genomic (transcription and post-transcription), binds to intracellular *VDR*, which subsequently heterodimerizes with another nuclear retinoid X receptor (*RXR*) and non-genomic mechanisms which may indirectly affect gene transcription via the regulation of intracellular signaling pathways that target transcription factors. *VDR* expressed has been detected in a variety of cultured human cell lines. In breast cancer, the protein levels of the *VDR* were elevated in sensitive cell lines upon $1{,}25OHD_3$ treatment, whereas resistant clones were unable to induce *VDR* (Jensen et al., 2002). The authors suggested that the levels of *VDR* in cancer might serve as a prognostic marker in cancer treatment with $1{,}25OHD_3$.

Calcitriol is a potent regulator of cell proliferation, differentiation and apoptosis in a variety of cell types. Calcitriol and its analogs induce apoptosis in tumor cells through the activation of a caspase cascade (Guzey et al., 2002; Weitsman et al., 2003). The caspases have been considered the pivotal executioner of all programmed cell death (Hengartner, 2000). However, calcitriol may induce apoptosis in cancer cells through another novel cascade- and *p53*-independent pathway that can be inhibited by *Bcl*-2 (Mathiasen et al., 1999). Calcitriol and its analogs may cause apoptosis in cancer cells directly by increasing intracellular free calcium ([Ca2+]i) (Vandewalle et al., 1995) and indirectly through the activation of a calcium-dependent cysteine protease, *μ-calpain* (Berry et al., 1999; Mathiasen et al., 2002). Furthermore, calcitriol stimulates membrane phospho-inositide breakdown in human colon cancer cell line, causing translocation of protein kinase C to the membrane, and increasing $[Ca^{2+}]_i$ by both releasing calcium stores and promoting calcium influx (Wali et al., 1992). Calcitriol and it analogs are potent inducers of both active and latent forms of transforming grow factor beta (TGFβ), which participates in the regulation of cell growth, phenotype, and differentiation in various tissues (Koli & Keski-Oja, 1995; Laiho & Keski-Oja, 1992).

Calcitriol has been shown to mediate a G_2/M cell cycle progression and induce cell death in a number of cancer cell lines via direct induction of $GADD_{45a}$, which is a *DNA*-induced and *p53*-regulated gene that plays an essential role in cell cycle control and *DNA* repair (Jiang et al., 2003; Akutsu et al., 2001). By contrast, the anti-proliferative functions of *VDR* are associated at the G_0/G_1 stage of the cell cycle, coupled with upregulation of a number of cell cycle inhibitors, kinase inhibitors $p21^{(waf1/cip1)}$ (Saramäki et al., 2006). However, paricalcitol arrested in G_1/G_0 phases and G_2/M phases in leukemia cell lines, in G_1G_0 in myeloma cells, and induced the expression of $p21^{(waf1/cip1)}$ and $p27^{(Kip1)}$, and down –regulation of $p45^{SKP2}$ (Wang et al., 1996; Munker et al., 1996; Jiang et al., 1994; Lin et al., 2003).

Angiogenesis has been suggested as an indicator of neoplastic transformation. Calcitriol has been reported a potent inhibitor of tumor cell-induced angiogenesis (Shokravi et al., 1995; Majewski et al., 1996). Calcitriol inhibits hypoxia inducible factor-1(HIF-1)/VEGF pathway in human cancer cells (Ben-Shoshan et al., 2007). Increased levels of HIF-1 activity are often associated with increased tumor aggressiveness, therapeutic resistance, and mortality (Semenza, 2003). VEGF stimulates endothelial cells to proliferate, migrate, and organize into capillary beds (Polverini et al., 2002). DBP-maf inhibited VEGF signaling by decreasing VEGF-mediated phosphorylation of VEGFR-2 and ERK1/2, a downstream target of the VEGF signaling cascade (Kalkunte et al., 2005). Calcitriol and its analogs have been demonstrated to inhibit tumor invasion and metastasis by reducing the expression of serine proteinases, metalloproteinases (MMP-2 and MMP-9), VEGF and parathyroid hormone related peptide (*PTHrP*) in lung carcinoma cell lines (LLC-GFP cells) (Nakagawa et al., 2005a). The metastatic growth of LLC-GFP cells was remarkably reduced in response to calcitriol (Nakagawa et al., 2005b).

Calcitriol and its analogs induced the expression of tumor suppressor gene *PTEN* (phosphatase and tensin homolog deleted on chromosome 10) (Liu et al., 2005; Kumagai et al., 2003). Overexpression of *VDR* stimulated the activity of *PTEN* promoter and also enhances the *PTEN* protein level (Pan et al., 2009). The *PTEN* phosphatase can block phosphoinositide 3-kinase/AKT (PI3K/Akt) signaling pathway, which contribute to both cell death and the inhibition of cell proliferation (Cantley & Neel, 1999). *PTEN* mutations have been found in many human cancers (Tamura et al., 1999). In colon cancer cells, calcitriol and its analogs increase the expression of *E-cadherin*, a transmembrane protein located in intercellular adherent junctions, which make cells more adherent to each other (Pálmer et al., 2001). Loss of *E-cadherin* expression is a common even during the transition from adenoma to carcinoma (Perl et al., 1998). *E-cadherin* is a tumor suppressor gene, and its decrease in expression is associated with poor prognosis in patients with prostate cancer (Umbas et al., 1994). Vitamin D also suppresses *tenascin-C*, which promotes growth, invasion, and angiogenesis during tumorigenesis (Gonzàlez-Sancho et al., 1998).

The induction of ornithine decarboxylase (ODC) may be an essential process in the mechanism of tumor promotion (O'brien et al., 1975), and calcitriol has been reported to inhibit tumor promoter-induced ODC expression in the skin, stomach, colon, and liver in animals (Hashiba et al., 1987). Calcitriol, however, did not induce epidermal ODC activity, but inhibited the induction of ODC by the tumor promoters 12-0-tetradecanoylphorbol-13-acetate (TPA) and teleocidin, suggesting that it is an anti-promoter rather than a promoter in mouse skin carcinogenesis (Chida et al., 1984).

Calcitriol has been reported to regulate the transcription of the tumor necrosis factor alpha (TNF-α) without affecting translation in leukemia cell line (Steffen et al, 1988), may increase the sensitivity of cancer cells to TNF-α and potentiates the cytotoxic effect of the cytokine (Yacobi et al., 1996), which is an important factor in immunological anti-cancer therapy. TNF-α potentiates the effect of $1{,}25OHD_3$ in inducing of differentiation of human myeloid cell lines (Trinchieri et al., 1987).

Prostaglandins (PGs) have been shown to play a role in the development and progression of many cancers. Calcitriol has been reported to regulate the expression of several key genes involved in the PG pathway causing a decrease in PG synthesis (Moreno et al., 2005). Cyclooxygenase (COX) participates in the conversion of arachidonic acid to PGs. COX-2 has been reported to increase in various malignancies (van Rees et al., 2001; Ristimaki et al., 2002). Calcitriol and its analogs decreased expression of COX-2 in colon cancer cells (Kumagai et al., 2003). Selective COX-2 inhibitor reduces the polyp in patients with familial adenomatous polyposis (Steinbach et al., 2000). 15-hydroxy-prostaglandin dehydrogenase (15-PGDH) is the enzyme that catalyzes the conversion of PGs to their corresponding 15-

keto derivatives; 15-PGDH has been demonstrated as an oncogene antagonist and plays a tumor-suppressive role in colon cancer (Yan et al., 2004). Calcitriol increases 15-PGDH *mRNA* and protein expression in various prostate cancer cells (Moreno et al., 2005). Calcitriol has also found to regulate COX-2 and 15-PGDH expression in other cells (Pichaud et al., 1997; Aparna et al., 2008). Calcitriol and its analogs can significantly decrease intestinal tumor load in *Apc*^{Min} mice (Huerta et al., 2002). Vitamin D and its metabolites have been known to inhibit cell proliferation in human rectal mucosa and a colon cancer cell line (Thomas et al., 1992).

The human peroxisome proliferator-activated receptor delta (*PPARδ*) and *VDR* signaling pathways regulate a multiple of genes that are of importance for a multiple of cellular functions including cell proliferation, cell differentiation, immune response and apoptosis. The provided link between *VDR* and *PPAR* may play an important role in treatment in prostate cancer and melanoma (Peehl & Feldman, 2004; Sertznig et al., 2009). *PPARδ* expression was reported to be increased by 1.5–3.2-fold after a 3-h stimulation of breast and prostate cancer cell lines with 1,25OHD$_3$ (Dunlop et al., 2005). *PPARδ* has been reported to regulate lung cancer cell growth (Fukumoto et al., 2005) and it also may attenuate colon and skin carcinogenesis (Hartman et al., 2004; Marin et al., 2006; Kim et al., 2004). In addition, *PPARδ* deficiency does not suppress intestinal tumorigenesis in *Apc*$^{Min/+}$ mice (Reed et al., 2004).

Hypercalcemia is a common complication of paraneoplastic syndromes and is a contributor to the morbidity of cancer patients; in most cases, hypercalcemia is mediated by *PHTrP*. The *PTHrP* production has been suppressed by 1,25OHD$_3$ and its analogs in cancer cell line via down-regulation and suppression of epidermal growth factor (ECF)-induced *PTHrP* gene expression (Kremer et al., 1996; Kunakornsawat et al., 2002; Fazon et al., 1998). Calcitonin has been known to secrete in response to high calcium level and C cell of the human medullary carcinoma and was suppressed by calcitriol (Telenius-Berg et al., 1975; Zabel & Dietel, 1991).

4. Conclusion

Vitamin D certainly has a role in the prevention and treatment of cancer. It is necessary to check serum 25OHD$_3$ and parathyroid hormone (PTH) status in cancer patients. Serum levels of PTH have been reported to correlate with PSA levels and colorectal cancer (Skinner & Schwartz, 2009; Charalampopoulos et al., 2010). Some authors proposed that, in patients with normal calcium levels, the serum 25OHD$_3$ levels should be stored to > 55ng/ml in cancer patients (colon, breast, and ovary) (Garland et al., 2007). Calcitriol, 1,25OHD$_3$, is best used for cancer treatment, because of its active form of vitamin D$_3$ metabolite, suppression of PTH levels (acted as cellular growth factor), and their receptors presented in most of human cells. However, monitor of serum 25OHD$_3$ after taking calcitriol is not necessary because calcitriol inhibits the production of serum 25OHD$_3$ by the liver (Bell et al., 1984; Luong & Nguyen, 1996). The main limitation to the clinical widespread evolution of 1,25OHD$_3$ is its hypercalcemic side-effects.

5. References

Agarwal, KS; Mughal, MZ; Upadhyay, P; et al. (2002). The impact of atmostpheric pollution on vitamin D status of infants and toddlers in Delhi, India. *Arch Dis Child.* Vol.87, pp.111-113.

Anderson, MG; Nakane, M; Ruan, X; et al. (2003). Expression of VDR and CYP24A1 mRNA in human tumors. *Cancer Chemother Pharmacol.* Vol.57, pp.234-240.

Albertson, DG; Ylstra, B; Segraves, B; et al. (2000). Quantitative mapping of amplicon structure by array CHG identifies CYP24 as a candidate oncogene. *Nat Genet.* Vol.25, pp.144-146.

Aparna, R; Subhashini, J; Roy, KR; et al. (2008). Selective inhibition of cyclooxygenase-2 (COX-2) by 1alpha-,25-dihydroxy-16-ene-23-yne-vitamin D_3, a less calcemic vitamin D analog. *J Cell Biochem.* Vol.104, pp.1832-1842.

Autier, P and Gandini, S (2007).Vitamin D supplementation and total mortality: a meta-analysis of randomized controlled trials. *Arch Intern Med.* Vol.167, pp.1730-1737.

Barger-Lux, MJ; Heany, RP. (2002). Effects of above average summer sun exposure on serum 25-hydroxyvitamin D and calcium absorption. *J Clin Endocrinol Metab.* Vol.87, pp.4952-4956.

Beer, TM; Lemmon, D; Lowe, BA; et al. (2003). High-dose weekly oral calcitriol in patients with a rising PSA after prostatectomy or radiation for prostate carcinoma. *Cancer.* Vol.97, pp.1217-1224.

Beer, TM; Venner, PM; Ryan, CW; et al. (2006). High dose calcitriol may reduce thrombosis in cancer patients. *Br J Hematol.* Vol.135, pp.392-394.

Bektas-Kayhan, K; Unür, M; Yaylim-Eraltan, I; et al. (2010). Association of vitamin D receptor Taq1 polymorphism and susceptibility to oral squamous cell carcinoma. *In Vivo.* Vol.24, No.5, pp.755-759.

Ben-Shoshan , M; Amir, S; Dang, DT; et al. (2011). 1α,25-dihydroxyvitamin D_3 (calcitriol) inhibits hypoxia-inducible factor-1/vascular endothelial growth factor pathway in human cancer cells. *Mol Cancer Ther.* Vol.6, No.4, pp.1433-1439.

Bell, NH; Shaw, S; and Turner, RT. (1984). Evidence that 1,25-dihydroxyvitamin D_3 inhibits the hepatic production of 25-hydroxyvitamin D in man. *J Clin Invest.* Vol.74, pp.1540-1544.

Berry, DM and Meckling-Gill, KA. (1999). Vitamin D analogs, 20-epi-22-oxa-24a,26a,27a-trihomo-1α,25$(OH)_2$-vitamin D_3, 1,24$(OH)_2$-22-ene-24-cyclopropyl-vitamin D_3 and 1α,25$(OH)_2$-lumisterol$_3$ prime NB4 leukemia cells for monocytic differentiation via nongenomic signaling pathways, involving calcium and calpain. *Endocrinology.* Vol.140, pp.4779-4488.

Blanke, CD; Beer, TM; Todd; et al. (2009). Phase II study of calcitriol-enhanced docetaxel in patients with previously untreated metastatic or locally advanced pancreatic cancer. *Investigational New Drugs.* Vol. 27, No.4, pp.374-378.

Bower, M; Colston, KW; Stein, RC; et al. (1991). Topical calcipotriol treatment in advanced breast cancer. *Lancet.* Vol.337, No.8743, pp.701-702.

Buyru, N; Tezol, A; Yosonkaya-Fenerci, E; Dalay, N. (2003). Vitamin D receptor gene polymorphisms in breast cancer. *Exp Mol Med.* Vol.35, pp.550-555.

Cantley, LC and Neel, BG. (1999). New insights into tumor suppression: PTEN suppresses tumor formation by restraining the phosphinositide 3-kinase/AKT pathway. *Proc Natl Acad Sci USA.* Vol.96, pp.4240-4245.

Charalampopoulos, A; Charalabopoulos, A; Batistatou, A; et al. (2010). Parathormone and 1,25$(OH)_2D_3$ but not 25$(OH)D_3$ serum levels, in an inverse correlation, reveal an association with advanced stages of colorectal cancer. *Clin Exp Med.* Vol.10, pp.69-72.

Chen, TC; Wang, L; Whitlatch, LW; et al. (2003). Prostatic 25-hydroxyvitamin D-1alpha-hydroxylase and its implication in prostate cancer. *J Cell Biochem.* Vol.88, pp.315-322.

Chen, W; Clements, M; Rahman, B; et al. (2010). Relationship between cancer mortality/incidence and ambient ultraviolet B irradiance in China. *Cancer Causes Control.* Vol.21, No.10, pp.1701-1709.

Chen, G; Kim, SH; King, AN; et al. (2011). CYP24A1 is an independent prognostic marker of survival in patients with lung adenocarcinoma. *Clin Cancer Res.* Vol.17, No.4, pp.817-826.

Chida, K; Hashiba, H; Suda, T; et al. (1984). Inhibition by 1α,25-dihydroxyvitamin D_3 of induction of epidermal ornithine decarboxylase caused by 12-0-tetradecanoylphorbol-13-acetate and teleocidin B. *Cancer Res.* Vol.44, pp.1387-1391.

Császá, A and Abel, T. (2001). Receptor polymorphisms and diseases. *Eur J Pharmacol.* Vol.414, pp.9-22.

de Lyra, EC; da Silva, IA; Katayama, ML; et al. (2006). $25(OH)_2D_3$ serum concentration and breast tissue expression of 1alpha-hydroxylase, 24-hydroxylase and vitamin D receptor in women with and without breast cancer. *J Steroid Biochem Mol Biol.* Vol.100, No.4-5, pp.184-192.

Dalhoff, K; Dancey, J; Astrup, L; et al. (2003). A phase II study of the vitamin D analogue Seocalcitol in patients with inoperable hepatocellular carcinoma. *Br J Cancer.* Vol.89, pp252-257.

Diffey, BL. (1991). Solar ultraviolet radiation effects on biologic systems. *Phys Med Biol.* Vol.36, pp.299-328.

Dogan, I; Onen, HI; Yurdakul, AS; et al. (2009). Polymorphisms in the vitamin D receptor gene and risk of lung cancer. *Med Sci Monit.* Vol.15, No.8, pp.BR232-242.

Dong, LM; Ulrich, CM; Hsu, L; et al. (2009). Vitamin D related genes, *CYP24A1* and *CYP27B1*, and colon cancer risk. *Cancer Epidemiol Biomakers Prev.* Vol.18, No.9, pp.2540-2548.

Dunlop, TW; Väisänen, S; Frank, C; et al. The peroxisome proliferator-activated receptor delta gene is a primary target of 1α,25-dihydroxyvitamin D_3 and its nuclear receptor. *J Mol Biol.* Vol.349, pp.248-260.

Falzon, M; and Zong, J. (1998). The noncalcemic vitamin D analogs EB 1089 and 22-oxacalcitriol suppress serum-induced parathyroid hormone-related peptide gene expression in a lung cancer cell line. *Endocrinology.* Vol.139, pp.1046-1053.

Ferrero, D; Campa, E; Dellacasa, C; et al. (2004). Differentiating agents + low-dose chemotherapy in the management of old/poor prognosis patients with acute myeloid leukemia or myelodysplastic syndrome. *Haematologica.* Vol.89, pp.619-620.

Fukumoto, K; Yano, Y; Virgona, N; et al. (2005). Peroxisome proliferator-activated receptor delta as a molecular target to regulate lung cancer cell growth. *FEBS Lett.* Vol.579, pp.3829-3836.

Garland, CF and Garland, FC. (1980). Do sunlight and vitamin D reduce the likelihood of colon cancer? *Int J Epidemiol.* Vol.9, pp.227-231.

Garland, CF; Grant, WB; Mohr, SB; et al. (2007). What is the dose-response relationship between vitamin D and cancer risk? *Nutr Rev.* Vol.65, No.8, Pt.2, pp.S91-S95

Giovannucci, E; Liu, Y; Rimm, EB; et al. (2008). Prospective study of predictors of vitamin D status and cancer incidence and mortality in men. *J Natl Cancer Inst.* Vol.98, pp.451-459.

González-Sancho, JM; Alvarez-Dolado, M; Muñoz, A. (1998). 1,15-dihydroxyvitamin D_3 inhibits tenascin-C expression in mammary epithelial cells. *FEBS Lett.* Vol.426, pp.225-228.

Grant,WB. ((2009). How strong is the evidence that solar ultraviolet B and vitamin D reduce the risk of cancer. *Dermato-Endocrinology.* Vol.1, No.1, pp.17-24.

Gregory, KJ; Zhao, B; Bielenberg, DR; et al. (2010). Vitamin D binding protein-macrophage activating factor directly inhibits proliferation, migration, and uPAR expression of prostate cancer cells. *PLos One.* Vol.5, No.10, p.213428.

Guzey, M; Kitada, S; Reed, JC; et al. (2002). Apoptosis induction by 1alpha,25-dihydroxyvitamin D_3 in prostate cancer. *Mol Cancer Ther.* Vol.1, pp.667-677.

Hartman, FS; Nicol, CJ; Marin, HE; et al. (2004). Peroxisome proliferator-activated receptor delta attenuates colon carcinogenesis. *Nat Med.* Vol.10, pp.481-483.

Hashiba, H; Fukushima, M; Chida, K; et al. (1987). Systemic inhibition of tumor promoter-induced ornithine decarboxylase in 1α,25-dihydroxyvitamin D_3-treated animals. *Cancer Res.* Vol.47, pp.5031-5035.

Hengartner, MO. (2000). The biochemistry of apoptosis. *Nature.* Vol.407, pp.770-776.

Hershberger, PA; Yu, WD; Modzelewski, RA; et al. (2001). Calcitriol (1,25-dihydroxycholecalciferol) enhances paclitaxel antitumor activity in vitro and in vivo and accelerates paclitaxel-induced apoptosis. *Clin Cancer Res.* Vol.7, pp.1043-1051.

Hollick, MF. (1995), Environmental factors that influence the cutaneous production of vitamin D. *Am J Clin Nutr.* Vol.61(suppl), pp.638S-645S.

Holt, SK; Kwon, EM; Peters, U; et al. (2009). Vitamin D pathway gene variants and prostate cancer risk. *Cancer Epidemiol Biomarkers Prev.* Vol.18, No.6, pp.1928-1933.

Holt, SK; Kwon, EM; Koopmeiners, JS; et al. (2010). Viamin D pathway gene variants and prostate cancer prognosis. *Prostate.* Vol.70, No.13, pp.1448-1460.

Hosseinpanah, F; Hashemi pour, S; Heibatollahi. M; et al. (2010). The effects of air pollution on vitamin D status in healthy women: A cross section study. *BMC Pub Health.* Vol.10, p.519.

Hsu, JY; Feldman, D; McNeal, JE; et al. (2001). Reduced 1alpha-hydroxylase activity in human prostate cancer cells correlates with decreased susceptibility to 25-hroxyvitamin D_3-induced growth inhibition. *Cancer Research.* Vol.61, pp.2852-2856.

Huerta, S; Irwin, RW; Heber, D; et al. (2002). 1alpha,25$(OH)_2$-D_3 and its synthetic analogue decrease tumor load in the Apc^{min} mouse. *Cancer Res.* Vol.62, No.1, pp.741-746.

Hutchinson, PE; Osborne, JE; Lear, JT; et al. (2000). Vitamin D receptor polymorphisms are associated with altered prognosis in patients with malignant melanoma. *Clin Cancer Res.* Vol.6, pp.498-504.

Jiang, H; Lin, J, Su, ZZ; et al. (1994). Induction of differentiation in human promyelotic HL-60 leukemia cells activates p21, WAF1/CIP1, expression in the absence of p53. *Oncogene.* Vol.9, pp.3397-3406.

Jensen, SS; Madsen, MW; Lucas, J; et al. (2002). Sensitivity to growth suppression by 1alpha,25-dihydroxyvitamin D_3 among MCF clones correlates with vitamin D receptor protein induction. (2002). *J Steroid Biochem Mol Biol.* Vol.81, pp.123-133.

Kalkunte, S; Brard, L; Granai, CO; Swamy, N. (2005). Inhibition of angiogenesis by vitamin-D binding protein: characterization of anti-endothelial activity of DBP-maf. *Angiogenesis.* Vol.8, pp.349-360.

Kim, DJ; Akiyama, TE; Hartman, FS; et al. (2004). Peroxisome proliferator-activated receptor beta (delta)-dependent regulation of ubiquitin C expression contributes to attenuation of skin carcinogenesis. *J Biol Chem.* Vol.279, pp.23719-23727.

Kimlin, MG; Olds, WJ; Moore, MR. (2007). Location and vitamin D synthesis: is the hypothesis validated by geographical data? *J Phochem Photobiol B.* Vol.86, pp.234-239.

Kinley, AM; Janda, M; Auster, J; Kimlin, M. (2010). In vitro model of vitamin D synthesis by UV radiation in an Australian urban environment. *Photochem Photobiol.* First published online: 2010 Dec 22. DOI: 10.1111/j.1751-1097.2010.00865.x

Kloss, M; Fischer, D; Thill, M; et al. (2010). Vitamin D, calcidiol and calcitriol regulate vitamin D metabolizing enzymes in cervical and ovarian cancer cells. *Anticancer Res.* Vol.30, No.11, pp.4429-4434.

Ko, LJ and Prives, C. (1996). p53: puzzle and paradigm. *Genes Dev.* Vol.10, pp.1054-1072.

Koli, K and Keski-Oja, J. (1995). 1,25-dihroxyvitamin D_3 enhances the expression of transforming growth factor β1 and its latent form binding protein in cultured breast carcinoma cells. *Cancer Res.* Vol.55, pp.1540-1546.

Köstner, K; Denzer, N; Müller, CS; et al (2009). The relevance of vitamin D receptor (VDR) gene polymorphisms for cancer: a review of the literature. *Anticancer Res.* Vol.29, No.9, pp.3511-3536.

Kremer, R; Shustik, C; Tabak, T; et al. (1996). Parathyroid-hormone-related peptide in hematologis malignancies. *Am J Med.* Vol.100, No.4, pp.406-411.

Kumagai, T; O'Kelly, J; Said, JW; et al. (2003). Vitamin D_2 analog 19-nor-1,25-dihroxyvitamin D_2: antitumor activity against leukemia, myeloma, and colon cancer cells. *J Natl Cancer Inst.* Vol.95, No.12, pp.896-905.

Kunakornsawat, S; Rosol, TJ; Capen, CC; et al. (2002). Effects of 1,25-dihydroxyvitamin D_3 [$1,25(OH)_2D_3$] and its analogs (EB1089 and analog V) on canine adenocarcinoma (CAC-8) in nude mice. *Biol Pharm Bull.* Vol.25, pp.642-647.

Ma, Y; Yu, WD; Trump, DL; et al. (2010). Enhances antitumor activity of gemcitabine and cisplatin in human bladder cancer models. *Cancer.* Vol.116, pp.3294-3303.

Mahmoudi, T; Mohebbi, SR; Pourhoseingholi, MA; et al. (2010). Vitamin D receptor gene Apa1 polymorphism is associated with susceptibility to colorectal cancer. *Dig Dis Sci.* Vol.55, No.7, pp.2008-2013.

Majewski, S; Skopinska, M; Marczak, M; et al. (1996). Vitamin D3 is a potent inhibitor of tumor cell-induced angiogenesis. *J Invest Dermatol Symp Proc.* Vol.1, No.1, pp.97-101.

Manicourt, DH and Devogelaer, JP. (2008). Urban tropospheric ozone increases the prevalence of vitamin D deficiency among Belgian postmenopausal women with outdoor activities during summer. *J Clin Endocrinol Metab.* Vol.93, pp.3893-3899.

Marin, HE; Peraza, MA; Billin, AN; et al. (2006). Ligand activation peroxisome proliferator-activated receptor delta inhibits colon carcinogenesis. *Cancer Res.* Vol.66, pp.4394-4401.

Mathiasen, IS; Lademann, U; Jäättelä, M. (1999). Apoptosis induced by vitamin D compounds in breast cancer cells is inhibited by Bcl-2 but does not involve known caspases or p53. *Cancer Res.* Vol.59, pp.4848-4856.

Mathiasen, IS; Sergeev, IN; Bastholm, L; et al. (2002). Cacium and caplain as key mediators of apoptosis-like death induced by vitamin D compounds in creast cancer cells. *J Biol Chem.* Vol.277, pp.30738-30745.

McCarthy, K; Laban, C; Bustin, SA; et al. (2009). Expression 25-hydroxyvitamin D_3-1α-hydroxylase, and vitamin D receptor mRNA in normal and malignant breast tissue. *Anticancer Res.* Vol.29, No.1, pp.155-157.

Meggouh, F; Lointier, P; Pezet, D; Saez, S. (1990). Evidence of 1,25-dihydroxyvitamin D_3 in human digestive mucosa and carcinoma tissue biopsies taken at different levels of the digestive tract, in 152 patients. *J Steroid Biochem.* Vol.36, No.1-2, pp.143-147.

Mims, FM 3rd. (1996). Significant reduction of UVB caused by smoke from biomass burning in Brazil. *Photochem Photobiol.* Vol.64, pp.814-816.

Moreno, J; Krishnan, AV; Swami, S; et al. (2005). Regulation of prostaglandin metabolism by calcitriol attenuates growth stimulation in prostate cancer cells. *Cancer Res.* Vol.65, pp.7917-7925.

Morris, DL; Jourdan, JL; Finlay, I; et al. (2002). Hepatic intra-arterial injection of 1,25-dihydroxyvitamin D_3 in lipiodol: pilot study in patients with hepatocellular carcinoma. *Int J Oncol.* Vol.21, pp.901-906.

Munker, R; Kobayashi, T; Elstner, E; et al. (1996). A new series of vitamin D analogs is highly active for clonal inhibition, differentiation, and induction of WAF1 in myeloid leukemia. *Blood.* Vol.88, pp.2201-2209.

Nakagawa, K; Sasaki, Y; Kato, S; et al. (2005a). 22-Oxa-1alpha-25-dihydroxyvitamin D_3 inhibits metastasis and angiogenesis in lung cancer. *Carcinogenesis.* Vol.26, pp.1044-1054.

Nakagawa, K; Kawaura, A; Sato, S; et al. (2005b). 1 alpha,25dihydroxyvitamin D_3 is a preventive factor in the metastasis of lung cancer. *Carcinogenesis.* Vol.26, pp. 294-440.

Newcomb, PA;Kim, H;Trentham-Dietz, A; et al. (2002). Vitamin D receptor polymorphism and breast cancer risk. *Cancer Epidemiol Biomarkers Prev.* Vol.11, pp.1503-1504.

Ntais, C; Polycarpou, A; Ioannidis, JP. (2003). Vitamin D receptor gene polymorphisms and risk of prostate cancer: a meta-analysis. *Cancer Epidemiol Biomarkers Prev.* Vol.12, pp.1395-1402.

Laiho, M and Keski-Oja, J. (1992). Transforming growth factor-β: as regulators of cellular growth and phenotype. *CRC Crit Rev Oncogenesis.* Vol.3, pp.1-26.

Lin, R; Wang, TT; Miller, WH; et al. (2003). Inhibition of F-Box protein p45^{SKP2} expression and stabilization of cyclin-dependent kinase inhibitor p27^{KIP1} in vitamin D analog-treated cancer cells. *Endocrinology.* Vol.144, pp.749-753.

Liu, W; Asa, SL; Ezzat, S. (2005). 1α,25-dihydroxyvitamin D_3 target PTEN-dependent fibronectin expression to restore thyroid cancer cell adhesiveness. *Mol Endocrinol.* Vol.19, pp.2349-2357.

Liu, G; Hu, X; Chakrabarty, S; et al. (2010). Vitamin D mediates its action in human colon carcinoma cells in a calcium-sensing receptor-dependent manner: downregulates malignant cell behavior and the expression of thymidylate synthase and surviving and promotes cellular sensitivity to 5-FU. *Int J Cancer.* Vol.126, pp.631-639.

Lopes, N; Sousa, B; Martins, D; et al. (2010). Alterations in vitamin D signaling and metabolic pathways in breast cancer progression: a study of VDR, CYP27B1 and CYP24A1 expression in benign and malignant breast lesions vitamin D pathways unbalanced in breast lesions. *BMC Cancer*. Vol.10, p.483.

Lundin, AC; Söderkvist, P; Erichsson, B; et al. (1999). Association of breast cancer progression with a vitamin D receptor gene polymorphism. *Cancer Res.* Vol.59, pp.2332-2334.

Luo, WJ; Chen, JY; Xu, W; et al. (2004). Effects of vitamin D analogue EB1089 on proliferation and apoptosis of hepatic carcinoma cells. *Zhonghua Yu Fang Yi Xue Za Zhi*. Vol.38, pp.415-418. [article in Chinese]

Luo, W; Karpf, AR; Deeb, KK; et al. (2010). Epigenetic regulation of vitamin D 24-hydroxylase/CYP24A1 in human prostate cancer. *Cancer Res.* Vol.70, No.14, pp.5953-5962.

Luong, VQK and Nguyen, THL. (1996). Coexisting hyperparathyroidism and primary hyperparathyroidism with vitamin D-deficient osteomalacia in a Vietnamese immigrant. *Endocrine Practice*. Vol.2, pp.250-254.

Luong, VQK and Nguyen, THL. (2010). The beneficial role of vitamin D and its analogs in cancer treatment and prevention. *Crit Rev Oncology/Hematology*. Vol.73, pp.192-201.

O'Brien, TG; Simsiman, RC; Boutwell, RK. (1975). Induction of the polyamine-biosynthetic enzymes in mouse epidermis and their specificity for tumor promotion. *Cancer Res.* Vol.35, pp.2426-2433.

Obara, W; Mizutani, Y; Oyama, C; et al. (2008). Prospective study of combined treatment with interferon-alpha and active vitamin D_3 for Japanese patients with metastatic renal cell carcinoma. *Int J Urol*. Vol.15, No.9, pp.794-799.

Oliveri, MB; Ladizesky, M; Mautalen, CA; et al. (1993). Seasonal variations of 25-hydroxyvitamin D and parathyroid hormone in Ushuala (Argentina), the southernmost city of the world. *Bone Miner*. Vol.20, pp.99-108.

Pálmer, HG; González-Sancho, JM; Espada, J; et al. (2001). Vitamin D_3 promotes the differentiation of colon carcinoma cells by the induction of *E-cadherin* and the inhibition of β-catenin signaling. *J Cell Biol.* Vol.154, No.2, pp.369-387.

Palmieri-Sevier, A; Palmieri, GM; Baumgartner, CJ; Britt, LG. (1993). Case report: long-term remission of parathyroid cancer: possible relation to vitamin D and calcitriol therapy. *Am J Med Sci.* Vol.306, No.5, pp.309-312.

Perl, AK; Wilgenbus, P; Dahl, U; et al. (1998). A causal role for *E-cadherin* in the transition from adenoma to carcinoma. *Nature*. Vol.392, pp.190-193.

Pichaud, F; Roux, S; Frendo, JL; et al. (1997). 1alpha,25-dihydroxyvitamin D_3 induces NAD^+-dependent 15-hydroxyprostaglandin dehydrogenase in human neotal monocytes. *Blood*. Vol.89, pp.2105-2112.

Pilz, S; Dobnig, H; Winklhofer-Roob, B; et al. (2008). Low serum levels of 25-hydroxyvitamin D predict fatal cancer in patients referred to coronary angiography. *Cancer Epidemiol Biomarkers Prev*. Vol.17, pp.1228-1233.

Polverini, PJ. (2002). Angiogenesis in health and disease: insights into basic mechanisms and therapeutic opportunities. *J Dent Educ*. Vol.66, pp.962-975.

Raina, V; Cunninham, D; Gilchrist, N; Soukop, M. (1991). Alphacalvidol is a nontoxic, effective treatment of follicular small-cleaved cell lymphoma. *Br J Cancer*. Vol.63, pp.463-465.

Reed, KR; Sansom, OJ; Hayes, AJ; et al. (2004). PPARdelta status and Apc-mediated tumorigenesis in the mouse intestine. *Oncogene.* Vol.23, pp.8992-8996.

Rehder, DS; Nelson, RW; Borges, CR. (2009). Glycosylation status of vitamin D binding protein in cancer patients. *Protein Science.* Vol.18, No.10, pp.2036-2042.

Ristimaki, A; Sivula, A; Lundin, J; et al. (2002). Prognostic significance of elevated cyclooxygenase-2 expression in breast cancer. *Cancer Res.* Vol.62, pp.632-635.

Saramäki, A; Banwell, CM; Campbell, MJ; Carlberg, C. (2006). Regulation of the human *p21*(waf1/cip1) gene promoter via multiple binding sites for p53 and the D_3 receptor. *Nucleic Acids Res.* Vol.34, pp.543-554.

Schwartz, GG; Eads, D; Rao, A; et al. (2004). Pancreatic cancer cells express 25-hydroxyvitamin D-1α-hydroxylase and their proliferation is inhibited by the prohormone 25-hydroxyvitamin D_3. *Carcinogenesis.* Vol.25, No.6, pp.1015-1026.

Semenza, GL. (2003). Targeting HIF-1 for cancer therapy. *Nat Rev Cancer.* Vol.3, pp.721-732.

Shokravi, MT; Marcus, DM; Alroy, J; et al. (1995). Vitamin D inhibits angiogenesis in transgenic murine retinoblastoma. *Invest Ophthalmol Vis Sci.* Vol.36, pp.83-87.

Skinner, HG, and Schwartz, GG. (2009). The relation of serum parathyroid hormone and serum calcium to serum levels of Prostatic-specific antigen: a population-based study. *Cancer Epidemiol Biomarkers Prev.* Vol.18, No.11, pp.2869-2873.

Slapek, CA; Desforges, JF; Fogaren, T; et al. (1992).Treatment of acute myeloid leukemia in the elderly with low-dose cytarabine, hydroxyurea, and calcitriol. *Am J Hematol.* Vol.41, pp.178-183.

Slattery, ML; Yakumo, K; Hoffman, M; Neuhausen, S. (2001). Variants of the VDR gene and risk of colon cancer (United States). *Cancer Causes Control.* Vol.12, No.4, pp.359-364.

Slattery, ML; Sweeney, C; Murtaugh, M; et al. (2006). Associations between vitamin D, vitamin D receptor gene and the and the androgen receptor gene with colon and rectal cancer. *Int J Cancer.* Vol.118, No.12, pp.3140-3146.

Slattery, ML; Curtin, K; Wolff, RK; et al. (2009). A compromise of colon and rectal somatic DNA alterations. *Dis Colon Rectum.* Vol.52, pp.1304-1311.

Slattery, ML; Wolff, RK; Herrick, JS; et al. (2010). Calcium, vitamin D, VDR genotypes, and epigenetic changes in rectal tumors. *Nutr Cancer.* Vol.62, No.4, pp.436-442.

Slebos, RJC; Hoppin, JA; Tolbert, PE; et al. (2000). K-ras and p53 in pancreatic cancer: association with medical history, histopathology, and environmental exposures in a population-based study. *Cancer Epidemiol Biomarkers Prev.* Vol.9, N0.11, pp.1223-1232.

Stambolsky, P; Tabach, Y; Fontemaggi, G; et al. (2010). Modulation of the vitamin D_3 response by cancer-associated mutant p53. *Cancer Cell.* Vol.17, No.3, pp.273-285.

Steinbach, G; Lynch, PM; Phillips, RK; et al. (2000). The effect of celecoxib, a cyclooxygenase-2 inhibitor, in familial adenomatous polyposis. *N Engl J Med.* Vol.342, pp.1946-1952.

Steffen, M; Cayre, Y; Manogue, KR; et al. (1988). 1,25-dihydroxyvitamin D_3 transcriptionally regulates tumour necrosis factor mRNA during HL-60 cell differentiation. *Immunology.* Vol.63, pp.43-46.

Stryd, RP; Gilbertson, TJ; Bruden, MN. (1979). A seasonal variation study of 25-hydroxyvitamin D_3 serum levels in normal human. *J Clin Endocrinol Metab.* Vol.48, pp.771-775.

Tamez, S; Norizoe, C; Ochiai, K; et al. (2009). Vitamin D receptor polymorphisms and prognosis of patients with epithelial ovarian cancer. *Br J Cancer.* Vol.101, pp.1957-1960.

Tangpricha, V; Flanagan, JN; Whitlatch, LW; et al. (2001). 25-hydroxyvitamin D_3-1α-hydroxylase in normal and malignant colon tissue. *Lancet.* Vol.357, pp.1673-1674.

Taylor, JA; Hirvonen, A; Watson, M; et al. (1996). Association of prostate cancer with vitamin D receptor gene polymorphisms. *Cancer Res.* Vol.56, pp.4108-4110.

Telenius-Berg, M; Almqvist, S; Wästhed, B. (1975). Serum calcitonin response to induce hypercalcemia. *Acta Med Scand.* Vol.197, No.5, pp.367-375.

Thomas, MG; Tebbutt, S; Williamson, RC. (1992). Vitamin D and its metabolites inhibit cell proliferation in human rectal mucosa and a colon cancer cell line. *Gut.* Vol.33, No.12, pp.1660-1663.

Ting, HJ; Hsu, J; Bao,BY; Lee, YF. (2007). Docetaxel-induced growth inhibition an apoptosis in androgen indepenpent prostate cancer cells are enhanced by 1alpha,25-dihydroxyvitamin D_3. *Cancer Lett.* Vol.247, pp.122-129.

Trinchierie, G; Rosen, M; Perussia, B. (1987). Induction of differentiation of human myeloid cell lines by tumor necrosis factor in cooperation with 1alpha,25-dihydroxyvitamin D_3. *Cancer Res.* Vol.47, pp.2236-2242.

Tumura, M; Gu, J; Tran, H; Yamada, KM. (1999). PTEN gene and integrin signaling in cancer. *J Natl Cancer Inst.* Vol.91, pp.1820-1828.

Umbas, R; Isaacs, WB; Bringuier, PP; et al. (1994). Decreased *E-cadherin* expression is associated with poor prognosis in patients with prostate cancer. *Cancer Res.* Vol.54, pp.3939-3933.

Wang, QM; Jones, JP; Studzinski, GP. (1996). Cyclin-dependent kinase inhibitor p27 as a mediator of the G1-S phase block induced by 1,25-dihydroxyvitamin D_3 in HL60 cells. *Cancer Res.* Vol.56, pp.264-267.

Wali, RK; Baum, CL; Bolt, MJ; et al. (1992). 1,25-dihydroxyvitamin D_3 inhibits Na^+-H^+ exchange by stimulating membrane phosphoinositide turnover and increasing cytosolic calcium in CaC0-2 cells. *Endocrinology.* Vol.131, No.3, pp.1125-1133.

Weitsman, GE; Ravid, A; Liberman, UA; et al. (2003). Vitamin D enhances caspase-dependent and independent TNF-induced breast cancer cell death: the role of reactive oxygen species. *Ann N Y Acad Sci.* Vol.1010, pp.437-440.

Welsh, JE; Zinser, LN; Mianecki-Morton, L; et al. (2011). Age-related changes in the epithelial and stromal compartments of the mammary gland in normocalcemic mice lacking the vitamin D_3 receptor. *PLoS One.* Vol.6, No.1, p.e16479.

Yacobi, R; Koren, R; Liberman, UA; et al. (1996). 1alpha,25-dihydroxyvitamin D_3 increases the sensitivity of human renal carcinoma cells to tumor necrosis factor alpha but not to interferon alpha or lymphokine-activated killer cells. *J Endocrinol.* Vol.149, pp.327-333.

Zabel, M and Dietel, M. (1991). Calcitriol decreases calcitonin secretion from a human medullary carcinoma cell line via specific receptor action. *Acta Endocrinol (Copenh).* Vol.125, No.3, pp.299-304.

Yan, M; Rerko, RM; Platzer, P; et al. (2004). 15-hydroxyprostaglandin dehydrogenase, a COX-2 oncogene antagonist, is a TGF-beta-induced suppressor of human gastrointestinal cancer. *PNAS.* Vol.101, pp.17468-17473.

Zinser, GM and Welsh, JE. (2004). Accelerated mammary gland development during pregnancy and delayed postlactational involution in vitamin D_3 receptor null mice. *Mol Endocrinol.* Vol.18, pp.2208-2223.

van Rees, BP and Ristimaki, A. (2001). Cyclooxygenase-2 in carcinogenesis of the gastrointestinal tract. *Scand J Gastrenterol.* Vol.36, pp.897-903.

Vandevalle, B; Hornez, L; Wattez, N; et al. (1995). Vitamin-D_3 derivatives and breast-tumor cell growth: effect on intracellular calcium and apoptosis. *Int J Cancer.* Vol.61, pp. 806-811.

2

Psychogenic Carcinogenesis

Oleg V. Bukhtoyarov and Denis M. Samarin
Center for Medical and Social Rehabilitation, UFSIN Russia of Kaliningrad Region
Russian Federation

1. Introduction

Scientific advances in understanding the cellular-molecular-genetic mechanisms of carcinogenesis (Coleman et al., 2006; Finn, 2008) and the impressive advances in the treatment of cancer in animal models clearly not correspond to the results of clinical studies (Knight et al., 2006). Cancer process is still uncontrollable and global forecasts are disappointing: in the world by 2050 will increase from 11 up to 24 million new cases and death rate – from 6 (in 1999) up to 16 million (Boyle et al., 2005). In addition, despite enormous progress in understanding biology of malignant tumors and mechanisms of carcinogenesis, the constant improvement of malignant tumor treatment methods the five years' survival rate of cancer patients has increased only by 14% - from 50% up to 64% over the past 30 years (Herbst et al., 2006). Obviously, there is a large gap between the cancer science and clinical oncology practice and it is constantly increasing as the molecular-genetic research technologies develop which lead scientists from a holistic vision of the person. Now considering the problem of cancer from the standpoint of experimental animal models and the three officially accepted types of carcinogenesis (chemical, physical & biological) is not enough.

We believe that there is the fourth type of carcinogenesis – psychogenic carcinogenesis (Bukhtoyarov & Samarin, 2009) the idea of the existence was generated during the clinical work with cancer patients. Thus, the multicenter anamnestic study of causes of cancer among 1200 cancer patients with 23 kinds of cancer from three regions of Russia and Kazakhstan showed that 50%-70% of cancer patients were determined by psychogenic factors (death of the close person, divorce, frequent family conflicts, change of residence, appearance of the disabled in family etc.), as the major ones in the appearance of malignant tumors (Bukhtoyarov & Arkhangelskiy, 2008). Understanding of psychogenic carcinogenesis would allow to find the new ways to solve many problems in modern oncology and to form the holistic approach to the cancer problem.

2. Psychogenic carcinogenesis: A new look at old problems

At present, a huge number of various scientific and clinical evidence was accumulated that can not be explained in terms of the existing views on the mechanisms of carcinogenesis. However, these facts can be explained by the pathogenetically meaningful participation of the psyche in the appearance, progression and recurrence of cancer. Ignoring this understanding explains much of uncontrollability and unpredictability of the flow of the cancer process in some cancer patients, and also explains the considerable difficulties in creating effective anti-cancer drugs. The main factor triggering the activation mechanisms of psychogenic carcinogenesis is a chronic debilitating psycho-emotional stress (CPS).

2.1 Chronic psycho-emotional stress and carcinogenesis

It is known that two interconnected processes are necessary for developing of a cancer under influence of chemical, physical or biological carcinogenic factors: genetic break/cell DNA damage and compromising of the immune system. However, these pathological processes can be generated without participation of exogenous carcinogens, i.e. can be induced psychogenically. Chronic psycho-emotional stress is capable to activate key carcinogenic mechanisms and to induce malignant tumor growth.

2.1.1 Chronic psycho-emotional stress and DNA damage

It is known that CPS leads to dysfunction of telomere (the ends of chromosomes) and to reduction of their length (Epel et al., 2004; Arehart-Treichel, 2005), which is accompanied by genome instability, acceleration of biological ageing (Simon et al., 2006), reduction of life expectancy (Kimura et al., 2008), formation of a lot of diseases including cardiovascular diseases and cancer (Anisimov, 2007). Short telomeres are biomarkers of cell ageing; they specify stressful history of a cell and cumulative action of a high level of oxidant stress on a cell (von Zglinicki & Martin-Ruiz, 2005). In its turn oxidant stress is capable to be activated in reply to CPS and damage DNA, lead to gene mutations by means of reactive oxygen and nitrogen species (RONS) that becomes critical event in activation of key tumorogenesis mechanisms (Gidron et al., 2006; Halliwell, 2007; Toyokuni, 2008). Person in condition of CPS is very sensitive to damaging action of various mutagens, spontaneous and induced levels of damage of DNA are more often registered (Dimitroglou et al., 2003). The chronic stress in model in vivo facilitates development of skin cancer almost in 3 times on a background of carcinogenic action of ultra-violet irradiation (Saul et al., 2006).

2.1.2 Chronic psycho-emotional stress and compromised immunity

Genetic damages are necessary but insufficient for the neoplastic transformation of the cells and tumor growth, cancer progressing or relapse as formation of tumor is impossible without infringements in immune system where stressful factors and mentality take an active part (Schussler & Schubert, 2001), that is a subject of studies psychoneuro-immunology and its sub-discipline – psychoimmunology of cancer (Lewis et al., 2002). On background of CPS decreased hypothalamo–pituitary–adrenal (HPA) and sympathetic–adrenal–medullary (SAM) axes responsiveness is observed that is accompanied with disregulation of neuromediator systems, infringement of hormonal expression and functions of immune system (Reiche et al., 2005; Ostrander et al., 2006).

At the cellular level stressed and depressed patients had overall leukocytosis, high concentration of circulating neutrophils, reduced mitogen-stimulated lymphocyte proliferation and neutrophil phagocytosis. At the molecular level high levels of serum basal cortisol, acute phase proteins, chemokines, adhesion molecules, plasma concentration of interleukins IL-1, IL-6, and TNF-alpha and a shift in the balance of Th1 and Th2 immune response towards humoral immunity. Both stress and depression were associated with the decreased cytotoxic T-lymphocytes and natural killer cell activities affecting the processes of the immune surveillance of tumors, the accumulation of somatic mutations and genomic instability. DNA damage, growth and angiogenic factors, proteases, matrix metalloproteinases and reactive oxygen species were also related to the chronic stress response and depression (Reiche et al., 2006). CPS induces apoptosis of lymphocytes and development of immune depression by means of glucocorticoid ways, participations of opiod systems (Wang et al., 2002), genes p53 and P13R/nuclear factor kappaB (Zhang et al., 2008).

In its turn oxidative stress also induced by CPS and depression supports immune suppression at malignant tumors (Corzo et al., 2007), and proinflamation cytokines, activated by mental depression, support a condition of mental depression (Dantzer et al., 2008), closing some vicious circles of psychogenically induced carcinogenesis.

2.1.3 Chronic psycho-emotional stress and chronic inflammation

It is necessary to notice that CPS supports the centers of not stopping chronic inflammation which are always available in an organism due to activation in them of proinflammatory cytokines (Miller et al., 2002). Generation of RONS in the centers of slow inflammation considerably exceeds their opportunities of neutralization and elimination. Therefore high levels of oxidative-nitrosative stress and DNA damage are always registered in these centers that associates with the raised risk of tumor genesis and the main substances transforming the center of inflammation in the center of a tumor, are prostaglandins and cytokines (Federico et al., 2007; Kundu & Surh, 2008). Therefore, chronic inflammation may play a key role in carcinogenesis by causing DNA damage (Kawanishi et al., 2006).

2.2 Chronic stress and cancer in vivo model

In vivo model chronic stress is accompanied by a hypermetabolic syndrome with the severe loss of lean body mass, hyperglycemia, dyslipidemia, increased aminoacid turnover and acidosis. This was associated with hypercortisolism, hyperleptinemia, insulin resistance and hyperthyroidism that lead to a significant reduction of power reserves, compensatory opportunities and abilities of an organism to cope with infection or cancer (Depke et al., 2008). Proof of chronic emotional stress connection with cancer development and progress was a result of experiments which have shown presence of IL-6-independent activation signal transducer and activator of transcription-3 through mediators of stress (norepinephrine and epinephrine), beta 1-/beta 2-adrenergic receptor and protein kinase A that has led to increased matrix metalloproteinase production, invasion and tumor growth (Landen et al., 2007). Besides chronic stress by means of beta-adrenergic activation induced the atrophy of thymus and the host resistance to tumors (Hasegawa & Saiki, 2005), and also induces resistance of tumoral cells to chemotherapy drugs through biological effects of adrenaline, alfa-2-adrenergic receptors and increase expression of a gene mdr1 which codes transport activity of plasma membrane ATPase, capable "to expel" molecules getting into a cell of cytostatic (Su et al., 2005). It is also impossible to exclude that chronic stress by means of p38/stress-activated protein kinase and endoplasmic reticulum stress promotes formation in an organism of dormant tumor cells based for many years and decades, refracted to the chemotherapy, participating in cancer metastasis formation and relapse (Ranganathan et al., 2006).

It is necessary to say that at animals high efficiency of treatment of a cancer is observed which unfortunately is not present at the person and results in vivo cannot be extrapolated on the person (Knight et al., 2006). Distinctions are hidden in absence at animals of the second signal system (mentality as a whole) which is the imperceptible factor interfering with an effective cancer treatment.

2.3 Stressful brain and cancer

Brain – the key body providing adaptive/disadaptive reactions of an organism on stress through involving vegetative, endocrine, immune mechanisms (McEwen, 2007). On the background of CPS, infringements HPA axis activity and glucocorticoids influences structural remodeling dendrite neurons of hippocampus, amygdala, prefrontal cortex occurs (Conrad, 2006), actually the atrophy of neurons in limbic structures of the brain responsible for processes of adaptation is observed, regulation of vegetative functions, generation of emotions and motivations, the organization of complete forms of behavior, etc (Morgan et al., 2005). It is worth noticing that reduction of cerebra metabolism in limbic structures of the brain in patients with various malignant tumors is observed (Tashiro et al., 1999). It is possible to assume that difficult to diagnose (subclinical) infringements of functions of limbic systems are formed in cancer patients before detection of new malignant growths on a background of CPS cumulative influence.

Besides, affective disorders (helplessness, depression) which are characteristic of cancer patients, are accompanied by dissociated changes in four major brain systems: (1) an unbalanced prefrontal-cingulate cortical system, (2) a dissociated HPA axis, (3) a dissociated septal-hippocampal system, and (4) a hypoactive brain reward system, as exemplified by a hypermetabolic habenula-interpeduncular nucleus pathway and a hypometabolic ventral segmental area-striatum pathway (Shumake & Gonzalez-Lima, 2003). Thus, behind a facade of serious somatic (neuroendocrine, immune) and psycho-emotional (anxiety, depression) disorders at cancer patients infringements of integrative functions of brain systems are presumably hidden which can be defined as brain disintegration syndrome (BDS). BDS is characterized by infringement of functions of suprasegmentar vegetative structures, descending tonic influences on sympathetic-adrenal and pituitary-adrenic devices that is shown by decomposition of activity of physiological systems at all levels of an organism.

Cancer is not only the pathology of genes it is the unique result of cumulative CPS influence with cumulative carcinogenic effect of catecholamines and glucocorticoids (Desaive & Ronson, 2008), serious infringement of antineoplastic activity of immune system and tissue morphofunctional homeostasis, actually, this is illness of a whole organism. However, the huge potential of brain is capable to supervise and modulate the processes connected with genesis and progression of a cancer (Mravec et al., 2008).

2.4 Mental depression and cancer

CPS is closely connected with formation of affective disorders, in particular due to changes in expression of a gene 5-HTTLPR responsible for transport of serotonin (Jacobs et al., 2006), therefore anxiety and depressive disorders often go together and are characteristic of cancer patients (Miller & Massie, 2006). Mental depression, serotonin system and proinflammatory cytokines are connected in uniform pathophysiological links participating in carcinogenic mechanisms (Cavanagh & Mathias 2008). For a long time there has been consent among a significant number of scientists and clinical physicians on depression as etiological factor in development of cancer (McGee et al., 1994). Comorbid depressive and/or anxiety disorders aggravate development of any chronic disease (Roy-Byrne et al., 2008), influence extremely negatively on immune basis of some infectious, autoimmune, cardiovascular diseases and malignant tumors (Spiegel & Giese-Davis, 2003; Irwin & Miller, 2007).

Depression promotes progress of cancer and is a signal of a short life of oncopatients however the fact of fatal association "depression-cancer" is practically ignored in strategy of preventive prophylaxis and treatment of a cancer (Lloyd-Williams et al., 2009). Adverse growth forecasts in cardiovascular diseases rate, malignant tumors and depression in the world should be paid attention to. By 2020 depression becomes the second leading reason of disease in the world after ischemic heart disease (Lopez & Murray, 1998). It is possible that depression is pathogenetically connected with development of the specified diseases and under certain conditions can act as the starting factor for psychogenic carcinogenesis.

2.5 Population data

Data of many population researches allow to see an opportunity of a psychogenic induction of malignant tumors. For example, depression and hopelessness can play the important role in etiology of breast cancer (BC) (Montazeri et al., 2004; Zhao et al., 2002). The people gone through massive stress or daily stress raise BC risk in 3.7 times (Kruk et al., 2004). Phenomena of a racial discrimination essentially raise BC rate among black women in the USA (Taylor et al., 2007). Population research of 10808 women who have gone through divorce or loss of a close person has shown sharp increase in risk of BC disease (Lillberg et al., 2003). In one of provinces of Poland the high level of malignant neoplasms has been connected with psychological stress on a background of social and economic transformations in 80 and 90th years of the last century (Tukiendorf, 2005). Death in war of 6284 sons led to increase at parents' disease of malignant tumors of lymphatic and hematopoietic systems, melanoma and if the cancer had been diagnosed before loss the risk of death has considerably increased (Levav et al., 2000).

Population research in Italy has shown that occurrence in children tumors of the central nervous system and Hodgkin's lymphoma has been essentially connected with the subsequent development in their mothers' cancer of the respiratory tract and among mothers of leukemic children cancers of the lymphohematopoietic system and BC were observed (Zuccolo et al., 2007). It has been collected a lot of similar data, however mechanisms of interrelations "mind-cancer" remain unclear.

2.6 Children psychogenic carcinogenesis

Greene and Miller informed about possible links of psychoemotional stress with development of cancer in children 50 years ago in their work (Greene & Miller, 1958), later researchers also paid attention to these links (Jacobs & Charles, 1980). Extremely negative influence of prenatal psychological stress and depression on mother–child symbiosis has been established up to an arrest of development of fetus and poor birth outcomes (Newport et al., 2002; Coussons-Read et al., 2006). Death of one parent during pregnancy is connected with high risk of development in the born children four tumor types: childhood acute lymphoblastic leukemia, Hodgkin's disease, embryonic carcinoma of the testis, and appendiceal carcinoid tumors (Bermejo et al., 2007). Family psychological stress is associated with infringement of children immune system functioning and increase in frequency of their disease (Wyman et al., 2007).

There is an impression that the fetus, neonatus and child even are more sensitive to CPS damaging influence in a continuum mother–child and parent–child than adults because of full dependence from mother/parent and absence of antistressful strategy of reaction to real or alleged dangers. It creates real conditions for a psychogenic induction of tumorogenesis in a developing children's organism.

2.7 Cancer in psychotic patients

The investigation of malignant tumors prevalence in psychotic illness has shown conflicting results, however, many authors have found the low level of morbidity and mortality from cancer in psychotic patients, except the patients with paranoid schizophrenia and manic-depressive psychosis in the period of depression, whose cancer rates are dramatically increased. For example, cancer patients with breast cancer increased morbidity 9,5 times (Damjanovic, A. et al. 2006). These patients are constantly in a state of emotional stress thinking about the ways to protect themselves from their persecutors, or loss of feeling of pleasure and meaning in life.

2.8 Spontaneous regression of cancer

The phenomenon of spontaneous regression of cancer is known for hundreds years and was observed in virtually all types of a cancer, but its mechanism remains unclear, confusing and controversial. Spontaneous regression of cancer is complete or partial, temporary or constant disappearance of all or some parameters of the diagnosed malignant disease in absence of medical treatment or treatment without sufficient explanation of regress. The various mechanisms of this were suggested: from infection and fever as the causes to the role of prayers. However, none of the proposed mechanisms independently alone explains the phenomenon of spontaneous regression of cancer. Moreover some researchers report about the changes in emotional state immediately before spontaneous regress of malignant tumors (Schilder et al., 2004).

2.9 Schema of psychogenic carcinogenesis

The basic parts of psychogenic carcinogenesis are presented in Figure 1. The schema allows to see participation of a hidden psychogenic component (a) in the development of known

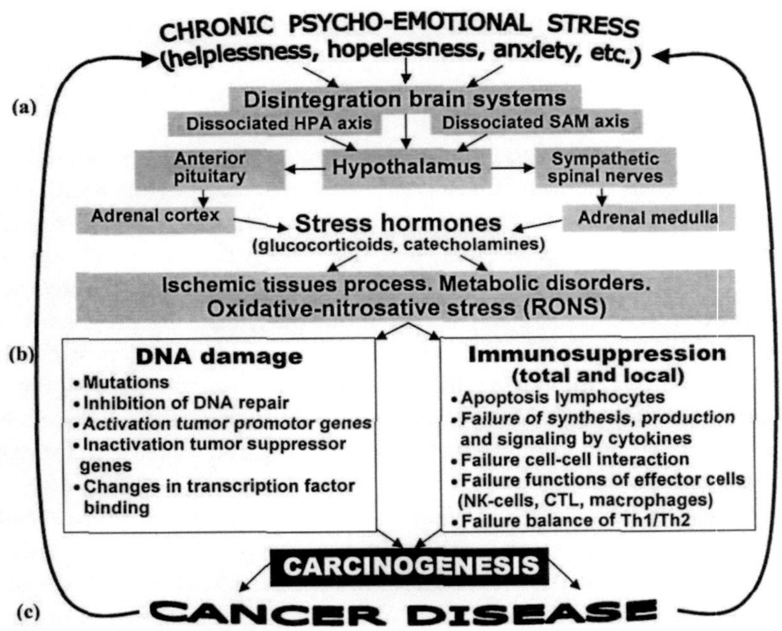

Fig. 1. Schema of psychogenic carcinogenesis.

key mechanisms of carcinogenesis (b) and formation of the cancer disease closing a vicious circle of carcinogenesis (c). Thus, chronic stressful dysfunction of the basic brain systems leads to descending tonic influences on pituitary-adrenal and sympathetic-adrenal systems, developing of ischemic, metabolic processes and activation of oxidative-nitrosative stress (reactive oxygen and nitrogen spices – endogenic carcinogens). Stress damage of the nuclear genetic apparatus of cells and oppression of supervising functions of the immune system, leading to emergence and growth of a malignant tumor. The formation of the cancer disease and inexhaustible emotional stress associated within as a personal reaction to a disease, close a vicious circle of carcinogenesis.

However, the main trigger factor of psychogenic carcinogenesis in a presented scheme remained completely undiscovered is a chronic debilitating psycho-emotional stress. How is this state formed, what does it mean for a man and what are its consequences? It is impossible to form holistic view about psychogenic cancer carcinogenesis without understanding the essence of the psychogenic factor. It is impossible to develop a pathogenetic approach in order to prevent, treat and rehabilitate the patients with psychogenic cancer. The answers to these and other important issues related to the functioning of a person during his life have been received in the concept of the dominant purpose of life.

3. Unity of mind and body: A new system view on health and human diseases (concept of life purpose dominant)

Problems of links between mind and body, ideal and material always attracted attention of the scientists and philosophers and within the framework of medicine there has always been a clear understanding of necessity in holistic perception of the patients however actually approach to the patients appears to be determinative. Unobviousness of influence of mind on a body and lack of a system view on psychosomatic links continuity have made modern practical medicine somatically focused. It is focused both in diagnostics of diseases and in their treatment and preventive maintenance. The scientific search is also mainly focused on study of somatic parameters of organism without the account of mind influences on them. The appearance of new research technology still carries scientists even more in depths of organism. The huge piles of fragmented facts are taken on a surface which are difficult to give the system analysis to. At the same time the huge amount of scientific data is kept showing extensive damaging influences of chronic psycho-emotional stress (CPS) on organism of animals in experiment and on human being in daily life (Ostrander et al., 2006; Gidron et al., 2006; Simon et al., 2006; McEwen, 2007; Spinelli, 2009). It is possible to state that CPS is an important an etiological and pathogenic factor in development of many somatic diseases including "diseases of civilization": atherosclerosis, cardiovascular disease (Knox, 2001; Dimsdale, 2008; Nemeroff, 2008; Shpagina et al., 2008; Roy-Byrne et al., 2008) and cancer (Adamekova et al., 2003; Reiche et al., 2005; Mravec et al., 2008). About that has been stated earlier in a hypothesis of psychogenic carcinogenesis. Psychogenic factor has always been and still remains essential component which mainly defines occurrence, development and outcome of human being diseases however in view of its idealness and unobviousness it is latent behind a facade of a clinical disease picture and as a rule is left untouched by pathogenic treatment. In connection with above stated there is one large, difficult and, at first sight, unsolved question: "How to see mind, biological, personal and social aspects of a healthy human and a patient in dynamic unity instead of considering only separate pathological process?"

3.1 The concept

The answer to this raised question would allow bringing in the proved and purposeful corrective amendments to scientific researches, diagnostic, medical and preventive measures in work with the patients. We offer the concept of life purpose dominant (LPD) which opens a system view on health of a human and process of any serious chronic disease formation with participation of mind and shows a possibility to control this pathological condition. On a basis of the offered by us LPD's concept lays inter-subject doctrine of a dominant as universal, biological principle of work of the nervous centers and vital functions of all living systems, general law of the intercentral relations in living organism (Ukhtomsky, 1927, 1966). The doctrine of a dominant was created by the academician A.A. Ukhtomsky (1884-1942) who is the largest thinker and ingenious scientist of the XXth century. However his doctrine has not received a due estimation and recognition neither during life of the author nor after his death. His scientific school existed simultaneously and in parallel with a school of the Nobel winner academician I.P. Pavlov that was recognized by the Soviet power as "sole correct scientific idea", therefore discovery of the ingenious scientist remained unnoticed for a long time. For the sake of justice it is necessary to tell that the basic rules of the doctrine of a dominant and a term "dominant" used in the works of scientists which have created a lot of the well-known theories: theory of human being motivation (Maslow, 1943), theory of installation (Uznadze, 1997), psychological theory of activity (Leont'ev, 1978), theory of movement behavior (Bernstein, 1967), theory of dynamic localization of mental functions (Luria, 1970), theory of the functional system (Anokhin, 1970), search activity concept (Rotenberg, 2009) and even a lot in Pavlov's doctrine of conditioned reflex appear to be component of the doctrine of a dominant. Really, uncountable set of reflexes in complete sense would blow up organism in the first instant of the existence if submission to their principle of a dominant when all reflexes work under the slogan "everybody for one, one for everybody". By the way, the formation of each conditional reflex under influence of conditional irritant is nothing else as the process of a dominant formation which preservation directly depends on supporting influences of conditional irritant.

3.2 Briefly about the doctrine of a dominant of the academician A.A. Ukhtomsky

Dominant, according to A.A. Ukhtomsky, it not any one topographic certain center of excitation in the central nervous system. It is certain constellation of the nervous centers with increased excitability in various departments of a brain and spinal marrow, in vegetative nervous system as well as it is a temporary association of the nervous centers for the solution of the certain task (Ukhtomsky, 1966). Spiral marrow and brain stem, conditional reflexes, processes of association, integrated images are equally subordinate to a principle of work of dominant reflexes of a spinal marrow where the environment as well as high nervous activity is perceived. The dominant is characterized with the following four features: 1) high excitability, 2) stability of the excitation, 3) ability to sum (accumulate) coming excitations and also 4) inertia (the dominant "insists on itself"). The condition of a dominant is not super excitation which would by all means be finished by braking and more or less long persistence of excitation "in one place and connected braking in the other". The dominant is capable to pull external irritants together that are not related to it, and do not prevent its development but strengthen it. The dominant represents prevailing need, motivation, and aim and is the powerful activator of activity. However, any dominant is always temporary and stops in the following cases: complete spontaneous end of dominant condition (for example, any of the biological acts), complete termination of reinforcement by adequate irritant and suppression by a more powerful competing dominant. It is necessary to pay special attention that at incomplete cancellation of adequate irritant, the dominant amplifies, aspires to keep itself. We shall return to this situation while considering treatment of human diseases.

A.A. Ukhtomsky paid special attention to cortical dominant - dominants of the high order which are the latent factors of psychological activity. All vital functions of a human being are dominant in their sense; they consist of a set of uncountable functional conditions of organism consistently changing each other - current dominants. However, there is the main dominant of a human to which all current dominants (more precisely subdominants) are subordinated, which holds in its power a whole field of spiritual life, defines "spiritual anatomy" and a vector of human existence. We dared to name it the life purpose dominant (LPD).

3.3 Life purpose dominant in a human

LPD is a non-material construction with material expression, which is formed in mental sphere and is shown by the maximal integration of mental and somatic processes, subordination of the current subdominants of a human being, maximal sanogenetic and adaptive possibilities of organism that allows him to resist to constant pressure of the environmental factors successfully. LPD is formed extremely under influence of a complex of verbal and not verbal suggestive irritants (processes of education and training, skills development, models of other people behavior etc.) which defines the life purpose that a human being aspires to achieve. A vivid example of an exclusive role suggestive irritants play in formation of life aims and personality is the well known phenomenon of Homo ferus ("Mowgli Syndrome") (Yousef, 2008) when children who have been brought up by animals completely acquire all behavior stereotypes of animals. In view of suggestive basis of LPD, life purpose and its loss can not be clearly realized by a human. For achievement of long-term, instead of momentary goal whole organism appears in subordination to its main conductor - LPD. LPD provides coordination of asynchronous work of organs and systems, mental and somatic processes, defines a vector of apparent chaos of numerous reflexes of organism, current subdominants (biological, mental, social etc.) and trajectory of everyday behavior of a human being. The LPD has certain similarity to work of ants carrying construction material in an anthill when the vectors of movement of separate ants are multidirectional and even opposite, but the resulting vector of their movement allows moving construction material in an anthill (Perelman, 2008). LPD defines not only functional condition of the central nervous system, high nervous activity and vector of behavior of a human being, it defines a functional condition of a whole organism at all its levels - from subcellular up to organismic. Let us notice, that at the adult human LPD has the most various contents but in a fetus, neonatus and a child LPD is shown by aspiration to safety. However, in process of development of a personality which represents a set of already holding suggestions, LPD is filled with other suggestive by the contents, that stability of LPD depends on.

3.4 Interrelations between a life purpose dominant and current subdominants of a human

LPD has supporting influences from numerous current subdominants, which do not have any direct attitude to it at all. However, there are basic subdominants among numerous LPD subdominants - "subdominants of health", its reinforcement and strengthening, which are actively created only by human being despite of constant action of external irritants (unfavorable environmental factors), competing subdominants, menacing formation and capable to occupy a place of LPD or even to destroy it. For example, a scientist is overcoming inconceivable number of obstacles in search of the truth or an actor is constantly aspiring to improve himself to be in demand, to feel love of the spectators and to receive the worthy fee. If these people terminate to create basic subdominants, their dominants of life purpose by all means will disappear that threatens with heavy mental and somatic consequences, we shall speak below about. Restriction of possibilities to create supporting basic subdominants is observed among refugees, disabled, prisoners and other people who lost life prospect. At the same time use of the minimal possibilities to reinforce LPD allows a human to keep his/her health even in conditions of massive chronic psycho emotional stress. For example, during the Second World war, some war prisoners in concentration camps died quickly and others planned their lives after concentration camps, they washed, had a shave, cared for others every day and being in inhuman conditions of existence they did not even catch colds at all (Rotenberg & Arshavsky, 1984). There is a great variety of examples of huge LPD force in a world history, in daily life and in clinical practice.

We have to mention numerous situations connected with achievement of life purpose, the termination of basic subdominants formation and natural LPD loss. A good example is the people with the most favorable financial, economic and social status who have achieved the life purpose and any possible well-being but imperceptibly appeared in "without dominant" condition - condition of chronic psycho-emotional stress with the subsequent development of heavy diseases.

3.5 Life purpose dominant at an animal

Proceeding from universality of the doctrine about a dominant for all living systems LPD should exist at an animal too. We consider that unlike a human being, LPD at an animal is biologically predetermined, formed in the central nervous system, constant at any age and is the dominant of safety - filled with aspiration to safety. Unlike human being, the animal practically is unable to show own activity in creation of strengthening basic LPD's subdominants. At wild animals the strengthening LPD occurs by a natural image under action of short-term subdominants - functional condition of an organism arising as a result of reactions on acute stressful irritants. At domestication and training of an animal human being becomes main irritant in formation of a unique basic subdominant strengthening an animal dominant of safety. This understanding is important, as it allows in experimental models on animals to simulate loss of LPD, similar to loss of LPD at a human.

3.6 Role of suggestions in occurrence and loss of a human's life purpose dominant

From above stated there is a clear exclusive role of suggestions in life of a human, as LPD and personality are a product of systematic suggestive influences. From all variety of irritants influencing a human being during his life suggestive influence are capable to destroy LPD directly and to become a leading though invisible pathogenic part in development of many diseases. In contrast to animal at which the acute stress always strengthens LPD, at a human everything depends on various results of intrapsychic processing of suggestive information of acute stress. For example, if the threat to life of an animal is finished with flight and LPD reinforcement, the threat to life of a human can both support LPD and be finished with its loss and development of disease, for example, post traumatic stress disorder. Besides, suggestive influence can in some minutes deprive a human being of life purpose and result in his death how an academician V.M. Bekhterev informed in the work describing experiment on a criminal sentenced to a death penalty (Bekhterev, 1998).

3.7 Diseases as dominant conditions

Any disease of a human being contains all features of a dominant therefore it can be considered as pathological dominant condition which is formed under influence of somatogenic and/or psychogenic irritants – etiological factors. The dominant dies away and disappears according to the doctrine of dominant after termination of adequate irritant. However, human diseases as pathological dominant condition do not disappear at complete termination of etiological irritants, but become chronic, as are supported by others already pathogenic irritants. In this connection, chronic diseases, as pathological dominant condition, have the supporting influences on the part of numerous current subdominants. Please note that there are pathological basic subdominants among them – "subdominants of disease" which are formed under influence of hetero- and autosuggestive irritants. Actually, they are pathological reflexes, for example, bronchial asthma attack, spasm of colon, arrhythmia attack or more complex cascade of reflex disorders at a relapse of a multiple sclerosis or cancer generated in a result of psycho-emotional shocks. These basic pathological subdominants (pathological reflexes) become a basis psychogenic component of chronic diseases.

3.8 Psychogenic component of disease as the basic part of pathogenesis

Psychogenic component of disease is an indispensable reaction of the person to disease with a complex of emotional, intellectual and volitional disorders connected to comprehension, experience and attitude of the patient to the condition and also with vegetative component which naturally interweaves with a structure of clinical displays of disease that gives it qualitatively new features. We consider that namely psychogenic component in human being defines development and outcome of human diseases as its basic pathogenic role consists of a distortion or blocking of sanogenesis mechanisms. There are no human diseases without psychogenic component and this is the cardinal difference of human diseases from diseases of animals. It is possible to state that the body does not suffer at influence of the unfavorable environmental factors but the mind is always injured, i.e. psychogenic factor can not be etiological but it is becomes pathogenic. Psychogenic component cannot be missed, deliberately ignored and waved away from it. On the contrary, it is necessary to see psychogenic component of disease to reveal pathological basic subdominants, i.e. to understand and control it to use successfully during treatment of the patients.

Thus utter elimination of pathological dominant condition, i.e. the patient's recovery, assumes elimination of not only a set of known etiological and pathogenic irritants supporting a pathological dominant but also requires indispensable elimination of a psychogenic component of disease. Otherwise, the incomplete elimination of irritants will indeed strengthen a pathological dominant of disease, which becomes more active, progressing and/or resistant therapy. Unfortunately, this phenomenon is quite often observed in clinical practice.

3.9 The characteristic of basic integrated human functional conditions

The basic integrated functional conditions of a human organism are defined by the contents of his main dominant that allows marking out 5 integrated functional conditions which replace each other during a whole life of a human in direct and opposite directions as a result of constant pressure of the various factors (irritants) of an environment:

i. "Ideal health dominant" is a functional organism condition which is characterized by LPD presence with its basic subdominants, maximum integration of psychosomatic processes, maximum and adaptive organism possibilities and lack of any chronic diseases.
ii. "Relative health dominant" is a functional condition of organism which is characterized by LPD presence with basic subdominants, sufficient integration of psychosomatic processes, sufficient sanogenetic and adaptive organism resources, allowing compensating any available chronic diseases.
iii. "Without dominant condition" is a transitive functional condition of organism deprived of basic subdominants and LPD which is characterized by disintegration of brain systems, psychosomatic processes, progressing reduction of sanogenetic and adaptive organism resources, formation of any psychosomatic pathology or decompensation of already available chronic diseases.
iv. "Disease dominant" is a pathological functional condition of organism which is characterized with occurrence of a dominant of any psychosomatic or soma psychic disease instead of LPD with formation of pathological basic subdominants supporting disease.
v. "Self-destruction dominant" is a pathological functional condition of organism which is characterized by occurrence of a dominant condition instead of LPD described by aspiration to death - a dominant of death with numerous pathological basic subdominants, maximal disintegration of brain systems and psychosomatic processes, failure of sanogenetic and adaptive of processes conducting to organism destruction.

3.10 Dynamics of the integrated human functional conditions within a life span

The dynamic links and change of the basic integrated functional condition of a human organism on a background of constant pressure of the environmental factors (irritants) are presented in figure 2. To visualize the dynamic presentation of complex psychosomatic processes each integrated condition of a human being is shown as "iceberg of psychosomatics" where the surface part - soma, underwater part - mind (psychogenic component) and central place in each condition is occupied with predominant dominant subordinating numerous current subdominants. All subdominants are formed in the central nervous system, in mental sphere, but have obligatory manifestations in soma and the speed of these manifestations depends on lag effect of somatic processes (nervous reactions, vascular reaction, hormone reaction, exchange processes in bones etc.). In figure 1: the small black circles are various current subdominants (meals, dream, walking etc.), black triangles - basic LPD subdominants, black squares - pathological basic subdominants of disease.

"Ideal health dominant" (see Figure 2, I) which is met in a smaller part of the population and more often among young people, turns into "relative health dominant" condition (see Figure 2, II) under influence of the unfavorable (pathogenic) factors of an environment (trauma, infections, stresses etc.). Thus pathogenic factors (irritants) do not destroy predominant dominant - LPD but result in occurrence of some chronic diseases (rather serious ones) which appear to be compensated because they become the current subdominants subordinate to LPD, and psychogenic component of these diseases carries out not pathogenic and sanogenic role. The people with disabilities participating in Paralympic Games or keen people living with HIV/AIDS, elderly people conducting an active lifestyle, i.e. actively creating and supporting basic "subdominants of health" can serve as an example. The reverse transition from condition II in a condition I seem to be difficult. In case of LPD (sense, life purpose) loss under pressure of the environmental factors, a human being appears in transitive "without dominant condition", in power of daily subdominants (see Figure 2, III) that is characterized by a condition of chronic consumptive psycho-emotional stress with its mental and somatic manifestations. For example, loss of the close person with whom the plans for the future are connected or loss of any life prospects as a result of social shocks (war, terrorism, financial and economic crisis, acts of nature etc.) and also others psycho-traumatic situations. A person can stay in a condition "without dominant" from several minutes up to several years. Under favorable conditions (the life purpose appearance) a person comes back in a condition of "relative health dominant" (see Figure 2, II) otherwise he/she stays in power of "disease dominant" (see Figure 2, IV) or "self-destruction dominant" (see Figure 2, V).

"Dominant of serious chronic disease" is represented in some serious chronic disease which has arisen in the period of "without dominant condition" (chronic psycho-emotional stress), with formation of pathological basic subdominants which make a basis psychogenic component of disease. They are manifested both in mental sphere (anxiety, depression, phobias etc.), and in somatic sphere (vegetative, neuroendocrinal, neuroimmune disorders, etc.) deforming psychosomatic relation and actively participating in pathogenesis of disease. There are numerous examples of occurrence of the most various diseases on a CPS background including development of malignant tumors (Levav et al., 2000) or multiple sclerosis (Li et al., 2004) after loss of the close person.

"Self-destruction dominant" (see Figure 2, V) always occurs from "without dominant condition" (see Figure 2, III) which in turn can arise from "disease dominant" (see Figure 2, transition IV in III). Psychogenic component "self-destruction dominant" contains a significant number of pathological basic subdominants that makes "self-destruction dominant" very strong and complicates reverse transition in "without dominant condition". Psychogenic component of "self-destruction dominant" is always brightly painted and clinically is shown through depressive symptomatology, phenomena of feebleness, hopelessness, down to catatonoid state with complete refusal of a human of the further life prospects and from the life itself, it is psychological capitulation (phenomenon "given-up/giving-up") under pressure of the environmental factors with active or passive aspiration to death. Somatogenic component "self-destruction dominant" is frequently shown through expressed somatic by disorders connected mainly to heavy frustration intimate - of vascular system (cardiac arrhythmias, weakness of cardiac activity etc.). A vivid example of "self-destruction dominant" is a known phenomenon "voodoo death" or psychogenic death (Lester, 2009) which was studied by us in oncological practice (Bukhtoyarov & Arkhangelsky, 2006). Psychological capitulation on a background of depression results in suicides precedes and accelerates approach of death of the patients with diseases of heart (Surtees et al., 2008; Seymour & Benning, 2009), cancer patients (Lloyd-Williams et al., 2009; Rodin et al., 2009) and patients with other diseases (Grossardt et al., 2009). By the way, self-liquidating behavior of some fans, sectarians or suicide attacker also is caused by "self-destruction dominant" arisen under influence of the external unfavorable mainly suggestive factors.

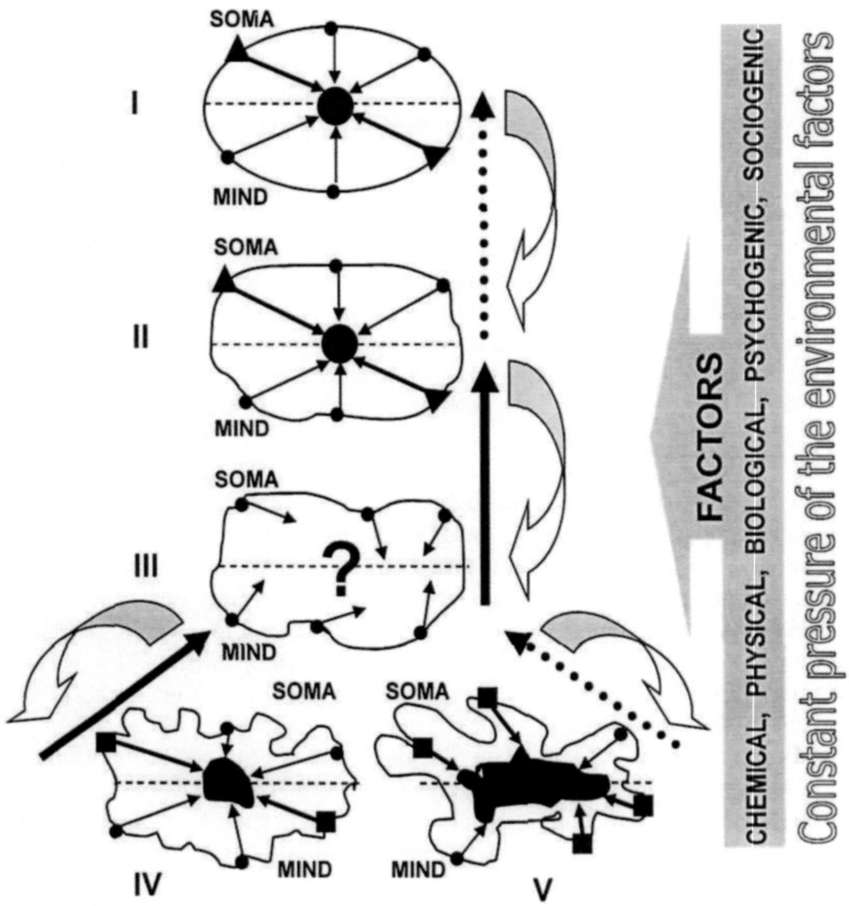

Fig. 2. "Iceberg psychosomatics": dynamics of the basic integrated functional conditions of the human organism within the life span under constant pressure of the environmental factors. ● - life purpose dominant (LPD); •- current subdominants; ▲- basic subdominants LPD; ■ - pathological basic subdominants of illness; ☗ - dominant of serious chronic disease; ✱ - self-destruction dominant. (I) Condition "ideal health dominant": LPD presence and its basic subdominants, orderliness of psychosomatic processes, absence of illnesses; (II) Condition "relative health dominant": LPD presence and its basic subdominants, equilibrium of psychosomatic processes ensuring remission of any chronic diseases; (III) "without dominant condition": LPD absence, disorder of subdominants, disintegration of psychosomatic processes, chronic psycho-emotional stress, possibility of transition into condition II; (IV) Condition "disease dominant": Occurrence instead of LPD dominant of serious chronic disease supported by pathological basic subdominants, deep disintegration of psychosomatic processes, opportunity of return into condition III. (V) Condition "self-destruction dominant": occurrence of death dominant instead of LPD with numerous pathological basic subdominants, practically irreversible disintegration of psychosomatic of processes, failure of sanogenesis mechanisms leading to death.

3.11 View of an animal from positions of a life purpose dominant concept

The main differences between a human and an animal are the second signal system (speech) and ability to abstract thinking, which defines existence of psychogenic component at a human only. The set of integrated functional condition of animal's organism within a life span is sharply narrowed because of absence of a psychogenic component (see Figure 3).

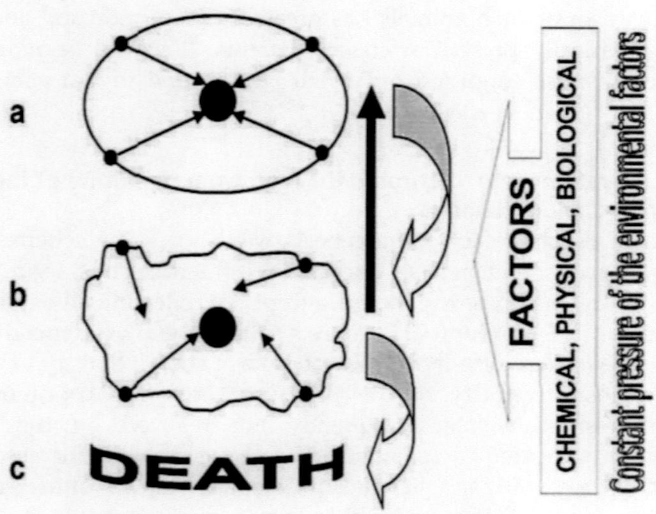

Fig. 3. Dynamics of the basic integrated functional conditions of an animal organism within a life span on a background of constant pressure of the environmental factors. ● - "safety dominant" (SD), • - current subdominants (CD). (a) Condition "dominant of life": presence SD, supported CD, integration nervous-somatic processes; (b) Condition "chronic stress dominant": presence of SD but CD mismatch, increasing but convertible disintegration of nervous-somatic processes; (c) Disappearance of SD on a background of irreversible disintegration nervous-somatic processes conducting to inevitable animal destruction.

A unique (sole) integrated functional condition with the maximum integration of nervous and somatic processes, maximum adaptive and sanogenetic resources is the condition when an animal LPD (safety dominant) is kept. We named this integrated condition of an animal organism "life dominant" where all current subdominants are subordinated to an animal LPD (see Figure 3a). For a wild animal the acute stresses and for a pet is a human being are the irritants, which strengthen their LPD. In situations of long influence of unfavorable irritants (chemical, physical, biological) there is a threat of LPD loss with chaos of the current subdominants, increasing disintegration of nervous and somatic processes, reduction of adaptive and sanogenic resources of organism. We named this integrated condition of an animal organism "chronic stress dominant" (see Figure 3b) that has a certain similarity with "without dominant condition" of a human described also by a CPS condition. LPD does not disappear in this condition only at an animal as its disappearance is equivalent to death. "Chronic stress dominant" is supported only by external irritants and is capable to reverse transition in "a life dominant" only after the termination of exogenous influences. Otherwise, there will be irreversible disorders in organism with LPD loss and subsequent destruction of an animal (see Figure 2c).

The stated representations show that the experimental models on animals can not precisely correspond to real events in human organism and require very careful preparation of experiments. For example, it is incorrect to run experimental approbation of anti-cancer drugs on animals that are in an integrated condition of "life dominant" and/or exposed to acute stress as organism of such animals has greatest sanogenetic and adaptive resources, which can not be basically present at cancer patients. It would be more correct to put animals into chronic stress condition on which background to test action of anti-cancer drugs.

3.12 Example of a system view of chronic disease from positions of the concept life purpose dominant - Cancer disease

In the hypothesis of psychogenic carcinogenesis was shown the scheme of formation of basic pathogenic parts of carcinogenesis under CPS influence. Thus, term "chronic psycho-emotional stress" has remained only general concept not reflecting all depth of its origin but from positions of the LPD concept CPS genesis with its known damaging influences on organism becomes clear. Our long-term researches have shown that up to an actual making out a cancer diagnosis, majority of the patients were in a condition of feebleness, hopelessness, helplessness despair (frequently not realized by the patients) which characterize LPD loss, appeared CPS. Statistic data prove dramatic increase in possibility of malignant tumors diseases with age (Jemal et al., 2008). It may be connected with loss of life prospects and plans for the future of an elderly person, in fact this is LPD loss with all ensuing negative psychosomatic consequences. Making out diagnosis of a cancer is in turn a powerful iatrogenic (suggestive) influence closing a vicious circle of carcinogenesis with formation of new additional pathological basic subdominants, supporting and strengthening the main pathological dominant - cancer dominant, which strongly occupies a LPD place. Modern somatic focused therapy of a cancer does not take into account and does not pay due influence to psychogenic component of cancer disease which defines development and outcome of a cancer in human. Somatic approach to cancer therapy is not capable to explain uncontrollability of carcinogenesis. The reasons for uncontrollability of cancer process during somatically focused therapy become clear from positions of the LPD concept (see Figure 4).

The modern complex therapy of cancer (surgery, chemotherapy, radiotherapy) results in incomplete elimination of irritants supporting cancer dominant and on the whole pathologically integrated condition of organism "disease dominant", i.e. carries out correction of its somatic component only (see Figure 4b) that can even strengthen manifestations of cancer disease. Besides, maintenance of psychogenic component of cancer dominant and "disease dominant" on the whole creates sufficient conditions for complete reflex restoration of its somatic component, i.e. occurrence of a recurrent cancer or occurrence of cancer of other tissue localizations at repeated reminding influence of psychogenic irritants (see Figure 4c) even after many years of the first cancer incident. In this connection, in pathogenically proved complex approach to cancer treatment the effective influences on psychogenic component of cancer disease should be stipulated.

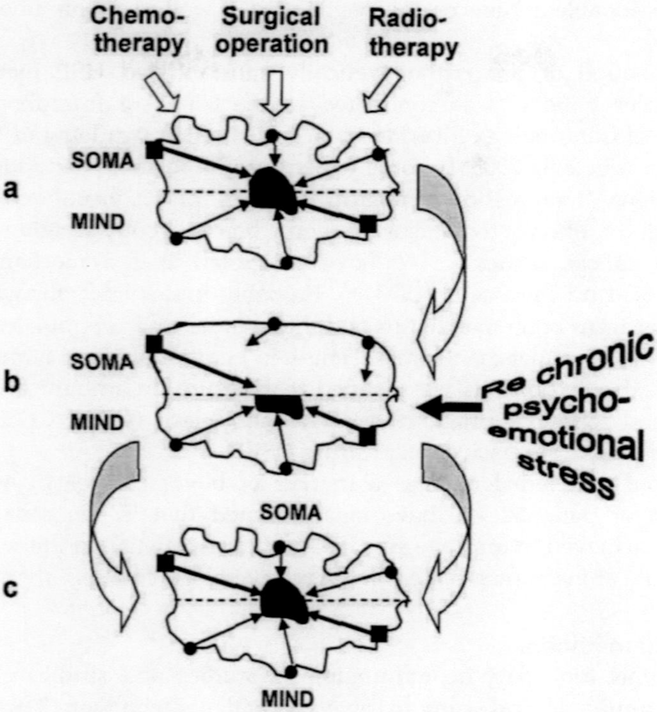

Fig. 4. The "Iceberg psychosomatics": schema of psychogenic reproduction of a cancer disease (cancer relapse). ● – cancer dominant (CD), •– current subdominants, ■ – pathological basic subdominant CD. (a) Influence of standard anticancer treatment on somatic component CD and in general "disease dominant"; (b) "Reconstructed soma" with previous psychogenic component (c) Complete reflex reproduction of CD and in general "disease dominant" (cancer relapse) during repeated reminding chronic psycho-emotional stress.

4. Psychogenic carcinogenesis: possibilities of psychotherapy in the re-integration of the immune system and increase survival for cancer patients

The immunopathology disorders are basis of malignant neoplasms and evident dysfunction in cellular immunity, control and differentiation cells mechanism abnormalities, immunological tolerance and effective immune reaction impossibility to growing tumor (Kim et al., 2007; Finn, 2008). A logical using of various methods of immunotherapy in modern oncology was a new step in a cancer treatment but was not as effective as was expected (Korman et al., 2006; Chouaib et al., 2006). According hypothesis of psychogenic carcinogenesis chronic psycho-emotional stress is always accompanied by immunosuppression and relates to a high risk of development and progression of malignant tumors. In this case an application of pathogenetically substantiated psychotherapeutic methods for correction of immunological dysfunctions is quite logical. Basing on our 20 years old experience of hypnosuggestive psychotherapy (HSP) in stressed and post stressed psychic and psychosomatic disorders treatment we have been developing a method of HSP for pathogenic reasonable influences on psychic state as well as on immune system of cancer patients.

A clinical approbation of our pathogenetically substantiated HSP method in complex treatment of cancer patients was conducted in the Clinic of Immunopathology of the Institute of Clinical Immunology Siberian branch of Russian Academy of Medical Sciences, Novosibirsk, Russia in 2002-2005. In some patients with melanoma and kidney cancer after HSP a clinical signs of regression biological age was found: visual acuity enhancement, increase vitality and motion activity as well as grey hair and body weight reduction without connection with cancer cachexia. We have suggested that a mechanism of revealed phenomena is based on stem cells (CD34+). Probably under HSP impact these cells start actively migrating from bone marrow to peripheral areas and repopulate different tissues. Perhaps we will discover that the telomere length in peripheral blood lymphocytes becomes longer. To check this hypothesis we planned to measure an amount of stem blood cells (CD34+CD38-) and stem cell progenitors of lymphopoiesis (CD34+CD38+) in peripheral blood from patients with stomach cancer during HSP.

We also measured telomere length as a marker of biological age in lymphocytes from peripheral blood of patients. We have also assumed that in the case of HSP method efficiency will be achieved to improve survival of cancer patients. In this context we studied 5-year survival rate of melanoma patients who received HSP course.

4.1 Materials and methods

In total, 98 patients took part in immunological studies and studies of cancer patients survival. In the immunological study involved 56 patients who were 3 groups: two groups were composed of patients with biopsy-diagnosed stomach cancer (n=18) and another one was composed of healthy donors (n=38). (1) Psychotherapeutic group (n=9) – patients with stomach cancer after surgical treatment but without chemo- and radiotherapy: 3 men and 6 women aged from 51 to 68 years, mean age 57,1±2,16 years, with stage III – 8 patients, stage II – 1 patient. (2) Control group (n=9) – patients with stomach cancer before surgical treatment and without any types of treatment: 5 men and 4 women aged from 51 to 71 years, mean age 62,1±2,52 years, all patients with stage III. (3) Healthy donors (n=38) were from 4 to 60 years old with mean age 33,2±12,49 years. It should be noted that all the cancer patients did not receive any additional treatment during the study period.

In the study of 5-year survival was attended 42 melanoma patients which constituted 2 groups. (1) Psychotherapeutic group (n=21): 7 men and 14 women, average age 46,1 ± 1,7 years, with stage IV – 11 patients , stage III – 6 patients and stage II – 4 patients. Level of functional activity (Karnofsky index) was not less than 70% (82,9 ± 2,41%). (2) Control group (n=21) consisted of melanoma patients which was not carried out HSP: 6 men and 15 women, mean age 46,8±1,9 years, with stage IV – 5 and stage III – 16 patients, Karnofsky index 86,2 ± 1,86. Evaluation of survival in melanoma patients with was carried out since the beginning of the observation patients.

4.1.1 CD34+ count, apoptosis and telomere length measurement

Count of CD34+ cells from patients' peripheral blood was measured by flow cytometry on FACS Calibur (Becton Dickinson, USA) with mouse anti-CD34+ and anti-CD38+ human antibody (Becton Dickinson, USA). Apoptosis and telomere length in peripheral lymphocytes were measured by Flow-FISH method using Cell Quest^{PRO}. Relative count cells

with hypodiploid DNA content (apoptotic cells) were measured by fluorescence of intracellular DNA dye 7-AAD on FL3 channel from lymphocyte gate. The measurement of the absolute telomere length was made using relative length, by formula y=2041,656 + 280,987×X ("y" is an absolute length (bp), and "X"- is a relative length in per cents). This formula was obtained by converting relative telomere length through absolute length for 5 donors. The telomere length of 5 donors was measured using Flow-FISH and Southern Blotting and then the correlated line was plotted, p=0,0008.
In the psychotherapeutic group of patients with stomach cancer CD34+ count in peripheral blood was measured before and after 4th key session HSP (after 4 weeks) and telomere length and apoptosis in peripheral blood lymphocytes was measured before HSP, and after 3, 5, 7, 9 and 11 weeks after 4th key session of HSP. In control group patients only telomere length was measured before surgical treatment.

4.1.2 Method of hypnossugestive psychotherapy

The method of HSP is based on strict successive, interconnected, figurative, pathogeneticaly substantiated suggestive influences in hypnotic states. This method was described in detail previously (Bukhtoyarov & Arkhangelskiy, 2008). This method includes: 1) Establishment of hypno-rapport between patient and physician; 2) Hypnotic de-actualization of psycho-traumatic emotions and experience including a fact of cancer diagnosis; 3) Hypnotic lockout of dreams connected with known stress situations which are regularly reproduced in the sleep with the corresponding psycho-vegetative reactions. It is needed for the subject's exhaustion of psychogenies and to prevent lingering course.
4) Hypnotic reproduction of a personal "health standard" or "health syndrome" - a key session of the whole course of HSP. This "syndrome" is based on using widely known phenomenon of hypnotic hypermnesia (increased memory under hypnosis) generally used for restoration of psychogenic abnormalities of memory. However, it is possible to restore memory of heart beat, respiratory rate, glycemic rate, enzyme reaction activity, and stereotype of digestive system functions etc. from a specific time in the past (Arkhangelskiy, 1999). The patient recollects the concrete day (date, month, year) from the past - "model, standard" of his health when there was no tumor and he felt well, mentally and physically. In a hypnotic state suggestions were conducted using the images that are required to retrieve from the memory of cancer patients the ' records" that are well known to the body as "health standard". It should be noted that in this key session HSP hypnotic suggestions related to the activation of a great desire, the need for further self-realization in their lives were conducted. In fact, these suggestions were aimed at restoring the lost of dominant purpose in life.
5-6) The last two HSP sessions have been focused on patients' education of self-hypnosis under hypnosis. Then patients were given detailed instructions to use autohypnosis for prolongation of the medicinal effect, as well as keeping psychic and vital tone of cancer patients.

4.1.3 Statistical analysis

Statistical calculations were made by methods of descriptive, parametric and non-parametric statistics (Mann-Whitney U test and Wilcoxon matched pairs test) using STATISTICA 6.0 (StatSoft, Inc. USA). An estimate of difference of value was by Student's test for depended sample. A significant difference was in p level less 0,05. Cancer patients survival was assessed using the Kaplan-Meier method.

4.2 Results

All patients felt significantly better after HSP in spite of the somatogenic component of the disease. Significant clinical changes in health, such as stable elevated mood, appetite, and night sleep, as well as increased psychic and locomotor activity and even regression of gastric dumping syndrome after gastric surgery were observed within 3-4 weeks after 4th session of HSP.

4.2.1 Stem cells dynamic during hypnosuggestive psychotherapy

In the same period (3-4 weeks after 4th session of HSP) a stem cell level (CD34+) in peripheral blood stomach cancer patients was changed (see Table 1).

Patients	Gender	Age	Stage	Before HSP			In a month after HSP		
				CD34+38-	CD34+38+	∑CD34+	CD34+38-	CD34+38+	∑CD34+
1 (Ani-kin)	M	52	III	0,19	0,11	0,30	3,03	0,98	4,02
2 (Vart-sh)	F	57	III	0,18	0,08	0,26	0,42	0,26	0,68
3 (Bak-ov)	M	52	III	0,38	0,28	0,66	0,36	0,17	0,53
4 (Stya-na)	F	51	III	0,30	0,30	0,60	0,84	0,47	1,31
5 (Mar-ov)	M	51	III	0,10	0,16	0,26	1,79	0,47	2,26
6 (Gur-va)	F	68	III	0,07	0,05	0,12	0,56	0,21	0,77
7 (Gas-ko)	F	67	III	0,25	0,11	0,36	0,93	0,11	1,04
8 (Vag-va)	F	56	III	0,11	0,09	0,20	0,82	0,23	1,05
9 (Mas-va)	F	55	II	0,27	0,23	0,50	0,55	0,31	0,86

Table 1. The level of stem cells in stomach cancer patients after hypnotherapy session, %.

Stem cell counts of CD34+CD38- were increased from 2 to 17,9 times and CD34+CD38+ from 1,3 to 8,9 times. A dynamic of middle values were in the following: CD34+CD38- cell counts before HSP was 0,21±0,03 % and in a month after 4th session was 1,03±0,29 % ($p<0,01$); CD34+CD38+ cell counts before HSP was 0,16±0,03 % and in a month 0,36±0,09 % ($p>0,05$). A whole count of CD34+ before HSP was 0,36±0,09 % and after that becomes 1,39±0,37 % ($p<0,01$).

4.2.2 Telomere length in lymphocytes after hypnosuggestive psychotherapy sessions

In the psychotherapeutic group (average age is 57), before HSP, telomere length in peripheral lymphocytes was 5,97kbp but it normally should be 6,23kbp according to deduced formula. In the control group without operative treatment an average telomere length was 5,7 kbp (average age is 62) but an appropriate normal length should be 6,04 kbp. This data point in the control group with stomach cancer, without operative treatment, has the same telomere length in lymphocytes as another one with operative treatment (difference with control is 0,34kbp in both groups). In three weeks after 4th session of HSP telomere length became longer (6,42kbp) but without significant difference until the fifth week after HSP ($p>0,05$). But in seven weeks after HSP telomere length became significantly longer and had reached 7,06kbp ($p<0,05$ comparing with value before HSP) (see Figure 5).

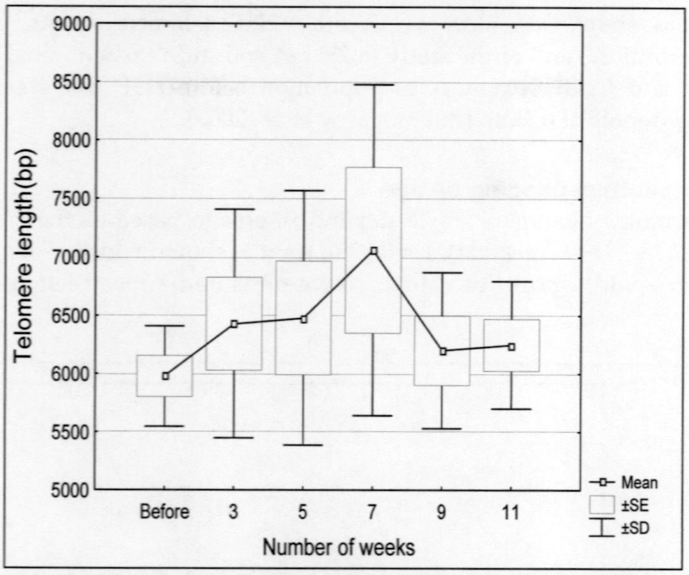

Fig. 5. The telomere length of lymphocytes in stomach cancer patients on the background of hypnotherapy.

4.2.3 Apoptosis level of lymphocytes after HSP sessions

In seven weeks after the 4th session of HSP we recorded another peak of immunological index regarding increased level of apoptotic lymphocytes to 1,7 times (comparing with value before HSP, $p<0,05$) (see Figure 6).

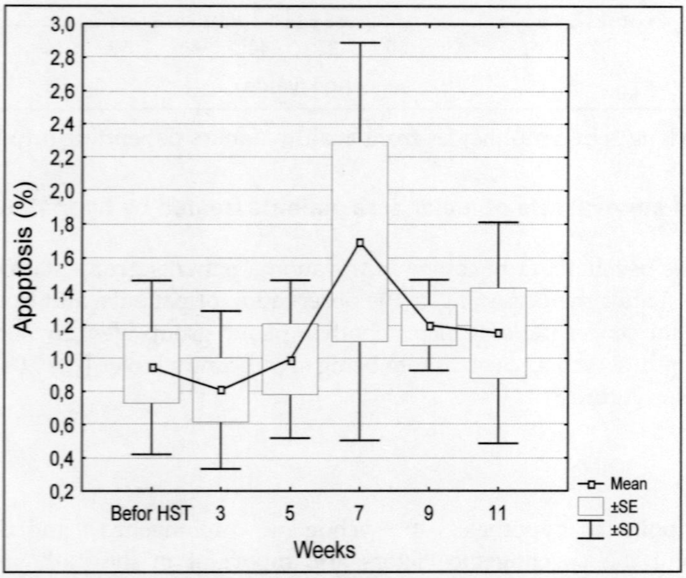

Fig. 6. The apoptosis level of lymphocytes in stomach cancer patients on the background of hypnotherapy.

Further dynamics show that nine weeks after HSP telomere length became 6,2kbp, remaining there until the end of the study (6,25kbp) and didn't reach initial level. Telomere length in CD4+ and CD8+ lymphocytes population before HSP was shorter of telomere length of healthy donors at 0,5kbp (Bukhtoyarov et al., 2008).

4.2.4 Telomere length depending on age

We derived a formula of telomere length dependent on age, based on the graphic: Telomere length (bp)=8312,18-36,64×Age(year), (p=0,023). As it is shown telomere length has a linear distribution with a wide spread of values, so we measured a mean telomere length value (see Figure 7).

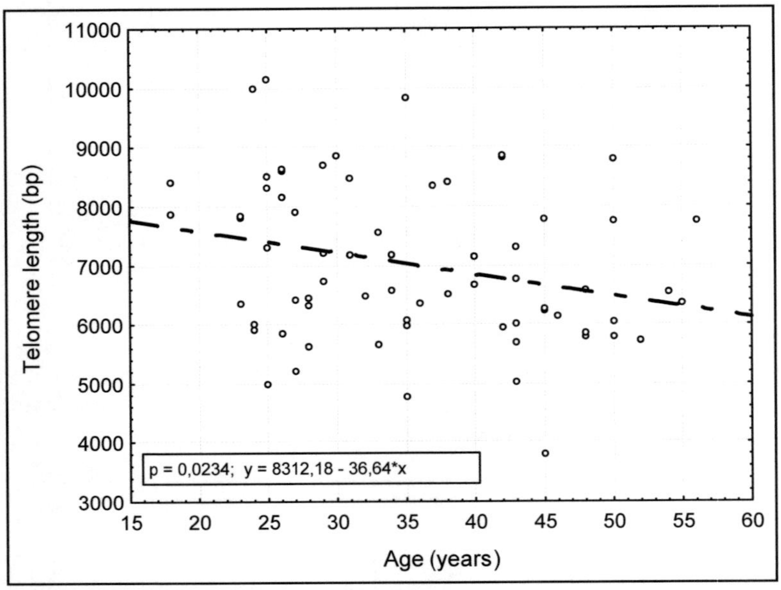

Fig. 7. Telomere length in lymphocytes from healthy donors depending on age (n=38).

4.2.5 Five-years survival rate of melanoma patients treated by hypnotherapy and autohypnosis

Hypnosuggestive psychotherapy course in melanoma patients group started almost 1 year (0,91 ± 0,17 years) after the beginning of the observation of patients, and from this point the survival curves for cancer patients of psychotherapeutic group went to "lethal crossroads" the control group in which a survival rate being significantly lower (p <0,05) within 5 years of observation (see Figure 8).

4.3 Discussion

From the standpoint of hypothesis of psychogenic carcinogenesis and the life purpose dominant concept the psychogenic factors are important in the pathogenic occurrence, development and recurrence of malignant tumors. It is logical to assume that psychogenic factors may act in the opposite direction, blocking the mechanisms of carcinogenesis.

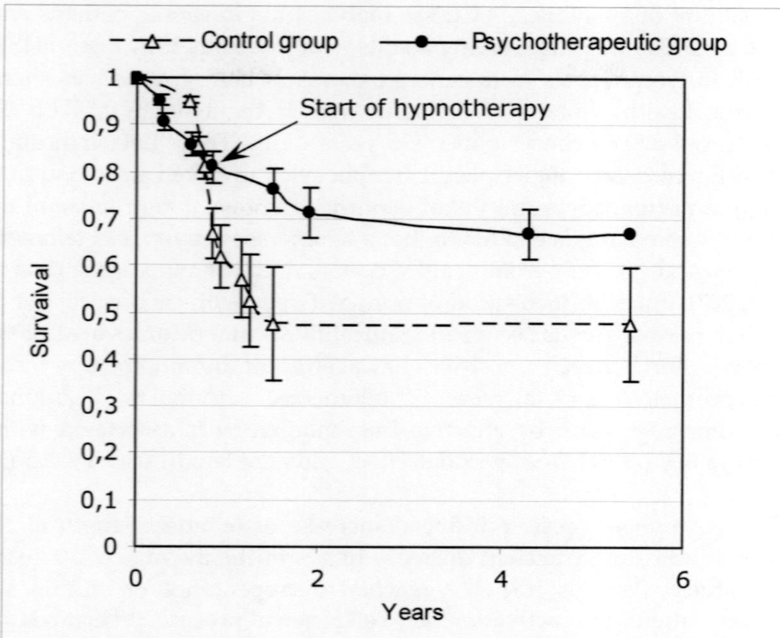

Fig. 8. The 5-year survival rate for melanoma patients after hypnotherapy (n=42).

In order to practice these assumptions, it was necessary to apply this method of psychological impact on cancer patients that would provide the most effective influence on psychogenic factors of carcinogenesis. From our own clinical experience, this method could be hypnotherapy, but with compulsory use of pathogenesis-related therapeutic suggestion. The use of hypnotherapy in oncology has a long history (Sacerdote, 1966), however, the therapeutic suggestion used for were exclusively symptomatic orientated (Marchioro et al., 2000; Montgomery et al., 2007; Jacobsen & Jim, 2008; Schnur et al., 2008; Monti et al., 2008). We purposefully developed the technique of hypnotherapy with the compulsory use of pathogenetically important therapeutic suggestions.

Thus, hypnosuggestive reproduction of a personal "standart of health" (4th session HSP) and the subsequent self-hypnosis sessions suggested that the positive changes in the immune system of cancer patients are possible in the case of sustained recovery in memory of the functional parameters of the body associated with the personal "standart of health" (when there no malignant tumor), positive changes in the immune system of cancer patients. A search for cellular-molecular mechanisms of biological age regression symptoms has found a hypnosuggestively induced mobilization of hematopoietic stem cells from bone marrow (immunofenotype CD34+CD38-) and lymphopoietic stem cells (immunofenotype CD34+CD38+) with initial gender-age average rates. Although it is known that in with breast cancer patients peripheral blood stem cell rates are 2,5 times lower than in healthy people (Rusé-Riol et al., 1984). No scientific publications reported earlier the possibility of hypnosuggestive mobilization of CD34+ cells. But there is data about hard mobilization of CD34+ in old people and cancer patients, especially with chemotherapy because of the inhibitive influence of high serum TGF-β concentration (McGuire et al., 2001). This feature excludes a possibility of spontaneous CD34+ mobilization in cancer patients and confirms no randomness of CD34+ mobilization in patients with psychotherapy due to HSP.

Telomere length in lymphocytes from cancer patients in both groups was shorter than in lymphocytes from healthy donors of the same age, at the average 0,34kbp (Fig. 7) and corresponding to cell age of cancer patients 5 years older. These data indicate an "earlier aging" and functional defect of peripheral lymphocytes involved in initiation, regulation and efficiency of anti-tumor immunity that confirms a known compromise of the immune system in cancer patients. It is well known that a telomerase activity and telomere length in T-, B-lymphocytes and NK-cells from healthy donors decrease with aging (Son et al., 2000; Ouyang et al., 2007), but after incubation of normal T-cells with cancer cells for 6 hours the telomere length in normal T-cells becomes significantly shorter (Montes et al., 2008). There is data about a connection between a positive clinical effect of immunotherapy by antigen and co-stimulating promotion and increase of telomerase activity in T-lymphocytes. For example, melanoma regression by effective immunotherapy is associated with increased telomere length to 6,3kbp, whereas without effect telomere length was 4,9kbp (Zhou et al., 2005).

The possibility of hypnosuggestive induced increase of telomere length at the average 1kbp (Fig. 5) and indicating transient decrease in age at the average of 10 years was first shown in this study. Perhaps HSP has reached disappearance of immunosuppression typical for cancer patients and activation of T cell renewal process. It becomes apparent by the increase of stem cells value and telomere length elongation. At the same time appearance of a new pool of lymphocytes should accompany the maintenance of a general number of lymphocytes. Therefore a mechanism of feed-back regulation for maintenance of cell homeostatic balance, such as a physiological death of cells by apoptosis, was activated. Actually, in patients with stomach cancer, at seven weeks, telomere length elongation in lymphocytes was simultaneous with lymphocyte apoptosis that increased to 1,7 times and confirmed the renewal process of lymphocytes after HSP. Data thus confirms a possibility of immune system reintegration in cancer patients by hypnosuggestive psychotherapy. It may happen at the expense of active acceleration of complex neuro-immuno-endocrinic regulation mechanisms, determinative stem cell mobilization from bone marrow, telomere length elongation, and renewal of circulating lymphocytes. The proposed mechanism of updating the immune system of patients with the stomach cancer on the background of our proposed method of hypnotherapy is shown in Figure 9. It is possible that the increase in the 5-year survival rate for melanoma patients has been associated with this mechanism.

Early in 2008, after the publication of preliminary results of our studies (Bukhtoyarov & Arkhangelskiy, 2008), in American colleges led by Elizabeth H. Blackburn, in his study, obtained similar results (Ornish et al., 2008). Thus, in 30 patients with biopsy-diagnosed low-risk prostate cancer during the course of the three-month comprehensive lifestyle changes showed the reduction of psychological distress associated with telomerase activity increased 29,84% in peripheral blood mononuclear cells. This confirms the existence of the possibility of non-pharmacological effects on the activity of telomerase, telomere length and indicates the reproducibility of our results that we received for the first time that increases their credibility. The research results show the particular importance of pathogenic significance of psychotherapeutic effects in treatment and rehabilitation of cancer patients.

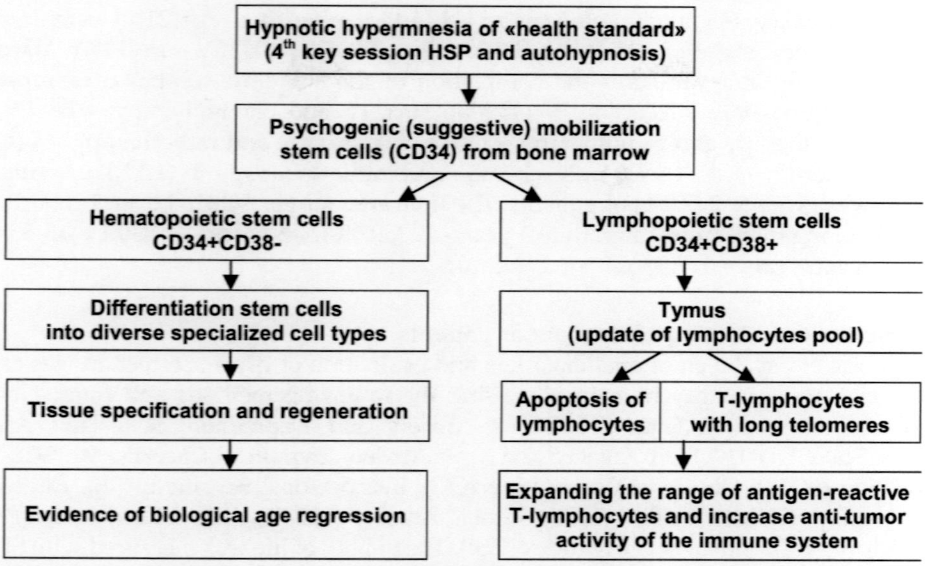

Fig. 9. The scheme proposed updates of the immune system of cancer patients on the background of hypnotherapy.

5. Psychogenic carcinogenesis: Possibilities of medication psycho-correction in the management of anti-tumor immunity of cancer patients

Despite the ancient history antiquity of hypnotherapy, we only consider it as a modern scientism method of clinical trials of sick human, cancer patients in particular, that yielded some interesting practical results based on our preliminary theoretical research. However, the main drawback of hypnotherapy is its complexity and the need for special training, which significantly limits its applicability in clinical practice. Thus, taking into account the previously obtained practical results of hypnotherapy, we hypothesized that the medication correction of psycho-emotional disorders, of cancer patients in combination with advanced special psychotherapy conversation will have positive effects on the anti-tumor activity of the immune system of cancer patients and provide for the cancer of anti-disease. Similar psycho-emotional disorders and the disorders of the same type of anti-tumor immunity regardless of the tissue localization of cancer are formed in cancer patients under psychogenic carcinogenesis. These assumptions, in combination with unknown prevalence of psychogenic carcinogenesis but compulsory psychogenic component of cancer disease in any type of human cancer allowed us to carry out psychoimmunology research of cancer patients in one group without separating them into separate nosology.

5.1 Materials and methods

The study was conducted in 2007-2010 in the Center for Psychoimmunology, Kaliningrad, Russia. 90 cancer patients, 78 women and 12 men aged: 30-40 years - 6 (6,7%), 41-50 years – 27 (30%), 51-60 years – 41 (45,5%), over 61-70 years – 11 (12,2%), 71-80 years – 5 (5,6%) patients, were involved in the study (smoking – 17 (18,9%), non-smokers – 73 (81,1%). The patients with 17 types of malignant tumors, predominantly, breast cancer – 34 (37,8%), ovarian cancer – 10 (11,1%); melanoma – 6 (6,7%), uterine cancer – 6 (6,7%), kidney cancer –

6 (6,7%), rectal cancer – 5 (5,6%), colon cancer – 4 (4,4%); other sites – 19 (21%) were involved in the study. Cancer stages: I – 15 (16%), II – 33 (35%), III – 26 (29%), IV – 16 (19%). All cancer patients randomly assigned after the completion of the standard combined treatment of malignant tumors: only surgery – 39 (43,3%), surgery and chemotherapy – 26 (28,9%), surgery, chemotherapy and radiotherapy – 14 (15,7%), surgery and radiotherapy – 4 (4,4%), only chemotherapy – 4 (4,4%), only chemo- and radiotherapy – 1 (1,1%) patients. No treatment was given to 2 (2,2%) of patients. The time after surgery varied from 1 month to 12 years and among them from 1 month to 1 year – 42 (50,6%), 1-3 years – 25 (30,1%), 3-5 year – 10 (12%); over 5 years – 6 (7,3%).

5.1.1 Psychometric testing of the cancer patients

The diagnosis of psycho-emotional disorders and evaluation of psychocorrection was carried out clinically and with psychometrically using the following methods and rates: Hospital Anxiety and Depression Scale (HADS) – Anxiety and Depression; State-Trait Anxiety Inventory Scale (STAI) – Stait Anxiety and Trait Anxiety; Symptom Checklist 90 (SCL-90) – Somatization (SOM), Obsessive-Compulsive (OC), Interpersonal Sensitivity (IS), Depression (DEP), Anxiety (ANX), Hostility (HOS), Phobic Anxiety (PHOB), Paranoid Ideation (PAR), Psychoticism (PSY), Global Severity Index (GSI). The quality of life was measured with SF-36 – Physical Functioning (PF), Role-Physical Functioning (RP), Bodily Pain (BP), General Health (GH), Vitality (VT), Social Functioning (SF), Role-Emotional (RE), Mental Health (MH).

5.1.2 Evaluation of specific anti-tumor activity of the immune system

Antitumor activity of the immune system was assessed by skin test of the delayed type hypersensitivity (DTH) reaction on the tumor-associated antigens, which were used as a lysed human melanoma cell line BRO in the amount of 25 thousand cells in a test. Human melanoma cell line BRO obtained at the Institute of Cytology RAS (St. Petersburg, Russia). As shown above (Wang, 1997), there are all kinds of tumor-associated antigens characteristic of solid tumors on the melanoma cells. The selected dose is not immunogenic, does not cause allergic reactions and other side effects and is diagnostic. Score samples (the diameter of redness in mm) were carried out in 12 hours (the peak response in most cases) after the intradermal administration on the forearm.

5.1.3 Measurement of plasma cortisol level

The measurement of plasma cortisol levels before and after medication psycho-correction carried out an enzyme-linked immunosorbent assay (ELISA) method for each cancer patient at 3.30 p.m.± 30 minutes with using a commercial kits (SteroidIFA-cortisol-01 ALKOR Bio, Saint-Petersburg, Russia). The normal range for afternoon blood cortisol levels in an adult human are 83 to 359 nmol/L.

5.1.4 Multiplex cytokine analysis (Human 30-Plex)

Storage of native plasma samples (at -80°C) each of cancer patients were obtained before and after medication psycho-correction. Multiplex testing service (Human Cytokine Panel 30-Plex, 96 Assay-Points) based on Luminex xMap-Technology: IL-1β, IL-1RA, IL-2, IL-2R, IL-4, IL-5, IL-6, IL-7, IL-8, IL-10, IL-12 (p40/p70), IL-13, IL-15, IL-17, TNF-α, IFN-α, IFN-γ, GM-CSF, MIP-1α, MIP-1β, IP-10, MIG, Eotaxin, RANTES, MCP-1, VEGF, G-CSF, EGF, FGF-basic, HGF, carried out in Microbionix GmgH (Franz-Josef-Strauss-Allee, 11, Raum D2.2.46, 93053 Regensburg, Institute of Medical Microbiology and Hygiene, Germany).

5.1.5 Medication psycho-correction of cancer patients

Mental disorders correction was carried out strictly individually with drug therapy using various anxiolytics, antidepressants, and their combinations. The following medications were used: afobazol, diazepam (microdoses), fluoxetine, coaxil, ixel, velaxin, paxil, valdoxan. The main goal of medication psycho-correction was the complete elimination of psycho-emotional disorders in cancer patients. In case of the absence of the clinical effect or the occurrence of side effects the drug and treatment scheme were replaced in the case the side effects did occur. 45 patients agreed to continue participating in the study after knocking mental disorders.

5.1.6 Statistical analysis

The statistical data processing was done using STATISTICA 6.0 (StatSoft, Inc. USA). The level of statistical significance used a p-value less than 0,05. Correlation analysis (Pearson's correlation coefficient) was used to study the relationship between psychometric and immunologic parameters, as well as to study the proposed immunomodulatory effect in the elimination of psychogenic immunosuppression during medication psycho-correction. In this case, the correlation is made between the «Before» (B) medication psycho-correction and derived quantity "After : Before" (A/B), reflecting the trends of indicators (Kozhevnikov et al., 2004). This method of statistical analysis was used because many parameters have changed by amounts exceeding the error of the method and direction of changes in the parameters is reversed.

5.2 Results and discussion

The anamnesis revealed that 79 cancer patients (87,8%) attributed the emergence of their disease with long-term psycho-emotional stress. Various mental disorders predominantly anxiety-depression spectrum were identified in 95,6% of cancer patients by clinico-psychiatric study that differs a great deal from commonly-accepted opinion concerning psychopathology at cancer patient (Miovic & Block, 2007). Most cancer patients have mental disorders regardless of types of malignant tumors. According to International Classification of Diseases (ICD-10) the disorders distribution was as follows: generalized anxiety disorder (F41.1) – 31 (36,0%), mixed anxiety and depressive disorder (F41.2) –10 (11,6%), prolonged depressive reaction (F43.21) – 10 (11,6%), mixed anxiety and depressive reaction (F43.22) – 28 (32,6%) and organic anxiety disorder (F06.4) – 7 (8,2)%, which in our opinion it was a complication chemotherapy. It is worth mentioning that work with such patients including the medication psycho-correction, contains difficulties that were determined by the peculiarities of psychical disorders within «chemo brain» phenomenon (Staat & Segatore, 2005). There were only 4 patients (8,9%) of 45 taking part in psycho-correction who required less than one month. 32 patients (71,1%) required 1 to 3 months, while 9 patients (20%) required 3 months psycho-correction. The time required for medication psycho-correction had no correlation ($p>0,05$) with disease stage, time after surgery and the severity of mental disorders. We came across the bad compliance at some cancer patients after the effective removing their psycho-emotional disorders. The patients felt very well and their further participation in their rehabilitation program considered useless. The dynamics of the tested parameters before and after medication psycho-correction of cancer patients are presented in Table 2.

Comparative analysis				
Parameters		Before (n=90) Mean (SD)	After (n=45) Mean (SD)	P
Hospital Anxiety and Depression Scale (HADS):				
Anxiety		9,5 (0,44)	4,4 (0,28)	0,0001
Depression		7,6 (0,46)	3,2 (0,34)	0,0001
State-Trait Anxiety Inventory Scale (STAI):				
Stait Anxiety		39,1 (1,17)	28,6 (1,28)	0,0001
Trait Anxiety		40,3 (1,14)	29,9 (1,26)	0,0001
Symptom Checklist 90 (SCL-90):				
SOM		1,31 (0,07)	0,90 (0,08)	0,0001
O-C		1,17 (0,07)	0,74 (0,06)	0,0001
I-S		0,97 (0,11)	0,60 (0,07)	0,025
DEP		1,38 (0,08)	0,82 (0,07)	0,0001
ANX		0,92 (0,06)	0,52 (0,11)	0,025
HOS		0,78 (0,06)	0,52 (0,07)	0,009
PHOB		0,47 (0,05)	0,26 (0,06)	0,012
PAR		0,69 (0,06)	0,56 (0,07)	>0,05
PSY		0,76 (0,06)	0,50 (0,06)	0,007
GSI		1,01 (0,05)	0,60 (0,04)	0,0001
SF-36:				
Physical Health	PF	69,2 (2,97)	80,0 (2,80)	0,011
	RP	29,4 (5,46)	56,8 (5,86)	0,001
	BP	51,8 (3,50)	71,4 (3,67)	0,0001
	GH	43,4 (2,99)	56,7 (3,19)	0,003
Mental Health	VT	46,3 (3,11)	66,7 (2,67)	0,0001
	SF	59,3 (4,18)	80,6 (2,78)	0,0001
	RE	34,2 (6,11)	68,6 (6,35)	0,0001
	MH	45,8 (2,96)	68,5 (2,19)	0,0001
Delayed type hypersensitivity reaction on the tumor-associated antigens:				
DTH reaction, mm		2,68 (0,39)	7,80 (0,96)	0,0001

Table 2. Dynamics of the tested parameters in cancer patients "Before-After" medication psycho-correction.

As it is shown in the table that the presence of mental disorders in cancer patients before medication psycho-correction have been identified clinically and confirmed by psychometric parameters. As a result, medication psycho-correction significant improvement occurred in almost all psychometric parameters and significantly improved quality of life for all indicators of physical and mental health SF-36 that led to an increase in DTH skin reaction on the tumor-associated antigens (p=0,0001), i.e increasing the specific antitumor activity of the immune system of cancer patients. The inverse correlations found between DTH skin reaction and psychometric parameters: Stait Anxiety (r= -0,34; p= 0,001) and Psychoticism (r= -0,21; p= 0,043). However, if the preliminary high indicators of DTH skin reaction (up to 15-16 mm) at cancer patients without psycho-emotional disorder (4 patients) are excluded, the true correlation connections have been discovered with great number of parameters of the psychical condition and the standard of living (see Table 3). It is possible, that these four cancer patients without psycho-emotional disorders their carcinogenesis was non-psychogenic. Thus, we can assume that effective medication psycho-correction and improvement of the quality of life of cancer patients can eliminate the psychogenic immunosuppressive effects on the immune system and create the conditions for controlling of specific anti-tumor immunity of cancer patients irrespective of the cancer types.

The results of Multiplex study (Human Cytokine Panel 30-Plex) during medication psycho-correction are paramount importance. The concentration of the following 14 cytokines: IL-1b, IFNα, IL-1RA, IL-2, IL-4, IL-5, IL-7, IL-10, IL-13, IL-15, IL-17, G-CSF, GM-CSF, IFN-γ was below lower limit of detection and they were excluded from the analysis. The significant multidirect changes took places as a result of effective medication psycho-correction among the determined concentration of cytokines. The statistically approved differences were not discovered (p>0,05) during the comparison of the average concentrations of cytokines.

Parameters		DTH skin reaction	
		r	p
SCL-90	OBS	-0,30	0,049
	DEP	-0,30	0,049
	HOS	-0,33	0,028
	PAR	-0,34	0,024
HADS	Anxiety	-0,97	0,0001
SF-36 (n=41)	PF	0,58	0,0001
	BP	0,49	0,0001
	GH	0,30	0,003
	VT	0,39	0,0001
	MH	0,56	0,0001

Table 3. Correlations between DTH skin reaction and tested parameters before medication psycho-correction (n=86).

Multidirects changes in the cytokine profile reflected the modulating influence of effective medication psycho-correction in relation to concrete cytokines participating in the processes inflammation, angiogenesis and cellular immunity. The negative coefficients of the correlations – rB/(A:B) indicated on the modulating effect of medication psycho-correction (when high the cytokine concentrations are reduced, and low concentrations are rising) (see Table 4).

Cytokines (pg/ml)	Before (n=90) Mean (SEM)	After (n=45) Mean (SEM)	Correlation analysis	
			$r_{B/(A:B)}$	P
VEGF	8,38 (0,94)	6,83 (0,80)	-0,56	0,005
FGF-basic	17,6 (4,06)	10,8 (1,19)	-0,74	0,034
IL-12p40/p70	59,1 (3,76)	54,8 (4,19)	-0,57	0,0001
RANTES	1732,5 (133,9)	1872,5 (190,8)	-0,53	0,001
MCP-1	635,6 (31,5)	605,9 (36,8)	-0,57	0,0001
IL-1RA	332,4 (51,3)	234,2 (17,7)	-0,72	0,013
IP-10	49,9 (5,08)	38,1 (3,94)	-0,37	0,015

Table 4. Modulating effects of medication psycho-correction on the plasma cytokine levels (Cytokine 30-Plex).

Where $r_{B/(A:B)}$ – correlation coefficients between the values «before» and the quotient of the «after : before».

In our opinion, multidirect individual changes in cytokines concentration at cancer patient reflected the peculiarities of intercellular interaction in the organism of every patient in respons to medication psycho-correction. It may be suggested that the discovered changes of the cytokine profile had anti-tumor direction at the background improving psycho-emotional state and increase specific anti-tumor activity of the immune system at cancer patients. Thus, for instance increase of cytokines, the concentration connected with the angiogenesis at some cancer patients may be connected with microcirculation improvement the tissues ischemisation decrease and the increase of their accessibility to the cells of immune system at the expense of angiogenesis activation. At the same time, the decrease of the initially high concentration of cytokines connected with angiogenesis at other cancer patients after medication psycho-correction may reflect the processes of neoangiogenesis suppression.

As another example multidirect changes of cytokines concentration participating in cell immunity mechanism can be provided. Thus, the increase of these cytokines concentration at a number of cancer patients after psycho-correction can point out at the activation cell immunity and anti-tumor immunity as well. At the same time, the decrease of these cytokines at some cancer patients after psycho-correction may evidence the cell immunity suppression and the activation of tissue reparation processes (fibroses, regeneration) that are in reciprocal correlations and accompany inflammation processes. It should be noted in particular that the normal reparation process of tissues is accompanied by physiological suppression cell-mediated immunity including anti-tumor immunity. An absences of suppression the cellular immunity processes slow down and distorted because the cells proliferation are eliminated as tumor transformed cells, because on the fact the proliferating cells express the differentiation and tumor-associating antigens. The reciprocal correlation of cellular immunity and reparation process are described as the balance between T-helper-1 and T-helper-2 lymphocyte subpopulations with the production the cytokines correspondent to them in the scientific literature. Resulting from the data received, we suggest that practically unique spectrum of molecular signaling, cytokine profile and genes expression at each cancer patients is formed on all stages of appearance and development of malignant tumor disease. That implies the lack of perspective in applying linear logic in the research of infinite molecular-genetic configuration that may be found at cancer patients. In particular, this is connected with the cases of psychogenic carcinogenesis, when pathological and sanogenetical processes, taking place on the cellular and molecular-genetic levels are secondary, effectory in the relation to central nervous system and higher nervous activity of man. It is obvious, that the linear logic with its attempts of isolated medication only on cellular, molecular and genetic levels aimed at governing malignant tumor processes will prove to be inappropriate in case of psychogenic carcinogenesis. This suggestion may be considered to be true concerning the use of any vaccine, immunomodulators on any other anti-cancer drugs because all of them will act in the conditions of suppression and distortion of the immune system reactions determined by the psycho-emotional disorders of cancer patients. The final result of such medication influence is connected with the danger of cancer process strengthening at the expense of even greater activation of distorted immune reactions at cancer patients.

Dwelling on the above presented scheme (see Figure 1), the stress hormones in particular cortisol that is the biologically active component of the HPA axis, turn out to be the essential phase psychogenic carcinogenesis. The mean values of cortisol plasma levels before and after medication psycho-correction of cancer patients had no differences (p> 0,05) and did not differ from the normal amounts. However, the initial levels of cortisol had backward correlations with the number of psychometric indexes: HADS – Anxiety (r= - 0,26; p= 0,014) and 5 parameters of Symptom Checklist 90 – OC (r= - 0,26; p= 0,014); DEP (r= - 0,20; p= 0,025); ANX (r= - 0,24; p= 0,026); PAR (r= - 0,32; p= 0,003); GSI (r= - 0,26; p= 0,014). Moreover, the direct correlation of cortisol and receptor IL-2R (r= 0,24; p= 0,022) that may be the indicator of quantity Treg cells suppressing the specific anti-tumor immunity has been discovered (Yang & Ansell, 2009; Fort & Narayanan, 2010). These data, to some extent, could clarify the mechanism of specific anti-tumor immunity suppression at cancer patients with psychogenic carcinogenesis. It would be appropriate first to effectively suppress the psycho-emotional disorders at cancer patients with psychogenic carcinogenesis that allows to remove the psychogenic immunodepressive influence from the central nervous system (higher nervous activity) and create the favourable conditions for using various immunological drugs, anti-tumor vaccines and other anti-tumor drugs. However, we failed to define and understand the cytokine mechanism of activation of specific anti-tumor immunity at canser patients after elimination of psycho-emotional disorders. Obviously, it is necessary to employ the other research techniques that could allow to find out the interconnections and supra-cytokine mechanism of management of anti-tumor immunity at cancer patients from the central nervous system.

6. Conclusion

It is obvious that the cancer problem become global long ago, the problem that affects the countries all over the world and all levels of the society. We have faced the amazing paradox – the illness and mortality from cancer are ever increasing with the rapid development of science. Which global carcinogenic factor effects the people all over the world in the way that simultaneously damages DNA cells and suppresses anti-tumor immunity? We believe that it is practically impossible to give the answer to this question taking into account three known types of cancerogenesis (chemical, physical, biological). The clinical practice, the results of numerous but various scientific research and the life itself pont out at the fourth mechanism of the carcinogenesis – psychogenic carcinogenesis. We assume that in case of formation of any tumors, psychogenic carcinogenic influences always take place and act both independently and in combination with the chemical, physical and biological carcinogens, essentially making their tumorogenic effect easier. In case of psychogenic carcinogenesis the cancerogenic factor is the chronic psychoemotional stress, the damaging influence of which is well known and can be noticed at all levels of the research of a human – from genic level to population one. The definite indicator of the existence of chronic psycho-emotional stress at man can be anxiety disorders and affective disorders, especially depression (subdepression) that has been considered the global problem of the modern society and world medicine (Daly, 2009). It is believed that cancer patients with depression have somato-psychic origin and is secondary in relation to somatic pathology.

However, earlier we obtained the results of multicentre anamnestic research of more than 1200 cancer patients with 23 types of cancer in which we discovered that about 70% of patients had the symptoms of anxious and depressive disorders during 1,5 years before they had been diagnosed the cancer disease (Bukhtoyarov & Arkhangelskiy, 2008). These psycho-emotional disorders occurred as a result of various psycho-traumatic events that led to the state of helplessness, hopelessness and formed the vision of impossibility of achieving personal aims and self-realization. In fact, these pathological states reflected the loss of objective and the meaning of life, that quite often are not realized by man. The analysis of the data obtained become the basis that allowed us to create of life purpose dominant concept describing the formation of the essential functional states of man during the life. We suggested that the cancer disease at some patients is the result of the consequent destruction of two essential closely connected with each other and perhaps "ancient" basic psychosomatic entities of the human organism purpose the meaning of life (i.e. life purpose dominant) and supervisory functions of the immune system. We believe that psychogenic carcinogenesis is the particular case of such disorders that is why other psychosomatic combinations are possible in case of other chronic diseases. The loss of the purpose and the meaning of life accompanied in the cascade of increasing disintegration processes at all levels of the organism that manifested the mosaic of the psycho-emotional disorders, metabolic and immunological disorders that form the basis of psychogenic carcinogenesis. The phenomena of disintegration, dissociation of functions and failure of cellular cooperation in cancer, create great difficulties in the scientific search of linear interconnections in the carcinogenic processes, in the formation of corrective conclusions only on the basis of cellular-molecular-genetic research. It is obvious that the holistic approach to the research of cancer problem at man requires to take it psychogenic compound in the compulsory account.

There exists a huge amount of facts in the scientific literature that point out at the close connection of positive emotional states (subjective well-being contributes) with the indicator of the good physical health: low blood pressure, high versus low density lipoprotein cholesterol, longer telomere length, age adjusted, rapid wound healing, renal and hepatic reserves and etc., but the conditions for reaching the stuble subjective well-being contributes up to now remain unknown (Diener & Chan, 2011). We consider that the main condition of subjective well-being contributes is the existence of life purpose dominant in man that ensures the maximum integration of psychic, somatic, sanogenetic processes, that creates the conditions for preserving good health and longer life expectancy. As far as the hypotheses of psychogenic carcinogenesis and life purpose dominant is concerned the direct correlation of the cancer desease and human aging to greater extent is explained by decreasing with the age the life perspectives, plans for the future and easiness with which the life purpose dominant is lost and thus results in chronic exhausting psycho-emotional stress.

The results of the current research have shown the close interconnection of psychical state with somatic processes at cancer patients regardless the type of cancer. At the background of the significant improvement of psychical state and life quality of cancer patients a number of previously unknown somatic phenomena has been described. They are as following: psychogenically caused stem cells mobilization, psychogenically caused increase of telomere length in lymphocytes, psychogenically caused increase of lymphocyte apoptosis, psychogenically caused modulation of cytokines in blood native plasma and psychogenically caused increase of specific anti-tumor activity of the immune system (increase of the delayed type hypersensitivity reaction on the tumor-associated antigens). We can assert that mind is the basis of generalization of the cancer process, mind is a promoter of cancer. Nevertheless, it is quite obvious that we have only made the first modest steps in psychogenic carcinogenesis research and the main difficulties of the research are connected with the complexity of the identification of the beginning of cancer process and individual "carcinogenic dose" of psycho-emotional stress. The share of psychogenic carcinogenesis in the whole structure of carcinogenesis also remains unclear. Dwelling on the results of the research, we suggest three clinical criteria of psychogenic carcinogenesis and the two of them are sufficient to suggest the existence of psychogenic carcinogenesis at a particular cancer patients: the presence of psychogenic anamnesis, psycho-emotional disorders and suppression of specific anti-tumor activity of the immune system. We strogly believe that the data of the presented research will prove useful both in the scientific search and in clinical practice with cancer patients.

7. Acknowledgment

The authors would like to thank Nikolay Tamodin (Moscow) and Alexey Palchevsky (Kaliningrad) for understanding the problem and providing the financial support for this scientific work. We express our great acknowlidgement to prof. Askold Arkhangelsky, who creatively developed the ideal of academician V.M. Bekhterev and showed us the way to holistic vision of man. We are very grateful to prof. Vladimir Kozhevnikov and the employes of his laboratory at the Institute of Clinical Immunology, Novosibirsk, and olso to Petr Tarasov (Rosneft Oil Company, Moscow). Our particular gratitude we express to our wives for their understanding, endless patience and support.

8. References

Adamekova, E.; Markova, M.; Kubatka, P.; Bojkova, B.; Ahlers, I. & Ahlersova, E. (2003). NMU-induced mammary carcinogenesis in female rats is influenced by repeated psychoemotional stress. *Neoplasma*, Vol. 50, pp: 428-432

Anisimov, V.N. (2007). Biology of ageing and cancer. *Cancer Control*, Vol. 14, pp: 23–31.

Anokhin, P.K. (1970). The theory of a functional system. *Uspekhi Matematicheskikh Nauk*, Vol. 1, pp: 19-54.

Arehart-Treichel, J. (2005). Can stress reduction fight some signs of ageing? *Psychiatric News*, Vol. 40, pp: 27.

Arkhangelskiy, A.E. (1999). *Pathology of nervous system and the pregnancy*. Military Medical Academy, SPb, Russia.

Bekhterev, V.M. (1998). *Suggestion and its role in social life*. Transaction Publishers, New Brunswick, USA.

Bernstein, N.A. (1967). *The coordination and regulation of movements*. Oxford: Pergamon Press, UK.

Bermejo, J.L.; Sundquist, J. & Hemminki, K. (2007). Risk of cancer among the offspring of women who experienced parental death during pregnancy. *Cancer Epidemiology, Biomarkers & Prevention,* Vol. 16, pp: 2204–2206.

Boyle, P. & Ferlay, J. (2005). Cancer incidence and mortality in Europe. *Annals of Oncology,* Vol. 6, pp: 481-488.

Bukhtoyarov, O.V. & Arkhangelsky A.E. (2006). Psychogenic death in oncology: study concept, pathogenesis, forms development, possibilities of prevention. *Voprosy oncology,* Vol. 52, No. 6, pp: 708-714.

Bukhtoyarov, O.V. & Arkhangelskiy, A.E. (2008). *Psychogenic cofactor of carcinogenesis: the possibility of using hypnotherapy.* Aletheia, St. Petersburg, Russia.

Bukhtoyarov, O.V. & Samarin, D.M. (2009). Psychogenic carcinogenesis: carcinogenesis is without exogenic carcinogens. *Medical Hypotheses.* Vol. 73, No. 4, pp: 531-536.

Bukhtoyarov, O.V.; Samarin, D.M.; Borisov, V.I.; Senyukov, V.V.; Kozhevnikov, V.S. & Kozlov, V.A. (2008). Immune system re-integration induced by hypnosuggestion in oncologIcal patients. *Medical Immunology,* Vol. 10, No. 6, pp: 527-534.

Cavanagh, J. & Mathias, C. (2008). Inflammation and its relevance to psychiatry. *Advances in Psychiatric Treatment,* Vol. 14, pp: 248–255.

Chouaib, S.; Hage, F.El.; Benlalam H. & Mami-Chouaib F. (2006). Immunotherapy of cancer: promise and reality. *Medical Science (Paris),* Vol. 22, No. 8-9, pp: 755-759.

Coleman, W.B. & Tsongalis, G.J. (2006). Molecular mechanisms of human carcinogenesis. *Experientia Supplementum,* Vol. 96, pp: 321-349.

Conrad, Ch.D. (2006). What is the functional significance of chronic stress-induced CA3 dendritic retraction within the hippocampus? *Behavioral and Cognitive Neuroscience Reviews,* Vol. 5, pp: 41–60.

Corzo, C.A.; Nagaraj, S.; Kusmartsev, S. & Gabrilovich, D. (2007). Role of reactive oxygen species in immune suppression in cancer. *Journal of Immunology,* Vol. 178, S: 85.

Coussons-Read, M.E.; Okun, M.L.; Schmitt, M.P. & Giese, S.T. (2005). Prenatal stress alters cytokine levels in a manner that may endanger human pregnancy. *Psychosomatic Medicine,* Vol. 67, pp: 625–631.

Daly, R. (2009). Depression biggest contributor to global disease burden. *Psychiatric News,* Vol. 44, No. 1, pp: 7.

Damjanovic, A.; Ivkovic, M. & Jasovic-Gasic, M. (2006). Comorbidity of schizophrenia and cancer: clinical recommendations for treatment. *Psychiatria Danubina,* Vol. 18, No. 1-2, pp: 55-60.

Dantzer, R.; O'Connor, J.C.; Freund, G.G.; Johnson, R.W. & Kelley, K.W. (2008). From inflammation to sickness and depression: when the immune system subjugates the brain. *Nature Reviews Neuroscience,* Vol. 9, pp: 46–56.

Depke, M.; Fusch, G.; Domanska, G.; Geffers, R.; Völker, U.; Schütt, C.H. & Kiank, C. (2008). Hypermetabolic syndrome as a consequence of repeated psychological stress in mice. *Endocrinology,* Vol. 149, pp: 2714–2723.

Desaive, P. & Ronson, A. (2008). Stress spectrum disorders in oncology. *Current Opinion in Oncology,* Vol. 20, pp: 378–385.

Diener, Ed. & Chan, M.Y. (2011). Happy people live longer: subjective well-being contributes to health and longevity. *Applied Psychology: Health and Well-Being,* Vol. 3, No. 1, pp: 1–43.

Dimitroglou, E.; Zafiropoulou, M.; Messini-Nikolaki, N.; Doudounakis, S.; Tsilimigaki, S. & Piperakis, SM. (2003). DNA damage in a human population affected by chronic psychogenic stress. *International Journal of Hygiene and Environmental Health,* Vol. 206, pp: 39–44.

Dimsdale, J.E. Psychological stress and cardiovascular disease. (2008). *Journal of the American College of Cardiology,* 51, pp: 1237-1246.

Epel, E.S.; Blackburn, E.H.; Lin, J.; Dhabhar, F.S.; Adler, N.E.; Morrow, J.D. & Cawthon, R.M. (2004). Accelerated telomere shortening in response to life stress. *PNAS,* Vol. 101, pp: 17312–17315.

Federico, A.; Morgillo, F.; Tuccillo, C.; Ciardiello, F. & Loguercio, C. (2007). Chronic inflammation and oxidative stress in human carcinogenesis. *International Journal of Cancer,* Vol. 121, pp: 2381–2386.

Finn, O.J. (2008). Cancer immunology. *New England Journal of Medicine,* Vol. 358, pp: 2704-2715.

Fort, M.M. & Narayanan, P.K. (2010). Manipulation of regulatory T-cell function by immunomodulators: a boon or a curse? *Toxicological Sciences,* Vol. 117, No. 2, pp: 253-262.

Gidron, Y.; Russ, K.; Tissarchondou, H. & Warner J. (2006). The relation between psychological factors and DNA-damage: a critical review. *Biological Psychology,* Vol. 72, pp: 291-304.

Greene, Jr. WA. & Miller, G. (1958). Psychological factors and reticuloendothelial disease. IV. Observations on a group of children and adolescents with leukemias: an interpretation of disease development in terms of mother-child unit. *Psychosomatic Medicine,* Vol. 20, pp: 124–144.

Grossardt, B.R.; Bower, J.H.; Geda, Y.E.; Colligan, R.C. & Rocca, W.A. (2009). Pessimistic, anxious, and depressive personality traits predict all-cause mortality: the mayo clinic cohort study of personality and aging. *Psychosomatic Medicine,* Vol. 71, pp: 491-500.

Gruzelier, J.H. (2002). A review of the impact of hypnosis, relaxation, guided imagery and individual differences on aspects of immunity and health. *Stress,* Vol. 5, No. 2, pp: 147-163.

Halliwell, B. (2007). Oxidative stress and cancer: have we moved forward? *Biochemical Journal,* Vol. 401, pp: 1–11.

Hasegawa, H. & Saiki, I. (2005). Psychosocial stress augments tumor development through b-adrenergic activation in mice. *Cancer Science,* Vol. 93, pp: 729–735.

Herbst, R.S.; Bajorin, D.F.; Bleiberg, H.; Blum, D.; Hao, D.; Johnson, B.E.; Ozols, R.F.; Demetri, G.D.; Ganz, P.A.; Kris, M.G.; Levin, B.; Markman, M.; Raghavan, D.; Reaman, G.H.; Sawaya, R.; Schuchter, L.M.; Sweetenham, J.W.; Vahdat, L.T.; Vokes, E.E.; Winn, R.J. & Mayer, R.J. (2006). Clinical cancer advances 2005: major research advances in cancer treatment, prevention, and screening – a report from the American Society of Clinical Oncology. *Journal of Clinical Oncology,* Vol. 24, pp: 190–205.

Hidderley, MA. & Holt, M. (2004). A pilot randomized trial assessing the effects of autogenic training in early stage cancer patients in relation to psychological status and immune system responses. *European Journal of Oncology Nursing,* Vol. 8, No. 1, pp: 61-65.

Hudacek, K.D. (2007). A review of the effects of hypnosis on the immune system in breast cancer patients: a brief communication. *International Journal of Clinical* and Experimental *Hypnosis,* Vol. 55, No. 4, pp: 411-425.

Irwin, M.R. & Miller, A.H. (2007). Depressive disorders and immunity: 20 years of progress and discovery. *Brain, Behavior, and Immunity,* Vol. 21, pp: 374–383.

Jacobs, N.; Kenis, G.; Peeters, F.; Derom, C.; Vlietinck, R. & van Os, J. (2006). Stress-related negative affectivity and genetically altered serotonin transporter function: evidence of synergism in shaping risk of depression. *Archives of General Psychiatry,* Vol. 63, pp: 989–996.

Jacobs, T.J. & Charles, E. (1980). Life events and the occurrence of cancer in children. *Psychosomatic Medicine,* Vol. 42, pp: 11–24.

Jacobsen, P.B. &, Jim, H.S. (2008). Psychosocial interventions for anxiety and depression in adult cancer patients: achievements and challenges. *Cancer Journal for Clinicians,* Vol. 58, No. 4, pp: 214-230.

Jemal, A.; Siegel, R.; Ward, E.; Hao, Y.; Xu, J.; Murray, T. & Thun, M.J. (2008). Cancer Statistics, 2008. *Cancer Journal for Clinicians,* Vol. 58, pp: 71-96.

Kawanishi, S.; Hiraku, Y.; Pinlaor, S. & Ma, N. (2006). Oxidative and nitrative DNA damage in animals and patients with inflammatory diseases in relation to inflammation-related carcinogenesis. *Biological Chemistry,* Vol. 387, pp: 365-372.

Kiecolt-Glaser, J.K.; Marucha, Ph.T. & Atkinson, C. (2001). Hypnosis as a modulator of cellular immune dysregulation during acute stress. *Journal of Consulting & Clinical Psychology,* Vol. 69, No. 4, pp: 674-682.

Kim, R.; Emi, M. & Tanabe, K. (2007). Cancer immunoediting from immune surveillance to immune escape. *Immunology,* Vol. 121, No. 1, pp: 1-14.

Kimura, M.; Hjelmborg, Jv.B.; Gardner, J.P.; Bathum, L.; Brimacombe, M.; Lu, X.; Christiansen, L.; Vaupel, J.W.; Aviv, A. & Christensen, K. (2008). Telomere length and mortality: a study of leukocytes in elderly danish twins. *American Journal of Epidemiology,* Vol. 167, pp: 799–806.

Knight, A.; Bailey, J. & Balcombe, J. (2006). Animal carcinogenicity studies: 2. Obstacles to extrapolation of data to humans. *Alternatives to laboratory animals,* Vol. 34, pp: 29–38.

Knox, S.S. (2001). Psychosocial stress and the physiology of atherosclerosis. *Advances in Psychosomatic Medicine,* Vol. 22, pp: 139-151.

Korman, A.J.; Peggs, K.S. & Allison J.P. (2006). Checkpoint blockade in cancer immunotherapy. *Advances in Immunology,* Vol. 90, pp: 297-339.

Kozhevnikov, V.S.; Konenkova, L.P.; Sizikov, A.E.; Zonova, E.V.; Korolev, M.A.; Pronkina, N.V.; Evsyukova, E.V.; Meniaeva, E.V.; Frolov, N.I. & Kozlov, V.A. (2004). The estimation of immunomodulatory effect of therapy with erythropoietin in rheumatoid arthritis patients. *Medical Immunology,* Vol. 6, No. 6, pp: 557-562.

Kruk, J. & Aboul-Enen, H.Y. (2004). Psychological stress and the risk of breast cancer: a case-control study. *Cancer Detection and Prevention,* Vol. 28, No. 6, pp: 399–408.

Kundu, J.K. & Surh, Y.J. (2008). Inflammation: gearing to the cancer. *Mutation Research,* Vol. 659, pp: 15–30.

Landen, C.N.; Lin, Y.G.; Pena, G.N.A.; Das, P.D.; Arevalo, J.M.; Kamat, A.A.; Han, L.Y.; Jennings, N.B.; Spannuth, W.A.; Thaker, P.H.; Lutgendorf, S.K.; Savary, C.A.; Sanguino, A.M.; Lopez-Berestein, G.; Cole, S.W. & Sood, A.K. (2007). Neuroendocrine modulation of signal transducer and activator of transcription-3 in ovarian cancer. *Cancer Research,* Vol. 67, pp: 10389–10396.

Leont'ev, A.N. (1978). *Activity, consciousness, and personality*. Prentice-Hall, Englewood Cliffs, USA.

Lester, D. (2009). Voodoo death. *Omega (Westport),* Vol. 59, pp: 1-18.

Levav, I.; Kohn, R.; Iscovich, J.; Abramson, J.H.; Tsai, W.Y. & Vigdorovich, D. (2000). Cancer incidence and survival following bereavement. *American Journal of Public Health,* Vol. 90, pp: 1601-1607.

Lewis, C.E.; O'Brien, R.M. & Barraclough, J. (2002). *The psychoimmunology of cancer.* Oxford Univ. Press, USA.

Li, J.; Johansen, C.; Brønnum–Hansen, H.; Stenager, E.; Koch–Henriksen, N. & Olsen, J. (2004). The risk of multiple sclerosis in bereaved parents: A nationwide cohort study in Denmark. *Neurology,* Vol. 62, pp: 726-729.

Lillberg, K.; Verkasalo, P.K.; Kaprio, J.; Teppo, L.; Helenius, H. & Koskenvuo, M. (2003). Stressful life events and risk of breast cancer in 10, 808 women: a cohort study. *American Journal of Epidemiology,* Vol. 157, pp: 415–423.

Lloyd-Williams, M.; Shiels, C.; Taylor, F. & Dennis, M. (2009). Depression – an independent predictor of early death in patients with advanced cancer. *Journal of Affective Disorders,* Vol. 113, pp: 127-132.

Lopez, A.D. & Murray, C.J.L. (1998). The global burden of disease, 1990–2020. *Nature Medicine,* No. 4, pp: 1241–1243.

Luria, A.R. (1970). The functional organization of the brain. *Scientific American,* Vol. 222, pp: 66-78.

Marchioro, G.; Azzarello, G.; Viviani, F.; Barbato, F.; Pavanetto, M.; Rosetti, F.; Pappagallo, G.L. & Vinante, O. (2000). Hypnosis in the treatment of anticipatory nausea and vomiting in patients receiving cancer chemotherapy. *Oncology,* Vol. 59, No. 2, pp: 100-104.

Maslow, A.H. (1943). A theory of human motivation. *Psychological Review,* Vol. 50, pp: 370-396.

McEwen, B.S. (2007). Physiology and neurobiology of stress and adaptation: central role of the brain. *Physiological Reviews,* Vol. 87, pp: 873-904.

McGee, R.; Williams, S. & Elwood, M. (1994). Depression and the development of cancer: a meta-analysis. *Social Science & Medicine,* Vol. 38, pp: 187–192.

McGuire, T.R.; Kessinger, A. & Hock, L. (2001). Elevated transforming growth factor beta levels in the plasma of cytokine-treated cancer patients and normal allogeneic stem cell donors. *Cytotherapy,* Vol. 3, No. 5, pp: 361–364.

Miller, G.E. & Cohen, S. (2001). Psychological interventions and the immune system: a meta-analytic review and critique. *Health Psychololology,* Vol. 20, No. 1, pp: 47-63.

Miller, G.E.; Cohen, S. & Ritchey, A.K. (2002). Chronic psychological stress and the regulation of pro-inflammatory cytokines: a glucocorticoid-resistance model. *Health Psychology,* Vol. 21, pp: 531–541.

Miller, K. & Massie, M.J. (2006). Depression and anxiety. *Cancer Journal,* Vol. 12, pp: 388–397.

Miovic, M. & Block, S. (2007). Psychiatric disorders in advanced cancer. *Cancer,* Vol. 110, No. 8, p:1665-1676.

Montazeri, A.; Jarvandi, S.; Ebrahimi, M.; Haghighat, S. & Ansari, M. (2004). The role of depression in the development of breast cancer: analysis of registry data from a single institute. *Asian Pacific Journal of Cancer Prevention,* Vol. 5, pp: 316–319.

Montgomery, G.H.; Bovbjerg, D.H.; Schnur, J.B.; David, D.; Goldfarb, A.; Weltz, C.R.; Schechter, C.; Graff-Zivin, J.; Tatrow, K.; Price, D.D. & Silverstein, J.H. (2007). A randomized clinical trial of a brief hypnosis intervention to control side effects in breast surgery patients. *Journal of the National Cancer Institute,* Vol. 99, No. 17, pp: 1304-1312.

Montes, C.L.; Chapoval, A.I. & Nelson, J. (2008). Tumor-induced senescent T cells with suppressor function: a potential form of tumor immune evasion. *Cancer Research*, Vol. 68, pp: 870-879.

Monti, D.A.; Sufian, M. & Peterson, C. (2008). Potential role of mind-body therapies in cancer survivorship. *Cancer*, Vol. 112, No. 11, pp: 2607-2616.

Morgan, P.J.; Galler, J.R. & Mokler, D.J. (2005). A review of systems and networks of limbic forebrain/limbic midbrain. *Progress in Neurobiology*, Vol. 75, pp: 143–160.

Mravec, B.; Gidron, Y. & Hulin, I. (2008). Neurobiology of cancer: interactions between nervous, endocrine and immune systems as a base for monitoring and modulating the tumorogenesis by the brain. *Seminars in Cancer Biology*, Vol. 18, pp: 150-163.

Nemeroff, C.B. (2008). Recent findings in the pathophysiology of depression. *Focus*, Vol. 6, pp: 3-14.

Newport, J.D.; Stowe, Z.N. & Nemeroff, C.B. (2002). Parental depression: animal models of an adverse life event. *American Journal of Psychiatry*, Vol. 159, pp: 1265–1283.

Ornish, D.; Lin, J.; Daubenmier, J.; Weidner, G.; Epel, E.; Kemp, C.; Magbanua, M.J.; Marlin, R.; Yglecias, L.; Carroll, P.R. & Blackburn, E.H. (2008). Increased telomerase activity and comprehensive lifestyle changes: a pilot study. *Lancet Oncology*, Vol. 9, pp: 1048–1057.

Ostrander, M.M.; Ulrich-Lai, Y.M.; Choi, D.C.; Richtand, N.M. & Herman, J.P. (2006). Hypoactivity of the hypothalamo-pituitary-adrenocortical axis during recovery from chronic variable stress. *Endocrinology*, Vol. 147, pp: 2008-2017.

Ott, M.J.; Norris, R.L. & Bauer-Wu, S.M. (2006). Mindfulness meditation for oncology patients: a discussion and critical review integrative cancer therapies. *Integrated Cancer Therapy*, Vol. 5, No. 2, pp: 98-108.

Ouyang, Q.; Baerlocher, G. & Vulto, I. (2007). Telomere length in human natural killer cell subsets. *Hematopoietic Stem Cells*, Vol. 1106, pp: 240-252.

Perelman, Ya. (2008). *Physics for entertainment. Book two*. Hyperion, New York, USA.

Ranganathan, A.C.; Adam, A.P.; Zhang, L. & Aguirre-Dhiso, J.A. (2006). Tumor cell dormancy induced by p38SARK and ER-stress signaling: an adaptive advantage for metastatic cells. *Cancer Biology and Therapy*, Vol. 5, pp: 729–735.

Reiche, E.M.; Morimoto, H.K. & Nunes, S.M. (2005). Stress and depression-induced immune dysfunction: implications for the development and progression of cancer. *International Review of Psychiatry*, Vol. 17, pp: 515–527.

Rodin, G.; Lo, C.; Mikulincer, M.; Donner, A.; Gagliese, L. & Zimmermann, C. (2009). Pathways to distress: the multiple determinants of depression, hopelessness, and the desire for hastened death in metastatic cancer patients. *Social Science & Medicine*, Vol. 68, pp: 562-569.

Rotenberg, V.S. & Arshavsky, V.V. (1984). *Search activity and adaptation.* Nauka, Moscow, USSR.

Rotenberg, V.S. (2009). Search activity concept: relationship between behavior, health and brain functions. *Activitas Nervosa Superior*, Vol. 51, pp: 12-44.

Roy-Byrne, P.P.; Davidson, K.W.; Kessler, R.C.; Asmundson, G.J.G.; Goodwin R.D.; Kubzansky L.; Lydiard, R.B.; Massie, M.J.; Katon, W.; Laden, S.K. & Stein, M.B. (2008). Anxiety disorders and comorbid medical illness. *Focus* Vol. 6, pp: 467-485.

Rusé-Riol, F.; Legros, M. & Bernard, D. (1984). Variations in committed stem cells (CFU-GM and CFU-TL) in the peripheral blood of cancer patients treated by sequential combination chemotherapy for breast cancer. *Cancer Research*, Vol. 44, pp: 2219-2224.

Sacerdote, P. (1966). The uses of hypnosis in cancer patients. *Annals of the* New York *Academy of Sciences,* Vol. 125, No. 3, pp: 1011-1019.

Saul, A.N.; Oberyszyn, T.M.; Daugherty, C.K.; Donna, J.S.; Jewell, S.; Malarkey, W.B.; Lehman, A.; Lemeshow, S. & Dhabhar, F.S. (2005). Chronic stress and susceptibility to skin cancer. *JNCI,* Vol. 97, pp: 1760–1767.

Schilder, J.N.; de Vries, M.J. & Goodkin, K. Psychological changes preceding spontaneous remission of cancer. (2004). *Clinical Case Studies,* Vol. 3, No. 4, pp: 288-312.

Schnur, J.B.; Bovbjerg, D.H.; David, D.; Tatrow, K.; Goldfarb, A.B.; Silverstein, J.H.; Weltz, C.R. & Montgomery, G.H. (2008). Hypnosis decreases presurgical distress in excisional breast biopsy patients. *Anesthesia & Analgesia,* Vol. 106, No. 2, pp: 440-444.

Schussler, G. & Schubert, C. (2001). The influence of psychosocial factors on the immune system and their role for the incidence and progression of cancer. *Zeitschrift fur Psychosomatische Medizin und Psychotherapie,* Vol. 47, pp: 6-41.

Seymour, J. & Benning, T.B. (2009). Depression, cardiac mortality and all-cause mortality. *Advances in Psychiatric Treatment,* Vol. 15, pp: 107-113.

Shpagina, L.A.; Ermakova, M.A.; Volkova, E.A. & Iakovleva, S.A. (2008). Clinical, functional and biochemical characteristics of arterial hypertension in military men under chronic stress. *Meditsina Truda i Promyshlennaia Ekologiia,* Vol. 7, pp: 24-29.

Shumake, J. & Gonzalez-Lima, F. (2003). Brain systems underlying susceptibility to helplessness and depression. *Behavioral and Cognitive Neuroscience Reviews,* No. 2, pp: 198-221.

Simon, N.M.; Smoller, J.W.; McNamara, K.L.; Maser, R.S.; Zalta, A.K.; Pollack, M.H.; Nierenberg, A.A.; Fava, M. & Wong, K.K. (2006). Telomere shortening and mood disorders: preliminary support for a chronic stress model of accelerated aging. *Biological Psychiatry,* Vol. 60, pp: 432-435.

Son, N.H., Murray, Sh. & Yanovski, J. (2000). Lineage-specific telomere shortening and unaltered capacity for telomerase expression in human T and B lymphocytes with age. *Journal of Immunology,* Vol. 165, pp: 1191-1196.

Spiegel, D. & Giese-Davis, J. (2003). Depression and cancer: mechanisms and disease progression. *Biological Psychiatry,* Vol. 54, pp: 269–282.

Spinelli, S.; Chefer, S.; Suomi, S.J.; Higley, J.D.; Barr, C.S. & Stein, E. (2009). Early-life stress induces long-term morphologic changes in primate brain. *Archives of General Psychiatry,* Vol. 66, pp: 658-665.

Staat, K. & Segatore, M. (2005). The phenomenon of chemo brain. *Clinical Journal of Oncology Nursing,* Vol. 9, No. 6, pp: 713-721.

Su, F.; Ouyang, N.; Zhu, P.; Ouyang, N.; Jia, W.; Gong, C.; Ma, X.; Xu, H. & Song, E. (2005). Psychological stress induces chemoresistance in breast cancer by upregulating mdr1. *Biochemical and Biophysical Research Communications,* Vol. 329, pp: 888–897.

Surtees, P.G.; Wainwright, N.W.J.; Luben, R.N.; Wareham, N.J.; Bingham, S.A. & Khaw, K-T. (2008). Depression and ischemic heart disease mortality: evidence from the EPIC-Norfolk United Kingdom prospective cohort study. *American Journal of Psychiatry,* Vol. 165, pp: 515-523.

Tashiro, M.; Kubota, K.; Itoh, M.; Yoshioka, T.; Yoshida, M.; Nakagawa, Y.; Bereczki, D. & Sasaki. H. (1999). Hypometabolism in the limbic system of cancer patients observed by positronemission tomography. *Psychooncology,* No. 8, pp: 283–286.

Taylor, T.R.; Williams, C.D.; Makambi, K.H.; Mouton, C.; Harrell, J.P.; Cozier, Y.C.; Rosenberg, L.; Palmer, J.R. & Adams-Campbell, L.L. (2007). Racial discrimination and breast cancer incidence in US black women: the black women's health study. *American Journal of Epidemiology,* Vol. 166, pp: 46–54.

Toyokuni, S. (2008). Molecular mechanisms of oxidative stress-induced carcinogenesis: from epidemiology to oxygenomics. *IUBMB Life,* Vol. 60, pp: 441–447.

Tukiendorf, A. (2005). Could socio-economic transformation and the resulting psychological stress influence cancer risk in Opole province, Poland? *Central European Journal of Public Health,* Vol. 13, pp: 125–131.

Ukhtomsky, AA. (1927). The dominant as a working principle of nervous centers. *Russkii Fiziologicheskii Zhurnal,* No. 6.

Ukhtomsky, AA. (1966). *The Dominant.* Nauka, Moscou, USSR.

Uznadze, DN. (1997). *The theory of installation.* Metsniereba, Tbilisi, Georgia.

von Zglinicki, T. & Martin-Ruiz C.M. (2005). Telomeres as biomarkers for ageing and agerelated diseases. *Current Molecular Medicine,* No. 5, pp: 197–203.

Wang, J.; Charboneau, R.; Barke, R.A.; Loh, H.H. & Roy, S. (2002). V-Opioid receptor mediates chronic restraint stress-induced lymphocyte apoptosis. *Journal of Immunology,* Vol. 169, pp: 3630–3636.

Wang, R.F. (1997). Tumor antigens discovery: perspectives for cancer therapy. *Molecular Medicine,* Vol. 3, No. 11, pp: 716-731.

Wood, G.J.; Bughi, S. & Morrison, J. (2003). Hypnosis, differential expression of cytokines by T-cell subsets, and the hypothalamo-pituitary-adrenal axis. *American Journal* of *Clinical Hypnosis,* Vol. 45, No. 3, pp: 179-196.

Wyman, P.A.; Moynihan, J.; Eberly, S.; Cox, C.; Cross, W.; Jin, X. & Caserta, M.T. (2007). Association of family stress with natural killer cell activity and the frequency of illnesses in children. *Archives of Pediatrics & Adolescent Medicine,* Vol. 161, pp: 228–234.

Yang, Z-Z. & Ansell, S.M. (2009). The role of Treg cells in the cancer immunological response. *American Journal of Immunology,* Vol. 5, No. 1, pp: 17-28.

Yousef, N. (2008). From the wild side. *History Workshop,* Vol. 65, pp: 213-220.

Zhang, Y.; Foster, R.; Sun, X.; Yin, Q.; Li, Y.; Hanley, G.; Stuart, C.; Gan, Y.; Li, C.; Zhang, Z. & Yin, D. (2008). Restraint stress induces lymphocyte through p53 and P13K/NF-kappaB pathways. *Journal of Neuroimmunology, V*ol. 200, pp: 71–76.

Zhao, C.; Fang, Q.; Tan, K. & Lu, X. (2002). Relationship among breast cancer and negative life event and cell immunity. *Zhonghua Yi Xue Za Zhi,* Vol. 82, pp: 1235–1236.

Zhou, J.; Shen, X. & Huang J. (2005). Telomere length of transferred lymphocytes correlates with In vivo persistence and tumor regression in melanoma patients receiving cell transfer therapy. *Journal of Immunology,* Vol. 175, pp: 7046-7052.

Zuccolo, L.; Pastore, G.; Pearce, N.; Mosso, M.L.; Merletti, F. & Magnani, C. (2007). Mortality from cancer and other causes in parents of children with cancer: a population based study in Piedmont, Italy. *European Journal of Cancer Prevention,* Vol. 16, pp: 390–395.

3

Rectal Cancer - Staging and Surgical Approach

Pramateftakis Manousos-Georgios, Papadopoulos Vasileios,
Michalopoulos Antonios, Spanos Konstantinos,
Tepetes Konstantinos and Tsoulfas Georgios
Aristotle University of Thessaloniki & University of Thessaly
Greece

1. Introduction

Pramateftakis MG

Worldwide, colorectal cancer is a major health problem. More than 1 million patients are diagnosed annually. It is the 3rd most common cancer type and about half a million people die of the disease each year. Incidence is higher in more developed than less developed regions suggesting that lifestyle, dietary habits and environmental exposures, beyond genetic background, are responsible for the disease in the industrialized world.

In recent years significant knowledge has been acquired and applied in everyday clinical practice as far as rectal cancer is concerned. The treatment of rectal cancer has changed over the last two decades as far as surgical techniques, chemotherapy and radiotherapy are concerned. Effective surgery and modern radiotherapy combined with cytotoxic chemotherapy have improved survival rates (Nicholls & Tekkis, 2008; Carlsen et al., 1998).

2. Rectal cancer staging

Pramateftakis MG, Papadopoulos V, Michalopoulos A

The assessment of a patient with rectal cancer involves the identification of disseminated disease and the locoregional staging of the tumor. Loco-regional factors which influence prognosis include T-stage, the lymph node status and the histological grade. Rectal cancer presents in 3 clinical categories. These are the early, the intermediate and the advanced lesions. The improvement of conventional diagnosis and the introduction of molecular screening advanced early diagnosis. Virtual colonoscopy, computed tomography (CT), magnetic resonance imaging (MRI), endorectal ultrasound (EUS) and positron emission tomography (PET) constitute a significant development to the diagnosis and staging of colorectal cancer (Kuhry et al, 2008). Endorectal ultrasound can demonstrate penetration of the rectal wall with high accuracy, but is poor at identifying the N stage. CT is useful for local extensive tumors particularly in identifying other organ involvement. MRI is accurate in determining the T stage but performs better in identifying the presence or absence of the circumferential margin involvement. In the last five years, preoperative staging has become more refined by advances in MRI imaging.

EUS seems to be an accurate method to stage rectal cancer preoperatively. The major drawback of EUS is that it is operator-dependent, but on the other hand it is easy and fast to perform, requires minimal patient preparation and it can be repeated without side effects. EUS based evaluation of rectal tumors provides an accuracy ranging from 62% to 92% for T staging and from 64% to 88% for N staging (Kim & Wong, 2005).

Pelvic CT staging of rectal cancer is inferior to EUS with the accuracy for T staging ranging from 53% to 94% and for N staging from 54% to 70% (Harewood, 2005). MRI, especially with the use of endorectal coil, seems to be superior to CT for locoregional rectal cancer staging, with accuracy for T staging ranging from 66% to 92% and that for N staging rising over 95% (Chen et al., 2005).

A recent meta-analysis showed that EUS and MRI had similar sensitivity for T staging (94%) but EUS had superior specificity compared to MRI (86% vs 69%). This study also showed that both EUS and MRI have poor sensitivity (67%) and specificity (77%) for N staging. However, there are reports in the literature stating that EUS may be overestimated, especially in small size series. Therefore, it seems that the accuracy of imaging methods for the N stage of rectal cancer needs further improvement (Harewood, 2005; Kwok et al., 2000).

PET scanning has been used preoperatively to rule out metastatic disease in selected cases and postoperatively for the detection of recurrence or to evaluate response to treatment. It is reported that PET scan alters the conventional preoperative stage in nearly 40% of cases leading to modification of therapeutic strategies in 17% of patients. Furthermore, there is evidence that PET is more sensitive than CT for the evaluation of the response to neoadjuvant treatment, able in some cases to 'predict' pathologic response. Currently, there are no large series with regards to the initial locoregional staging of rectal tumors using PET and the significance of this method is mainly identified in neoadjuvant protocols (Heriot et al., 2004).

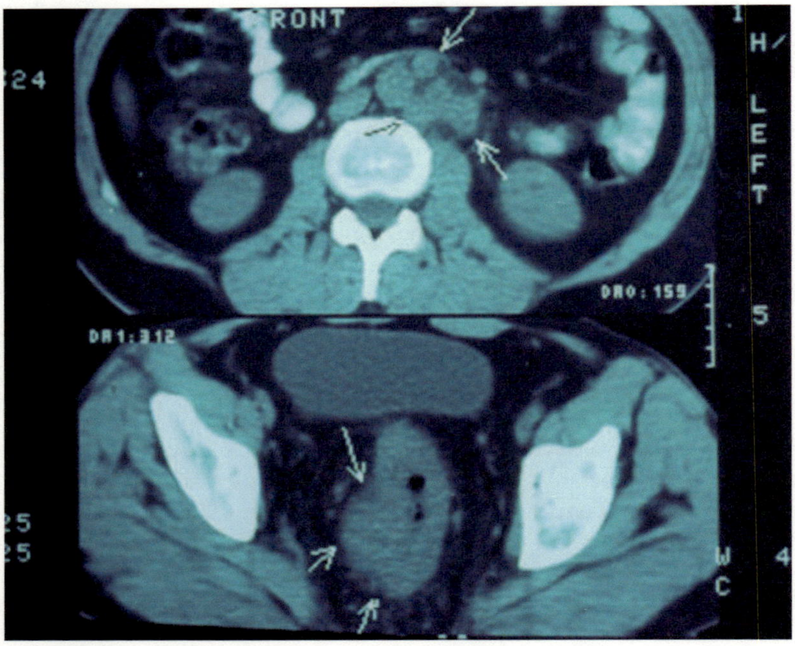

Fig. 1. Rectal mass identified on CT scan. Metastatic lymphnodes at the inferior mesenteric artery root.

3. Surgical approach to rectal cancer

Pramateftakis MG, Tsoulfas G

After the diagnosis and staging of a rectal tumor, a decision needs to be made with regards to the optimal method of surgical treatment. To save or not to save the sphincters is a common question. Is there a level below which an anastomosis should not be attempted? The optimal surgical technique for low rectal tumors remains controversial in the absence of randomized trials. Conversely, too often, in a fanatic effort to avoid a colostomy and to reestablish intestinal continuity, surgeons compromise on the margins of resection. The consequences are often tragic for the patient (recurrence, anastomotic obstruction, functional problems and pelvic pain).

The intention of oncologic surgery for rectal cancer is the removal of the primary tumour and regional lymphatics and the prevention of tumour cell spillage. Controversy still exists about the extent of lymphadenectomy, the importance of the Turnbull's no touch technique, the optimal free distal margin and the irrigation of the rectal stump. Whether complete retroperitoneal clearance of all lymphatic tissue ("pre-aortic strip") offers advantage to survival rates is still doubtful. There are no randomised clinical trials supporting the value of extended lateral internal iliac lymph node excision. Moreover, there is a high incidence of urinary and sexual complications because of autonomic nerve damage (Pramateftakis et al., 2010).

In 1981, Heald introduced the concept of total excision of the mesorectal adipose and lymphatic tissue for middle and lower rectal carcinomas, namely the Total Mesorectal Excision (TME). Apart from the TME, oncologic resection involves the mobilization of the splenic flexure, high ligation of the inferior mesenteric artery (IMA) and the sharp dissection under direct vision of the mesorectal tissues to the level of the levators. The fascia propria of the mesorectum and the nerve plexus must be preserved intact, leaving a smooth mesorectal surface. The middle rectal vessels must be cauterized. With this technique, all the lymphatic tissue surrounding the rectum is removed. The specimen may contain the tumor tissue, its intraluminal extent, the metastatic infiltrated lymph nodes, vessels and nodules. TME is now considered to be the 'gold standard' approach for the middle and low rectal cancers (Heald, 1982, 1992).

Hospital patients' volume seems to have an impact on colostomy rates, postoperative mortality and overall survival. In a series of 7257 patients diagnosed with Stage I–III rectal cancer between 1994 and 1997, there were statistically significant differences in colostomy rates (29.5% versus 36.6%), 30-day postoperative mortality (1.6% versus 4.8%) and in overall 2-year survival (83.7% versus 76.6%) in hospitals with higher patient volumes (>20 procedures per year) compared to those with fewer than 7 procedures annually. The ability for sphincter-sparing surgery is also affected by the hospital volume. In an adjuvant treatment trial of 1330 patients with Stage II or III rectal cancer, the rates of abdoperineal resections as opposed to low anterior resections were significantly higher in low-volume hospitals (46% versus 32%, respectively) (Meyerhardt et al., 2004).

The type of operation that can be offered to a patient with rectal cancer depends not only on tumour stage, but also on the location of the tumour in relation to the surgical anatomy. Surgical anatomy refers to the anatomic landmarks that determine resectability and sphincter preservation. The NCI consensus on rectal cancer recommended localizing the tumour relation to the anal verge, which is defined as starting at the intersphincteric groove. Another important landmark defining the upper limit of the anal canal is the anorectal ring.

From the surgeon's perspective, the top of the anorectal ring is the lower limit of a distal resection margin. A large, full-thickness cancer needs to be located high enough above the top of the anorectal ring to allow for an adequate distal margin if sphincter preservation is contemplated. If the dissection is to be carried lower towards the dentate line, then the tumor must be confined to the mucosa, submucosa, and superficial layer of the internal sphincter (Bleday & Garcia-Aguilar, 2007).

Quality surgery and adjuvant therapy have improved overall 5-year survival rates for colorectal cancer over the last decades. It is nowadays proven that a sphincter-sparing surgical approach does not sacrifice survival in selected patients when an adequate margin can be achieved (Bleday & Garcia-Aguilar, 2007).

In summary, aim of the technique chosen is the regional disease control, the radical tumor resection (R0) and the preservation of the sphincter mechanism (whenever possible). Therefore, depending on the tumor location, the surgical choices are the low anterior resection, the intersphincteric resection, the transanal resection and the abdominoperineal resection. All approaches will be discussed in detail in the following paragraphs.

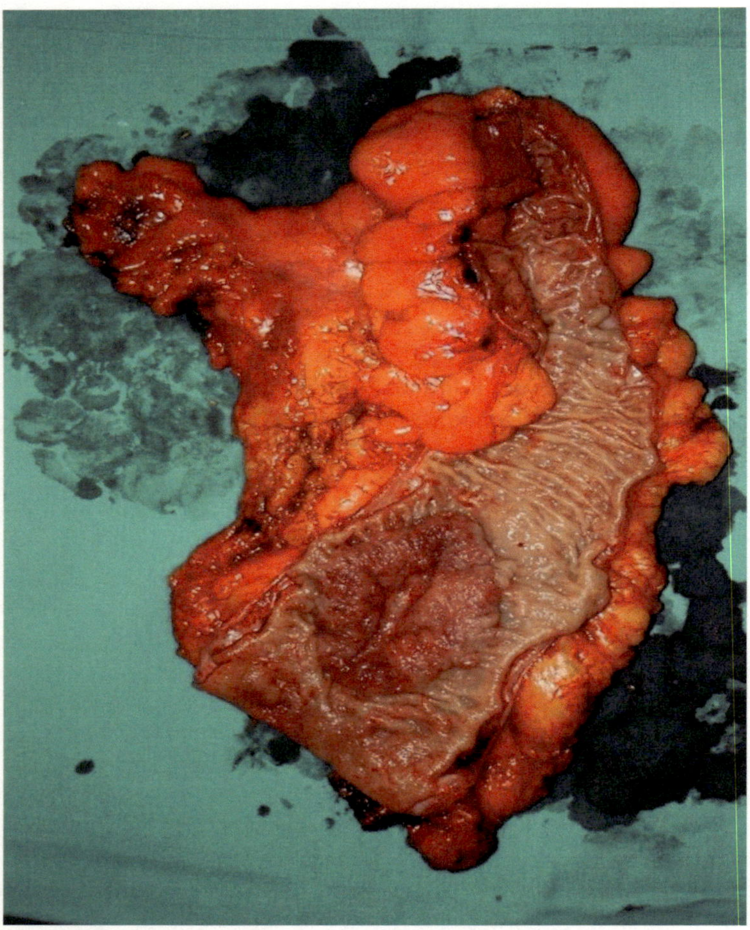

Fig. 2. Low anterior resection specimen with high ligation of the feeding vessels (IMA).

4. Low anterior resection for rectal cancer

Michalopoulos A, Papadopoulos V, Pramateftakis MG

A low anterior resection is undertaken in order to remove malignant tumors of the middle and lower rectum. For the radical excision of a rectal cancer, a "5-cm rule" distal free margin below the tumor has been an important issue. However, intramural spread exceeds 1–2 cm in a few occasions only and further increase of the distal margin beyond 2 cm does not improve the locoregional recurrence rate or survival. An established principle is that the mesorectum and the wall of the rectum should be transected at the same level (Williams et al., 1983). The resection concerns the intra- and extraperitoneal rectosigmoid and the anastomosis is conducted below the peritoneal reflection (<8 cm from the anal ring). The anastomosis is performed either manually (usually in an end-to-end manner) or by the use of automatic stapling devices, in which case it can be performed as an end-to-end, end-to-side or side-to-side anastomosis.

4.1 Technical considerations & controversies

4.1.1 Low anterior resection and coloanal anastomosis

In case of a very low anterior resection, the anastomosis is performed at the level of the dentate line, after excision of the upper half of the internal sphincter. The direct end-to-end anastomosis is performed either transanally, or by the York Mason technique, the Kraske technique, or even by the use of a circular stapler. A diverting ileostomy should also be performed (Pramateftakis et al., 2010).

4.1.2 Coloanal anastomosis with colonic J-pouch

A colonic J-pouch is recommended for carcinomas of the middle and lower rectum, large benign tumors of the lower rectum, heavy radiation orthitis and rectal Crohn's disease.

Contraindications for a J-pouch include the infiltration of the levator muscles by the tumor, inflammation and fistulas of the perineum and anal incontinence.

The rectal cancer excision is similar to the traditional very low anterior resection, with the addition of a colonic J-pouch construction. The descending colon is preferred to the sigmoid colon, because it is firmer and has better adaptability. For the safety of the low anastomosis, the operation must be supplemented by the creation of a temporary ileostomy, which is usually reversed after 2-3 months. Patients with a pouch have fewer stool evacuations per day, but some of them may need enemas or suppositories to evacuate. However, the anastomosis is considered safer and there is a lower incidence of the post-operative low anterior resection syndrome, nevertheless only in the early postoperative period. During the late postoperative period, there are no statistically significant advantages of a colonic J-pouch when compared to the simple coloanal anastomosis, as the intestine gradually seems to adapt (Jeng-Kai et al, 2005; Nicholls, 1991).

4.1.3 Low Colorectal anastomosis with ileocecal reservoir transposition

An alternative method of a colonic reservoir after a low anterior resection is the ileocecal transfer, in cases of inadequate left colic flexure mobilization. The cecum, along with the final part of the ileum and their blood supply (ileocolic artery) are transferred to the rectal stump. In this case, the cecum is used as a pouch, with the added effect of a valve mechanism (ileocecal valve) (Jeng-Kai et al., 2005).

4.1.4 Pull-through (coloanal anastomosis)

After removing the rectum, the anus is dilated and, using stay sutures to the rim of the rectal stump, the anus or the rectal stump is reversed and is delivered out of the anal ring, with the mucosa facing outwards. Then, through the inverted rectal stump, the sigmoid or the descending colon is pulled out for about 10 cm and the anastomosis is performed. Alternatively, a catheter can be placed into the sigmoid colon and the excessive intestine is excised 2 weeks later, after mucosal approximation with absorbable sutures (Bennett, 1986).

4.1.5 Total Mesorectal Excision (TME)

The posterior wall of the mesorectum is covered by the fascia propria, which is a part of the visceral fascia. The sacrum and the coccyx are covered by a strong aponeurotic fascia, which represents the continuation of Todd's fascia. The fascia of Waldayer is a thickening of this pelvic aponeurotic fascia and connects the rectal fascia to the pelvic sacral fascia. In the middle of the anterior wall, the rectum receives a reflection from the peritoneum of the posterior wall of the bladder in men or the uterus in women, creating the Douglas pouch, at a distance of 7-9 cm from the anus. This is usually deeper in women and divides the rectum in an intraperitoneal, covered by serosa in the front and sides and an extraperitoneal part, not covered by serosa, but by a thin layer of the visceral fascia, called Denonvillier's fascia (Heald, 1982).

The rectum is devoid of mesentery, but the fascia propria covers the lymphatic tissue and the lymphnodes of the rectum, the upper and mid rectal vessels, and lipoid tissue forming the "Mesorectum". The resection of the rectum and mesorectum with the lymph nodes and the preservation of the neural plexus is called a "total mesorectal excision" (TME). A correctly performed TME avoids complications from the urogenital system and the sphincters, since it does not damage the autonomic nerve plexus. Key step of the procedure is the identification and preservation of the pre-aortic superior sympathetic hypogastric plexus and the laterally located hypogastric nerves and sacral splanchnic nerves, forming the inferior hypogastric plexus (sympathetic-parasympathetic nerves S2-S4) on both sides of the pelvic wall. Intact nerves should look like a "fishbone" near the sacral promontory, after a proper dissection (Miles, 1971).

TME is currently recommended for distal mid- and lower rectal cancers, with complete excision of the visceral mesorectal tissue, down to the level of the levators. For upper third or rectosigmoid cancers a tumour specific mesorectal excision (TSME) should be preferred, performing perpendicular and circumferential excision of the mesorectum to a resection margin level of 5 cm distal to the tumour (Wibe et al., 2002).

4.1.6 Extent of distal resection margin for rectal cancer

Even though the intraluminal spread of colorectal cancer is accomplished through the lymphatics of the submucosa or those of the perirectal fat, the mucosal cancer spread rarely extends beyond the 4 cm, distally. In well differentiated, very low carcinomas a distal margin of 2 cm is considered satisfactory, since the 98% of tumour dispersion is in a distance less than 2 cm. This necessitates the preoperative identification of the degree of tumor cell differentiation and the proper measurement of the distal margin in the fresh specimen by the surgeon (Heald, 1982; Wibe et al., 2002).

4.1.7 High ligation of the inferior mesenteric artery (IMA)

High ligation of the inferior mesenteric artery is mandatory. The dissection and ligation of the IMA 1cm from the aorta, preserves the superior hypogastric plexus, formed by fibres of the sympathetic ganglia of the prevertebral sympathetic chain. In a study by Hohenberger et al, 14 patients with local recurrence after 'radical excision' of rectal carcinomas underwent a selective angiography of the inferior mesenteric artery. The remaining stamp of the IMA was found to be longer than 1cm in 11 cases (79%). Some authors report a 5-year survival improvement by 5,7% following a high IMA ligation, while others found no improvement in survival even in patients of stage Dukes C (Hohenberger et al., 1991).

4.1.8 Extensive lymphatic clearance

Extensive lymphatic dissection includes the excision of tissues and lymph nodes surrounding the aorta and iliac vessels reaching proximally to the duodenum, distally to the levator muscles and laterally to the ureters. It also includes the TME, the dissection of the thyroid spaces and the possible ligation of one of the internal iliac vessels. Even though 5-year survival is reported to increase from 2.3% to 10.4% after extensive lymph node dissection, this approach is accompanied by higher morbidity and increased risk of complications, such as damage to the ureters and cystic or sexual dysfunction (McDermott et al, 1982).

4.1.9 No-Touch Technique

This technique involves the early ligation of the inferior mesenteric vessels (first the inferior mesenteric vein distally to the lower border of the pancreas followed by the inferior mesenteric artery, flat to the aorta), before any handling of the tumor finds place. Following the vessel ligation, the colonic lumen is isolated proximally and distally to the cancer. In this way, the spillage of cancer cells during the operating manoeuvres is avoided.

Particularly for the rectal carcinoma, the intraluminal cancer cells apoptosis, spillage and implantation of tumour cells are considered to be important for the increase of the cancer relapses across the stapled line, following a low anterior excision. The technique of early luminal occlusion with a clamp or a rectal stapler distally, followed by complete TME and the intrarectal wash out with antiseptics and cytotoxic solutions, appears to reduce the local recurrences (Young-Fadok et al., 1998). However, in a randomized, prospective study by Wiggers et al., there was no significant difference in the 5-year survival rate between the two techniques (Wiggers et al., 1988).

4.1.10 Oophorectomy

The incidence of synchronous metastases to the ovaries in case of colon cancer is 2-8%. Colorectal carcinomas metastasize to the ovaries either by direct implantation or by lymphatic and haematogenous metastases, due to the pelvic lymphatics. Ovarian metastases seem to appear more frequently in postmenopausal women, while at the same time the risk of developing primary ovarian malignancy is referred to be 5 times higher when compared to the general population. However, prophylactic oophorectomy does not appear to offer any benefits to all colorectal cancer patients, because the risk of occult microscopic disease seems to be low (Young-Fadok et al., 1998). Bilateral oophorectomy is advised when one or both ovaries are grossly abnormal or involved with contiguous extension over the colon cancer. However, prophylactic oophorectomy is not recommended. (Level of Evidence Class II, Grade B) (Otchy et al., 2004).

4.2 Early complications following low anterior resection

4.2.1 Bleeding

Intraoperative bleeding is usually due to inadequate preparation of the rectal stump, an error in the performance of the purse string suture, poor haemostasis of the mesorectum, inadequate vascular ligations or a presacral plexus injury. Endo-rectal bleeding is considered to be due to the shape of the clips, forming a "B" after their closure and allowing gaps through which bleeding can occur. Bleeding may also be due to the capture of foreign tissue inside the circular stapler, such as the prostate and the vagina (Nesbakken et al., 2002).

4.2.2 Anastomotic leakage

Anastomotic dehiscence occurs more commonly in rectal and oesophageal anastomoses than in other parts of the alimentary tract. The main reasons are technical difficulties in dissection of these organs and their easily compromised blood supply. Leakage following a low anterior resection can cause a faecal fistula, pelvic peritonitis or generalized peritonitis. Subclinical leaks are often reported when a postoperative radiologic control is conducted (Kanellos I et al., 2004).

Systematic protective colostomy or ileostomy does not prevent the occurrence of the complication, but limits its consequences, as well as the postoperative hospitalization time. Elderly patients may develop delayed leakages, due to slower healing capabilities (Bittorf et al., 2003; Demetriades et al., 2004).

Anastomoses located 3 to 6 cm from the anal verge may lead to leak rates up to 17%. Some centres are now routinely fashioning a 'protective' diverting stoma. In a randomized multicentre trial, the overall rate of symptomatic leakage was reported to be 19.2%. Patients who had a defunctioning stoma had an anastomotic leakage at 10.3% of the cases and those without a stoma had leakage rates of 28% ($p \leq 0.001$). The necessity for an urgent re-operation was 8.6% in patients with a protective stoma and 25.4% in those without one ($p \leq 0.001$) (Matthiesen et al., 2007; Vrakas et al., 2010).

In another study comparing laparoscopic vs open TME, intestinal obstruction occurred in 5 cases in the laparoscopic group and in 3 cases in the open group. In the laparoscopic group, intestinal obstruction was in the majority of the cases (60%) caused by a problem at the ileostomy site. As a consequence, the loop ileostomy was abandoned as a mode of diversion in favour of the use of a loop transverse colostomy (Staudacher et al., 2007).

Whether a loop ileostomy or a loop colostomy is a better form of faecal diversion remains controversial. Two randomized studies that compare the two techniques and included only patients who had elective TME for rectal cancer reported controversial results. Nevertheless, a trend towards a higher anastomotic leak rate has been observed in patients in whom a stoma was not fashioned at the primary operation. Therefore, many surgeons who perform TME have now the policy to temporarily defunction almost all low anastomoses (Law et al., 2002; Rullier et al., 2003; Staudacher et al., 2007).

Subclinical (meaning non-symptomatic) anastomotic failure may occur in up to 51% of patients, associated with mortality rates ranging from 6% to 22%. Branagan & Finnis reported a 30-day mortality rate of 10% (Branagan & Finnis, 2005). Ptok et al found that patients with anastomotic leakage had a higher rate of immediate postoperative complications (50.8% vs 26.5%, $p \leq 0.001$) and longer hospital stay (29 vs 15 days, $p \leq 0.001$) (Ptok et al., 2007). Taflampas et al reported that male sex, smoking, alcohol abuse and preoperative malnutrition are all risk factors for anastomotic leakage. They also concluded that the distance of the anastomosis from the anal verge has a significant impact on anastomotic failure rates. They recommend the routine mobilisation of the splenic flexure and anastomosis of the descending colon, instead of the sigmoid, to the rectal stump (Taflampas et al., 2009).

The use of a colonic J-pouch seems to decrease the leakage rates after low anterior resection. The size and stage of the primary tumor, the type of the anastomosis (stapled or hand-sewn), omentoplasty, extraperitoneal positioning of the anastomosis, bowel preparation, the use of laparoscopy and the use of a pelvic drain do not reduce the leakage rates. The short scheme of radiotherapy is also not considered to be a significant risk factor. Collagen type and enzyme expression of the tissues, blood transfusions and the learning curve associated with the use of staplers are factors whose association and importance on anastomotic leakage is not yet clarified (Taflampas et al., 2009).

It is uncertain whether the long scheme of radiotherapy or the addition of chemotherapy increases the anastomotic leakage rate. The value of creating a protective stoma is debatable. It may be indicated for anastomoses lower than 6 cm from the anal verge, even though some suggest its elective use (Taflampas et al., 2009).

4.3 Late complications following low anterior resection

4.3.1 Anastomotic stricture

A stricture of the anastomosis is defined as the difficulty of passing the 19mm rectoscope through it. Possible reasons considered are reactive fibrosis to a foreign body (clips), or the consequence of a subclinical leakage. The first possibility is unlikely, while the latter is in contrast to the fact that since there are statistically more subclinical leakages in hand sewn coloanal anastomoses, they should therefore display more frequently strictures than the stapled ones; something that does not happen.

Other causes of strictures are ischemia caused by excessive devascularisation of the rectal stump and the use of small calibre staples (<28mm). Defunctioning colostomies are also thought to provoke strictures because of regression in the diameter of the distal colon (Rees et al., 2004).

4.3.2 Rectovaginal fistula

Rectovaginal fistulae may be a consequence of radiation therapy preceding or following rectal surgery, of inflammatory bowel diseases, such as ulcerative colitis and especially Crohn's disease, or as a complication following improper firing of the stapler. When creating a stapled anastomosis, the accidental capture of vaginal wall between the main body and the anvil of the stapler results in the creation of a rectovaginal fistula. Other causes for fistula creation are subclinical anastomotic dehiscence, haematoma, ischemia, or abscess. Incomplete or excessive rectal stump devascularisation can also lead to a rectovaginal fistula formation.

In cases of a fistula because of cancer recurrence, a lower anterior resection, or an abdominoperineal resection must be performed.

In other cases, a diverting colostomy may initially be conducted followed by a restorative operation at a later stage (transvaginal or transanal). Adhesive substances for eliminating the fistula have also been tried, with controversial results (Sugarbaker, 1996).

4.3.3 Urinary and sexual dysfunction

Postoperative impotence and/or retrograde ejaculation have been observed in 25%-75% of cases, particularly when lateral wall lymphadenectomy and splanchnic nerve resection are performed. In contrary, when TME with careful nerve-sparing dissection is performed, impotence occurs in only 10%-29% of cases (Bleday, 2007). Nevertheless, excessive dissection during TME may also lead to sexual dysfunction. During the dissection of the rectum inside the pelvis, the so called "lateral ligaments" should not be clamped and ligated, but cauterized instead. These ligaments contain small nerve branches of the inferior hypogastric plexus and minor vessels arising from the branches of the internal iliac artery, which pass to the mesorectum. These plexuses can be damaged by dissection and clamping. Great care also has to be taken during the lateral dissection of the Denonvillier's fascia, where the neurovascular bundle of Walsh rises from the inferior hypogastric plexus. That bundle runs along the posterolateral aspect of the prostate.

The clinical consequence of an isolated sympathetic nerve injury is retrograde ejaculation. Dissection beneath the presacral or pelvic fascia from the sacral promontory around to the lateral pelvic sidewall can injure both parasympathetic and sympathetic nerve fibres which can result in impotence and bladder dysfunction (Nesbakken et al., 2002).

4.3.4 Incontinence

It may be due to a disorder in the sensation for faecal evacuation (due to the rectal excision), damage to the pudendal nerves, destruction of nerve plexuses or damage to the sphincter mechanism (Bittorf et al., 2003; Rasmussen et al., 2003).

4.3.5 Post-operative low anterior resection syndrome

The low anterior resection syndrome characterizes the disturbance in the perception of continence of various degrees, the quality and frequency of evacuation, urgency, tenesmus, urinary and sexual dysfunction following a low anterior resection of the rectosigmoid. Continence, as well as normal bowel evacuation, is due to the integrity of sensory, motor and central nervous functions and anatomic formations (hypogastric plexuses, pudendal nerves, tension receptors of the pelvic floor etc.) Furthermore, the knowledge and acceptance of the coordination mechanism of continence and defecation (constipation, incontinence, continence and biofeedback and re-education) plays an important role.

Incontinence is due to:

a. Disorders of the rectal reservoir, eg. because of chronic inflammation (Crohn's disease, ulcerative colitis, radiation) or because of a very low anterior resection
b. Neurologic disorders, eg. damage of the CNS (CNS or spine injury), sensory receptor damage (Whitehead operation, pull-through excision) or damage to the motor transmission (perineal descent syndrome, age, childbirth)
c. Muscle damage, eg. due to sphincteric lesions (fistulas, episiotomy, accidents)
d. The low anterior resection syndrome (Rasmussen et al., 2003; Matzel et al., 2003)

Theories that have been reported to be associated with the low anterior resection syndrome are:

i. Theory of loss of the rectal pouch.
ii. Theory of loss of anal sensation.
iii. Theory of damage to the internal anal sphincter.
iv. Theory of the proximal intestine's lumen diameter (Lumen score, r^2).
v. Theory of sympathetic denervation (Rasmussen et al., 2003).

The Low Anterior Resection Syndrome is a multi-factorial condition (sympathetic denervation, rectal pouch capacity loss, sphincteric damage, colonic motility disorders and patient's psychopathology). Improvement is expected at 6 months after the operation, while the CNS may act unpredictably. The J-pouch construction is controversial and chemo-radiotherapy increases the degree of incontinence. Prognostic factors for the possibility of occurrence of post-operative incontinence are anal sensitivity testing, manometry, radiologic data and anorectal endosonography. However, the preservation of the nervic plexuses may contribute in minimizing the consequences of the Low Anterior Resection Syndrome. Low anterior resection may cause some degree of incontinence in 15-30%, but regardless of that, 70% of the patients are fully and 14% partially satisfied, post-operatively (Matzel et al., 2003; Rasmussen et al., 2003).

4.4 Local recurrence and survival after low anterior resection; the importance of TME

Total mesorectal excision rapidly became the "gold standard" for anterior resection of the rectum and a marked reduction of local recurrence rates has been seen. It is reported that the locoregional recurrence rate at 4 years by conventional techniques is 12-32%, in contrast to 6-9% following TME (Wibe et al., 2002).

Data from a randomized, prospective trial by the National Surgical Adjuvant Breast and Bowel Project, demonstrated no significant differences in survival or local recurrence when comparing distal rectal margins of <2cm, 2–2.9 cm and >3 cm (Heriot et al., 2006; Saito et al., 2009). As a result, a 2-cm distal margin is considered acceptable for resection of rectal carcinoma; even though a 5-cm proximal margin is still recommended for upper rectal cancers. The radial margin seems to be critical for local control. Macroscopic pathologic characteristics of completeness of mesorectal excision are (Vordermark et al., 1989):

Incomplete excision:	Little bulk to the mesorectum
	Defects in the mesorectum up to the muscularis propria
	Very irregular circumferential margin at transverse sectioning
Nearly complete excision:	Moderate bulk to the mesorectum
	Irregularity of the mesorectal surface with defects greater than 5 mm, but not up to the muscularis propria
	No area of visibility of the muscularis propria
Complete excision:	Intact bulk to the mesorectum with a smooth surface
	Only minor irregularities of mesorectal surface
	No surface defects greater than 5 mm in depth
	No 'coning' of the distal mesorectum
	Smooth circumferential margin at transverse sectioning

Local recurrence may result from an incomplete radial or circumferential margin. About 25% of cases may have unsuspected involvement of the radial margin after rectal excision, which may result in local recurrence from an incomplete radial resection rather than from an incomplete distal mesorectal excision. A positive circumferential (radial or lateral) margin increases the risk of local recurrence 3.5 times and doubles the risk of disease-related death. Completeness of the mesorectum in the specimen predicts both local recurrence and distant metastases. The mesorectal surface must be marked with ink before formalin fixation. Assessment of the distance between the tumor and the nearest radial margin is mandatory. Circumferential margin is scored as positive if the tumour is located 1 mm or less from the inked non-peritonealised surface of the specimen (Compton et al., 2000; Wibe et al., 2002).

The distance of the tumour from the proximal and distal margins should also be assessed in millimetres. Anastomotic recurrences are rare when this distance is ≥5 cm. For a lower rectal cancer, a 2 cm margin is considered adequate (Compton et al., 2000).

The R-classification indicates the completeness of a surgical excision, depending to a large part on the radial margin. R0 suggests complete tumor resection with all margins negative, R1 is an incomplete tumor resection with microscopic margin involvement and R2 is an incomplete tumor resection with macroscopic involvement of a margin and gross residual tumor.

Total mesorectal excision may reduce local recurrence rates from 20-30% to 8-10% or less, and may increase 5-year survival rates from 48% to 68%. There is strong evidence that sharp dissection under full visualisation is superior to a blunt and partly blind dissection technique and that one should avoid entering into the wrong dissection plane, keeping the fascial envelope intact (Compton et al., 2000).

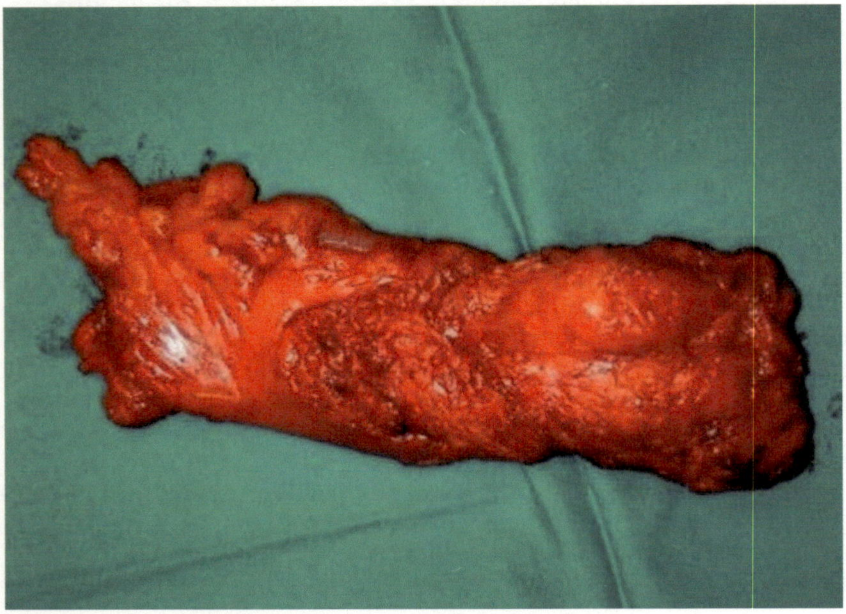

Fig. 3. TME on rectal resection specimen.

5. Intersphincteric resection for rectal cancer

Spanos K, Pramateftakis MG, Tepetes K

For technical and oncological reasons, the standard surgical treatment in very low rectal cancers is the abdominoperineal resection. Nevertheless, in recent years, intersphincteric resection (ISR) has been proposed to offer sphincter preservation in patients with such low lesions (Chamlou et al., 2007).

The principle of the ISR technique is based on an anatomic dissection plane between the internal anal sphincter (IAS) and the external anal sphincter (EAS). The technique incorporates a combined abdominal and perineal approach. During ISR, a transanal division of the rectum, with removal of part or the entire IAS is performed after TME, thus obtaining an adequate distal margin. Restoration of bowel continuity is achieved by performing a hand-sewn coloanal anastomosis. For tumors less than 3 cm from the dentate line, an ISR may be performed (Chamlou et al., 2007).

5.1 Indications

Inclusion criteria for performance of ISR include the following:

- Local spread restricted to the rectal wall or the IAS.
- Adequate sphincter function and continence.
- Absence of distant metastases.
- Distal margin potential of 2 cm for T2, T3 tumors.
- Distal margin potential of 1 cm for T1 tumors

Contraindications to the performance of ISR are the presence of fecal incontinence, T4 lesions, undifferentiated tumors, as well as tumors invading the puborectalis and the EAS.

The extent of local disease can be assessed with the use of MRI and/or endorectal ultrasound. Such studies greatly assist in selecting patients for performance of ISR. Patients with T1 and T2 lesions usually undergo ISR alone. For patients with T3 tumors and T2 tumors with IAS infiltration, neo-adjuvant radio-chemotherapy is recommended (Rullier et al., 2005; Yamada et al., 2009).

5.2 Short-term adverse events

The overall operative mortality associated with ISR is 1.6% and the anastomotic leak rate 10.5% (range 0-48%). Anastomotic stricture is reported at 5.8%.

Rates of clinically apparent anastomotic leakage following stapled anastomosis after anterior resection are in the range of 3-15%. Leakage rates rise significantly for more distally sited anastomoses. Anastomotic leakage is associated with postoperative anastomotic stricture, cancer recurrence, poor postoperative function as well as increased operative mortality. ISR can be performed with acceptable rates of anastomotic leakage and low operative mortality (Rullier et al., 1998; Tilney & Tekkis, 2007).

5.3 Oncologic outcomes

Radical surgical removal of the tumor is the only chance for permanent cure of rectal cancer, despite all progress in the development of oncologic therapy. Rullier et al reported a local recurrence rate of 2% in their series of 92 patients undergoing ISR (Rullier et al., 2005). Most patients (78%) had T3 lesions and 88% underwent long-course neo-adjuvant radiochemotherapy. The overall 5-year survival rate was 81%, with a 5-year disease-free survival of 70%.

Yamada et al reported a similarly low 2.5% cumulative 5-year local recurrence rate, a 5-year disease-free survival rate of 83.5% for stage II patients and 72% for stage III patients (Yamada et al., 2009).

Tilney and Tekkis performed a literature search to identify studies reporting outcomes following ISR. Twenty-one studies accumulating a total of 612 patients were identified (Tilney & Tekkis, 2007). The pooled rate of local recurrence was 9.5% with an average 5-year survival of 81.5%. Distant metastases occured in 9.3%.

Rates of local recurrence following low anterior resection for the treatment of rectal cancer are commonly reported in the range of 2.6-32% following surgery alone (Heriot et al., 2006). Preoperative chemoradiation therapy has led to local recurrence rates in the 6% range.

Therefore, the performance of ISR for the treatment of very low rectal cancer affords similar oncologic outcomes to those of conventional resections. Moreover, Saito compared outcomes of patients undergoing ISR with patients undergoing abdoperineal resection (APR). Similar local recurrence rates (ISR=10.6%, APR=15.7%, p=non-significant), and 5-

year disease-free survival (ISR=69.1%, APR=63.3%, p=non-significant) were reported (Saito et al., 2009). Patients undergoing ISR had significantly longer 5-year overall survival compared to patients undergoing APR (ISR=80%, APR=61.5%, $p<0.05$). As a conclusion, local and distant oncologic outcomes are not compromised with ISR. It is considered that the risk of local recurrence is more likely due to circumferential margin involvement than to distal margin involvement.

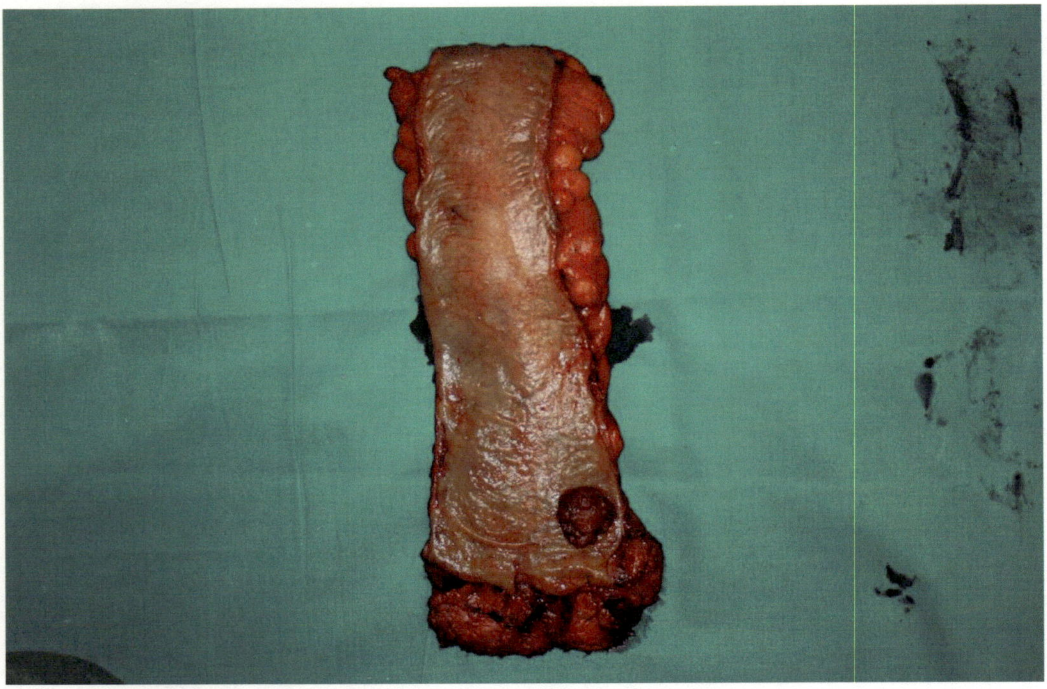

Fig. 4. Intersphincteric resection of low rectal cancer.

Risk factors for local and distant recurrence after ISR were reported by Akasu et al. Local recurrence rate was 6.7% and distant recurrence was 13% (Akasu et al., 2008). In the multivariate analysis, risk factors for local recurrence included positive microscopic resection margins, focal differentiation of tumor (tumor budding) and elevated preoperative levels of CA 19-9 (> 37 U/ml). The identified risk factors for distant recurrence were pN1 & pN2 disease, poor differentiation and the distance of tumor from the anal verge (2.5 cm).

5.4 Anorectal physiology

An important goal of sphincter-preserving surgery is to reach acceptable quality of life levels by preserving fecal continence. The main concern of the ISR technique is functional outcome. Physiologic studies have shown that the anal resting pressure is 55% due to the IAS, 15% due the hemorrhoidal plexus and 30% due to the EAS (Sangwan & Sola, 1998).

Total or partial excision of the IAS is bound to affect continence. Furthermore, preoperative radiation therapy may cause additional loss of sphincter function. Kohler et al reported a 29% reduction in resting anal pressure following ISR. Squeeze pressure recovered to preoperative levels after 12 months. Rullier et al compared outcomes in patients undergoing partial or subtotal IAS resection. Subtotal excision of the sphincter was associated with significant reduction in resting but not squeeze pressure after ISR (Kohler et al., 2000; Rullier et al., 1999).

5.5 Functional outcomes and quality of life

Bretagnol et al reported that faecal continence measured by both the Kirwan and Wexner scores was significantly worse after ISR. In addition, the need for anti-diarrheal medication was higher in patients undergoing ISR compared with patients which had undergone conventional coloanal anastomosis (Bretagnol et al., 2004).

Functional and continence score results were similar between patients undergoing partial ISR and total ISR. Frequency, urgency, the Wexner score and the Fecal Incontinence Severity Index (FISI) were shown to be significantly improved following colonic J-pouch reconstruction compared with straight coloanal anastomosis.

Regarding quality of life (QOL), Bretagnol et al used both the SF-36 and the Fecal Incontinence Quality of Life (FIQL) to compare QOL between patients undergoing ISR and conventional coloanal anastomosis. There was no difference in the QOL scores between ISR patients and conventional coloanal anastomosis patients in the physical and mental subscales of the SF-36.

Patients undergoing ISR with J-pouch reconstruction scored better in the domains of lifestyle, coping, depression and embarrassment at 3 months postoperatively but worse in the domain of embarrassment at the first postoperative year (Bretagnol et al., 2004).

6. Local excision for rectal cancer

Tepetes K, Pramateftakis MG, Spanos K

Local excision (LE) seems to be an attractive therapeutic option because of the minor morbidity, short recovery time and excellent postoperative functional results. There is, however, a significant issue regarding the long term oncological results because of the limited ability of the technique in controlling regional disease.

6.1 Indications

The ideal candidates for LE should theoretically be:

1. Low risk T1, T2 tumors
2. Patients with significant co-morbidities unable to undergo a radical procedure
3. Symptomatic patients with multi-organ distant metastatic disease
4. Well informed patients denying a radical procedure or a stoma

Generally, three approaches to local excision are reported: a) the transanal (conventional or Transanal Endoscopic Microsurgery), b) the transcoccygeal, and c) the transsphincteric. The transanal techniques have been customized for a long time throughout the world and for this reason they can be evaluated more reliably (Garcia-Aguilar et al., 2000).

Factors associated with either the efficacy or the safety of the transanal excisions are the macroscopic and microscopic characteristics of the lesions.

i. Macroscopic characteristics:
    1. T1, T2 lesions
    2. Lesions located within the distal 10-11 cm of the rectum
    3. Lesions smaller than 4 cm
    4. Lesions involving less than 40% of the lumen circumference.

ii. Microscopic characteristics:
   1. Tumor invasion (T): The local recurrence rate is strongly related to the depth of the initial mural invasion (T stage). It is not only the size of the tumor per se that makes the difference, but the lymph node involvement (N stage) as well, which is independently associated. T1 tumors have a 6-12% incidence of lymph node (LN) involvement, T2 tumors have positive lymph nodes (LNs) in 17-22% of the cases and T3 tumors have LN involvement in more than 66% of the cases. The aforementioned differences are reported to result in different 5-year local recurrence rates, namely 5% for T1 tumors, 18% for T2 tumors and 22-33% for T3 tumors (Bouvet et al., 1999).
   2. Lymph node involvement (N): The LN involvement is not only associated with the T stage. Well or moderately differentiated T1 and T2 lesions may present with positive LNs in 14% of the cases and they may have a 5-year local recurrence rate of 11%, whereas poorly differentiated same size tumors have positive LNs in 30% of the cases and a 5-year local recurrence rate of 33%. In addition, T1 and T2 tumors without vascular, lymphatic or perineural infiltration present positive LN stages in 4-17%, in comparison with same size lesions with vascular, lymphatic of perineural infiltration which have LN positive disease in 31-33% of the cases. Finally, it is reported that mucinous rectal cancers have positive LN stage in 52% of the cases, in comparison with the non-mucinous tumors which have LN positive stage in 30% of the cases (Bayar et al., 2002).

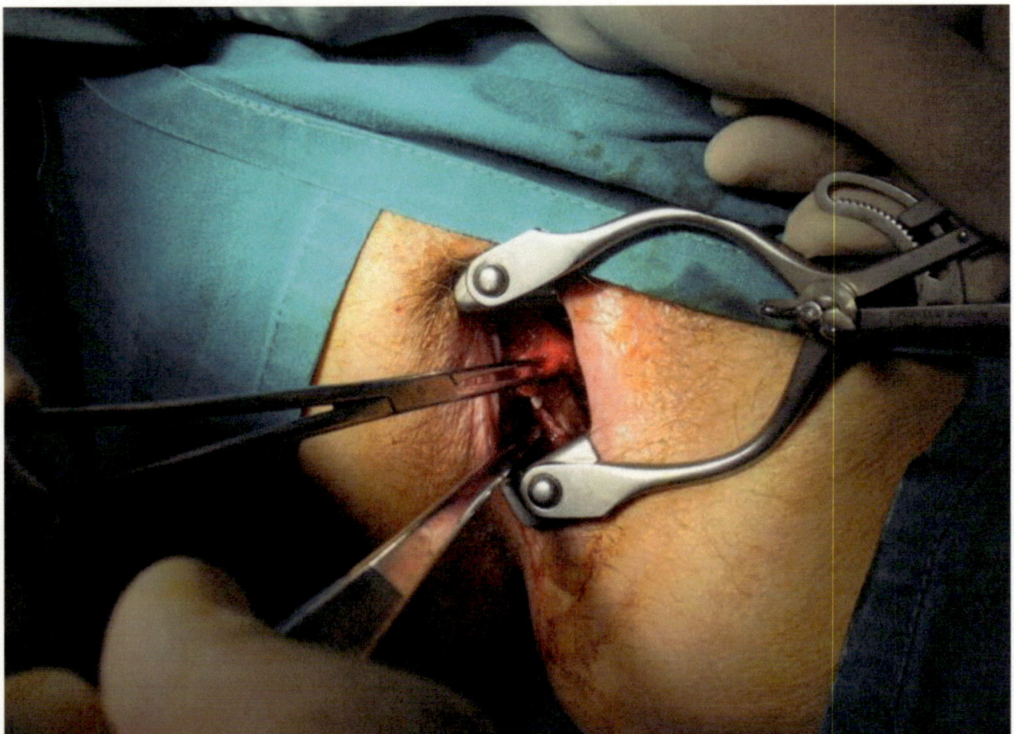

Fig. 5. Transanal excision of T1 lesion of the lower rectum.

6.2 Recurrence & survival

Local transanal excision of early rectal cancers (T1, T2) can be of value in well-informed patients. The locoregional recurrence rate for T1 tumors ranges from 4% to 29% and the 5-year survival rate ranges from 83% to 100%. The best results are reported to be achieved in well-differentiated, non-mucinous, non-ulcerative lesions without vascular, lymphatic or perineural invasion and negative N staging. Quite often though, there are discrepancies in reported patient series with regards to patient selection criteria, staging protocols, surgical techniques, adjuvant treatment or length of follow-up. The length of follow-up is of paramount importance, especially in old patients carrying high co-morbidity. In addition, tumor recurrence can be seen later than 5 years postoperatively and 28% of rectal cancer deaths occur later than this time interval. Thus, 10-year survival following local excision for T1 and T2 tumors drops to 74% and 72% respectively and the 10-year local recurrence rate is 17% to 26% (Chen et al., 2005; Garcia-Aguilar et al., 2000).

There are no randomized trials comparing radical surgery (RS) to local excision, but there are comparative data from retrospective studies originated in specialized centres with regards to T1 rectal cancers. In these reports, recurrence rates following LE are 2-fold to 5-fold higher. The cancer related survival rates of LE are also inferior to those of RS. The differences however are less prominent compared to those regarding recurrence, probably due to the short life expectancy of the older patients undergoing more often LE or ablative techniques. Another cause of discrepancy between groups is the proportion of patients undergoing salvage surgery in case of local recurrence. This rate varies significantly (50% to 80%) and the 5-year survival rates present a similarly wide range (30% to 88%). The long term results in these cases are poorer than those following initial RS. More than 50% of salvage surgery cases require extended pelvic dissection due to the size and the extent of recurrent disease. Thus, 6-year survival rate is reported to be 30% compared with the average 5-year survival which is over 50%. Generally, it seems that less than 25% of patients who develop recurrence following LE are eventually cured (Endreseth et al., 2005; Mellegren et al., 2000).

There is however a group of patients undergoing LE in the first place who can achieve survival and recurrence rates similar to those of patients undergoing initial RS. These are the patients who undergo early secondary radical resection (within 30 days following LE) because of high risk histological features in the excised specimens (positive margins, vascular invasion, etc.) The 5-year disease free survival of these patients is reported to reach 94%. Therefore, LE as a sole therapeutic intervention is associated with considerable long-term recurrence rates even for T1 rectal tumors. The main reason for these results seems to be the high incidence of regional LN metastases which may reach even 22% to 34% in T1 rectal cancer overall, in comparison with 3% to 10% in T1 cancers of the rest large intestine. Therefore, it seems that in order to have improved results from LE, this method should be included in a multi-modality therapeutic strategy (Balch et al., 2006; Garcia-Aguilar et al., 2000).

6.3 The role of radio-chemotherapy

The contribution of postoperative radiotherapy (RTx) following LE for T1 or T2 rectal tumors is difficult to be evaluated because of lack of large randomized trials and the large variation of reported doses (2,700-6,300 cGy) and techniques. The 5-year overall survival ranges from 67% to 80%, which lies close to survival following LE alone (Bittorf et al., 2003).

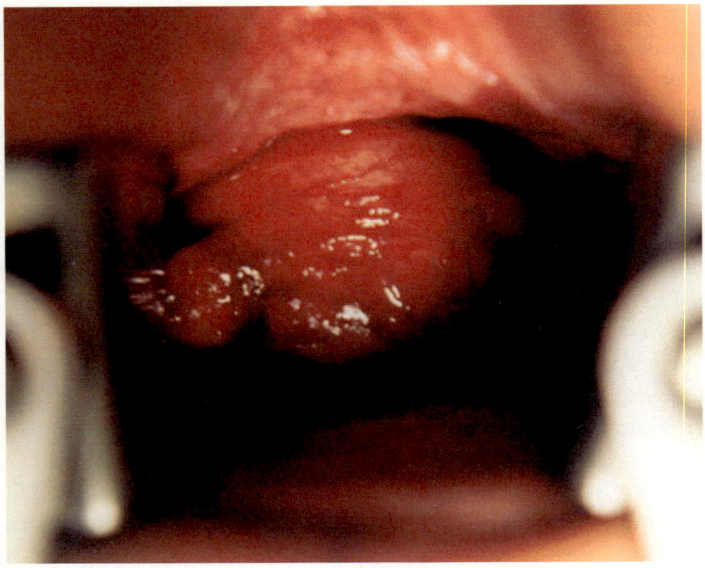

Fig. 6. Well-differentiated rectal tumor visible through the anal dilator during transanal resection.

The fact that it is usually patients with high risk prognostic features that undergo postoperative RTx and the lack of randomization explain in part the absence of improved results. The local control rate following postoperative RTx however is reported to reach 96% at 5 years, dropping to 57% at 8 years. Perhaps postoperative RTx following LE does not alter the natural history of the disease per se, but it rather seems to delay locoregional recurrence by approximately 1 year (Kurt et al., 2005; Wagman et al., 1999).

Preoperative radiotherapy or chemoradiation has been used to downstage rectal tumors and to facilitate sphincter-sparing surgery. In addition to the increased resectability of bulky rectal cancers, another benefit of neoadjuvant therapy seems to be the reduction of locoregional recurrence and the improved survival. It is reported that even T3N0 rectal cancer patients with complete clinical and pathologic response after neoadjuvant chemoradiation can achieve local recurrence and survival rates following LE equivalent to those following RS (Bonnem et al., 1999). The main limitation of suggesting conservative surgery for such patients is the accuracy of imaging methods (EUS, MRI) in restaging the original lesion, as well as the residual LN involvement following chemoradiation. Especially after radiotherapy, there is considerable difficulty to distinguish residual tumor and lymph node involvement from post radiation fibrosis. Nevertheless, 15-30% of patients seem to present reliable, complete clinical regression by endoscopic, imaging and serologic means, following neoadjuvant treatment (Mohiuddin et al., 2000).

In addition, most of these patients will show complete pathologic response as well in RS specimens. Therefore, these patients (especially elderly ones) may have the same long term results after LE. The pathologic T-stage following neoadjuvant chemoradiation and LE (YPT stage) seems to be a strong predictor of residual LN disease (YpN stage). Patients with complete pathologic T regression (ypT0) have 0-24% risk for LN disease. In fact, there are small series reporting overall recurrence rates from 0% to 13% in patients with ypT0 and ypT1 lesions (Bedrosian et al., 2004; Marakis et al., 2009).

It seems that the advances in staging technology and methodology, as well as the adoption of modern neoadjuvant multimodality strategies may provide reliable conservative surgical treatment options. Carefully selected patients (e.g. elderly ones) undergoing local excision of early rectal cancer may have similar outcome with the ones following radical surgery, when the appropriate adjuvant or neo-adjuvant treatment is applied.

7. Abdominoperineal resection for rectal cancer

Papadopoulos V, Michalopoulos A, Pramateftakis MG

In 1908, while investigating the pathogenesis of rectal cancer, Miles established the role of the lymphatic system in the spread of malignancy and emphasised the need for synchronous removal of the rectum and its "lymphatic drainage" with the abdominoperineal approach. Progress in medicine resulted in a decrease in post-operative deaths and allowed abdominoperineal resection (APR) to yield better long-term results as compared to trans-sacral procedures.

7.1 Indications

The question "Which patient with low rectal carcinoma is best treated by an APR?" has no simple answer. Many factors influence the decision to perform an APR for rectal cancer, as seen in Table 1. Surgeons have the responsibility to carefully weigh these factors, discuss all available options with the patient, and be knowledgeable and flexible in approaching those options individually for each patient (Rothenberger & Wang, 1992).

Tumor-related	Level from anal verge Depth of invasion Organ involvement Unfavourable characteristics for local treatment Metastases
Patient-related	Anal sphincter dysfunction Pre-existing GI tract dysfunction (eg diarrheal syndromes) Systemic diseases Concomitant conditions indicating/contraindicating colostomy Blindness Severe arthritis Mental incapacity Paraplegia / Quadriplegia Life expectancy
Technique-related	Inadequate clearance margins Body habitus Extended operation Intraoperative complications

Table 1. Factors that influence the decision of performing an APR.

The decision of the surgeon to reject sphincter-saving operations in favor of an APR should be based on a variety of variables, characteristic for the tumor and the patient. Therefore, the surgeon should make the final decision of operative technique upon completion of total mesorectal excision (TME), being certain of the absence of macro and microscopic evidence of cancer invasion in the circular and distal margin of expected resection ("rectum neck" in the area of junction to levator). An inadequacy of providing uninvaded margins can serve as an indication to perform APR.

Invasion of the dentate line or a free margin less than 1 cm is also an indication for an APR. Digital rectal examination and rigid proctosigmoidoscopy are typically required for accurate tumour assessment. It is undeniable that cancer of the lower rectum can serve as an indication for APR when the parietal fascia is involved, as well as when there are symptoms of lymphatic spread, regardless of the distal margin of the tumour from the dentate line.

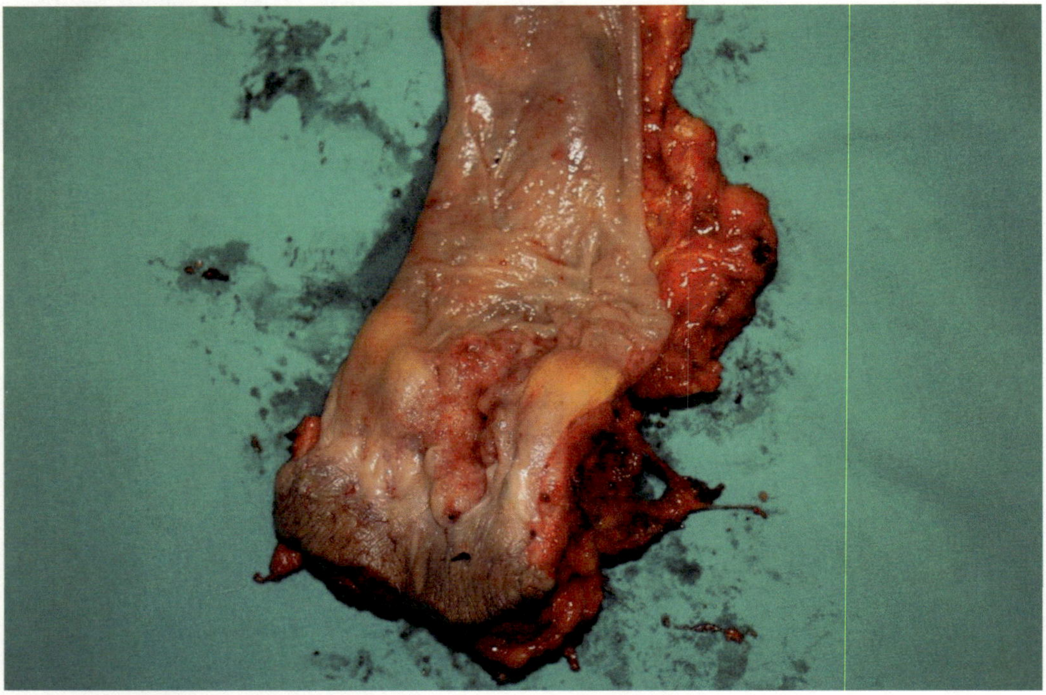

Fig. 7. Specimen following abdominoperineal resection of the rectum.

The variety of factors which can affect the surgeon's decision whether to perform resection of the rectum should include the condition of the anal sphincters, bowel function, patient's age, concomitant diseases and capability of self-care of stoma. Thus, in case of anal incontinence, for patients with adenocarcinoma located 1–2 cm from the dentate line, it is unreasonable to aim for intestine continuity, because incontinence can even deteriorate (Tsarkov, 2005).

7.2 Contraindications

Contraindications for the performance of APR include:

1. Low dimensional tumors (less than 2 cm in diameter)
2. Tumors characterized by a high or good degree of differentiation
3. Invasion of the tumor not exceeding the submucosal layer
4. Absence of lymphovascular invasion.

In all these cases it is reasonable to apply various other procedures such as transanal local excision, transanal endoscopic microsurgery, diathermocoagulation via anoscope, etc. At the same time, the T1 or T2 tumours without involvement of the internal sphincter and longitudinal muscle in case of well differentiated adenocarcinomas located 1–2 cm from the dentate line cannot be considered as an implicit indication for APR. These tumours should be judged from the viewpoint of the possibility of implementing resection of the rectum with subsequent formation of either ultralow stapled colorectal or hand-sutured colo-anal anastomosis.

7.3 Postoperative care, complications and mortality

Following pelvic dissection, there is some laxity of the anterior support as well as swelling and edema due to the procedure, which may lead to voiding difficulties in the first few days, particularly in male patients. The pelvic and abdominal drains are left in situ until they drain less than 50 ml daily.

The operative mortality after an abdominoperineal resection should be less than 2%. As with all forms of major abdominal surgery, improved anesthesia techniques and invasive perioperative monitoring have allowed the reduction in mortality from 42% reported by Miles in 1908 (Chiappa et al., 2006; Peparini et al., 2006). Today, the majority of operative mortality in reported series is related to cardiopulmonary and septic complications. While mortality is relatively low, morbidity varies from 15% to 35% (Nissan et al., 2001; Piso et al., 2004).

A prospective randomized trial demonstrated that laparoscopic-assisted APR offers better immediate outcomes in terms of faster return of bowel function, earlier mobilization and less analgesic requirements when compared with open surgery for low rectal cancer, but at the expense of longer operative times and higher cost. Oncological clearance and long-term survival are seemingly not jeopardized by the laparoscopic-assisted approach (Ng et al., 2008).

After rectal cancer surgery, postoperative general complications occur in 20-35% of all patients and postoperative hospital stay is 5-7 days. “Fast-track” rehabilitation has been shown to accelerate recovery, reduce general morbidity and decrease hospital stay after elective rectal surgery (Schwenk et al., 2006).

7.4 Complications of APR

The potential benefit of surgery should be measured against the morbidity associated with pre-existing conditions not related to the primary disease and which may jeopardize the surgical outcome. Complications are related to the patient’s fitness, the operative procedure, surgical technique and anaesthesia. Therefore the surgeon’s role, besides careful patient selection and preoperative optimisation of pre-existing medical conditions, extends to a level of knowledge and technical skill that should minimise early and late complications (Tsarkov, 2005).

7.4.1 Ureteric injury

The ureters are prone to injury in any pelvic operation. Such injuries can occur during either the abdominal or perineal phase of an APR. Care should be taken to identify and protect the ureters intra-operatively. During an APR for recurrent carcinoma and for very extensive rectal cancers, consideration may be given to the use of ureteric stents to aid the ureter identification. The incidence of ureteral injury in large published series has been variable. Eickenberg and colleagues reported ureteral obstruction in 7 out of 100 patients undergoing APR but could not distinguish whether this was due to intra-operative injury or other causes. The major morbidity from ureteric trauma is the unrecognized injury that presents later as an obstruction or fistula (Eickenberg et al., 1976).

7.4.2 Compartment syndrome

One of the concerns of placing the patient in the lithotomy position is its association with the development of a compartment syndrome. This occurs when elevated pressure in an osteo-fascial compartment compromises local perfusion. This can result in neurovascular damage and permanent disability, emphasizing the importance of prevention and early diagnosis. Intermittent, sequential compression of the lower limbs is strongly encouraged to prevent venous stasis (Boulos & O'Bichere as cited in Hakim & Papalois, 2007).

7.4.3 Abdominal Haemorrhage

Haemorrhage is either primary or secondary. Primary bleeding at the time of surgery or in the immediate postoperative period is the result of poor surgical technique and the failure to achieve satisfactory haemostasis. Clotting disturbances due to massive transfusions and restoration of blood pressure with fluid replacement or drug therapy may be contributing factors. Secondary haemorrhage occurring 7–10 days after surgery is attributed to a dislodged blood clot, dissolution of ligature materials or erosion of a vessel due to an intra-abdominal infection.

7.4.4 Pelvic Haemorrhage

In cases when there is locally advanced or recurrent cancer, previous pelvic surgery or pre-operative radiotherapy, pelvic dissection of the rectum should be undertaken with extreme care. Rarely, a middle sacral artery over the sacral promontory or a left common iliac vein is injured at the start of the pelvic dissection. The lower pelvic side walls may cause significant bleeding when the pelvic fascia is pulled medially by fibrosis or tumour tethering leading to dissection outside the fascia that may injure the internal iliac vessels. Dissection along the correct plane is avascular down to the lateral ligaments which are then divided by clamping or ligation.

Presacral haemorrhage is sometimes unavoidable when the presacral fascia (overlying the high pressure anterior venous plexus) is disrupted or if it is densely adhered to the mesorectal fat. Presacral haemorrhage can also occur from an injury to the anterior presacral plexus or the basivertebral veins during the placement of rectopexy sutures. Significant haemorrhage can occur if the basivertebral veins are divided at the level of the lower sacral foramina. These veins communicate with the internal vertebral venous system, a large valve-less venous system that communicates with the inferior vena cava. The rapid blood loss associated with this injury is related to high hydrostatic pressure in the depth of the pelvis accentuated in the lithotomy position, which increases venous pooling within the pelvis. In most instances bleeding can be controlled by packing, suture ligation, clips or cautery. These will be ineffective if the basivertebral veins are injured at the sacral foramina, due to the fact that these large veins tend to retract themselves into the sacral foramina when injured. Bone wax or thumbtacks are employed to occlude the foramina and stop the bleeding (Boulos & O'Bichere as cited in Hakim & Papalois, 2007).

7.4.5 Small bowel obstruction

Mechanical bowel obstruction that occurs early in the postoperative period is commonly caused by fibrinous adhesions before they become organised by the invasion of fibroblasts and sprouting capillaries to form permanent fibrous adhesions. It is less frequently a result of internal herniation, volvulus, anastomotic edema, intraperitoneal haematoma or abscess.

The appearance of a paralytic ileus is variable after abdominal surgery and is due to reflex inhibition of normal peristalsis. It is painless and lasts for a few days but is prolonged by visceral injury, abdominal sepsis or bleeding, immobility and some medications (atropine, ganglion blocking agents, diuretics).

7.4.6 Genitourinary complications

Other than operative trauma genitourinary complications comprise voiding and sexual dysfunction related to neurological damage during a pelvic dissection which might be unavoidable particularly in resections for advanced carcinomas. However with knowledge of the pelvic anatomy, surgical technique can be refined, exercising caution where nervous structures are particularly vulnerable, hence minimising the risk of these complications and improving the quality of life (Eickenberg et al., 1976; Tsarkov 2005).

7.4.7 Bladder injuries & voiding dysfunction

The bladder is exposed to injury during exploration via a lower incision of the abdomen or due to adhesions from previous surgery. An accidental cystotomy in the anterior surface of the bladder is easily repaired with two layers of continuous absorbable suture, and a urinary catheter is left in situ for 7 days. Injury to the posterior bladder wall can occur when mobilising an inflammatory or neoplastic recto-sigmoid mass or during perineal excision of the rectum. The repair of such an injury is more demanding, especially if the injury is at the base of the bladder. In that case, a urologist should be involved because of the risk of damaging the ureters during the repair. This can be carried out from inside the bladder through an anterior cystotomy, whereby ureteric stents are passed retrogradely to ensure their patency.

Undetected injuries will manifest as a vesicoperineal fistula or an enterovesical fistula. Vesicoperineal fistulae are recognised by the leakage of urine through the perineal wound. The diagnosis is confirmed by a cystogram. Small fistulae may close with urethral or suprapubic catheter drainage for a minimum duration of 6 weeks.

Urinary problems constitute the most frequent and troublesome complications following an APR. Urinary tract infections are very common, occurring in 6–32% of patients (Piso et al., 2004). Contributing factors include the use of urinary catheters and urinary stasis. While bladder neck or prostate angulations may be contributory, the majority of micturition disturbances are due to neurologic injuries. As voiding dysfunction following an APR is common and transitory, one can expect it to subside within three to six months post-operatively.

Fowler et al warned that if large volume retention in the post-operative period secondary to bladder denervation is not recognised and remains untreated, bladder rehabilitation and restoration of normal voiding may be impossible. Many authors advocate the use of urodynamic studies in order to identify patients at risk of developing urinary problems and to detect early post-operative voiding dysfunction (Fowler et al., 1978).

Urinary dysfunction is of particular interest in the evaluation of the nerve-preserving procedure effectiveness. The parasympathetic nerve supply is responsible for bladder contraction. Furthermore, the sympathetic nerve supply allows relaxation of the bladder wall and contraction of the bladder neck while the perineal branch of the pudendal nerve supplies the external urethral sphincter. Early complications are recognised on removal of the urinary catheter and include urinary retention, infection and incontinence due to posterior bladder displacement after abdomino-perineal excision of the rectum, neurologic injury and pre-existing outlet obstruction precipitated by epidural anaesthesia, general anaesthesia, prolonged bed rest and alpha-agonist and anticholinergic medication. Recatheterisation, antibiotics, withdrawing drugs that contribute to urinary retention and a trial of alpha-adrenergic blockers are simple but often effective measures.

Patients with urinary symptoms that continue for longer than 6 weeks after surgery should undergo urodynamic studies to determine the nature of the injury and differentiate it from a simple outlet obstruction requiring prostatectomy (Boulos & O'Bichere as cited in Hakim & Papalois, 2007; Eickenberg et al., 1976; Tsarkov 2005).

7.4.8 Sexual dysfunction

This is more common in males than females because of the anatomical relationship of the rectum to the nerves responsible for the sexual function and due to a better understanding of the male sexual response and disorders that follow pelvic surgery. Women suffer decreased libido, difficulty with orgasm and most commonly dyspareunia. Male dysfunction includes erectile difficulty, retrograde ejaculation and total impotence. Sexual dysfunction is more likely in patients of higher age and after resections for cancer than inflammatory bowel disease, due to the fact that dissection in this case is close to the rectal wall and perineal excision is performed in the intersphincteric plane.

Male sexual dysfunction is regulated by the autonomic nervous system via the pelvic plexus which lies posterolateral to the bladder. Sympathetic nerves are responsible for ejaculation, while parasympathetic nerves govern erection. 15% of patients with normal sexual function prior to an APR are expected to experience some kind of sexual dysfunction (Boulos & O'Bichere as cited in Hakim & Papalois, 2007).

7.4.9 Perineal complications

Wound infections, perineal hernias, delayed healing and very rare chronic perineal sinuses are complications occurring at the perineal site. Only few patients require surgical intervention for such complications. Perineal wound infection is associated with closure rather than with open packing of the perineal wound especially when excision of the rectum is complicated by faecal contamination. Treatment consists of wound opening and local care. Nevertheless, the wound might not heal and if it remains unhealed for more than six months it is then defined as a perineal sinus.

7.4.10 Stoma complications

An array of stomal complications can occur in patients undergoing APR, as seen in table 2. The majority of these are preventable by careful attention to site selection and operative technique. Complications are more frequently encountered in unplanned stomas, in obese patients and in elderly patients.

Stoma complications	Aetiology
Ischemia / Necrosis	Inadequate blood supply Excessive mesenteric stripping
Haemorrhage	Inadequate haemostasis
Abscess formation	Faecal spoilage / Haematoma Wall perforation by sutures
Stoma retraction	Excessive bowel tension
Stenosis	Ischaemia Inadequate skin aperture
Parastomal hernia Prolapse	Oversized abdominal wall aperture Inadequate fixation / repair Excessive stoma length Redundant sigmoid

Table 2. Complications following stoma formation for APR.

Skin problems such as skin irritation are usually the result of a flush or retracted stoma, an improperly placed stoma and allergy to adhesive materials on the bag. With strict hygiene, skin barriers and local antimicrobials the majority of these skin problems are easily manageable. A subcutaneous infection can lead to the formation of a fistula. The latter can be avoided by adjusting the size of the abdominal wall opening to the size of the bowel and by preserving the subcutaneous fat, in order to avoid creating dead space, prone to the formation of haematomas and infection.

Necrosis is the result of skeletonization of the terminal bowel and inadequate abdominal wall opening particularly if the mesentery is thickened due to fat or inflammation. A colour change of a stoma is more likely to be due to ischaemia rather than to venous engorgement or submucosal haematoma if the stoma does not feel warm and there is no arterial ooze from the mucosa on pin-prick. The level of necrosis should be determined by examining the stoma with a paediatric proctoscope or a flexible endoscope as this guides further management. The long-term result of superficial necrosis is stenosis and the stoma can be revised by local exploration. Necrosis below the fascia, therefore intraperitoneally, requires immediate exploration via a laparotomy. Tension on the stoma, improper construction or ischaemia are responsible factors. An abdominal opening that is wider than the bowel lumen causes tension on the mucocutaneous sutures which break and the stoma separates itself from the skin. Stoma retraction may occur as a late complication if a patient gains excessive weight.

Stenosis, often due to ischaemia, is a common cause of colostomy obstruction. The obstruction resolves spontaneously or by saline irrigation of the colostomy through a Foley catheter. Careful dilatation with the finger or graduated dilators can also be attempted in a stenosed stoma. If these measures fail to relieve obstruction, refashioning of the stoma is considered and this will probably require re-exploration, due to the fact that at this early stage local revision can be technically difficult and not safe due to inflammation and oedema at the stoma site. Stenosis identified at a later stage can be revised locally at least 3 months after the initial procedure, as fibrosis becomes established and the tissue planes are better defined to allow exteriorisation of a fresh segment of the bowel for fashioning of a new stoma.

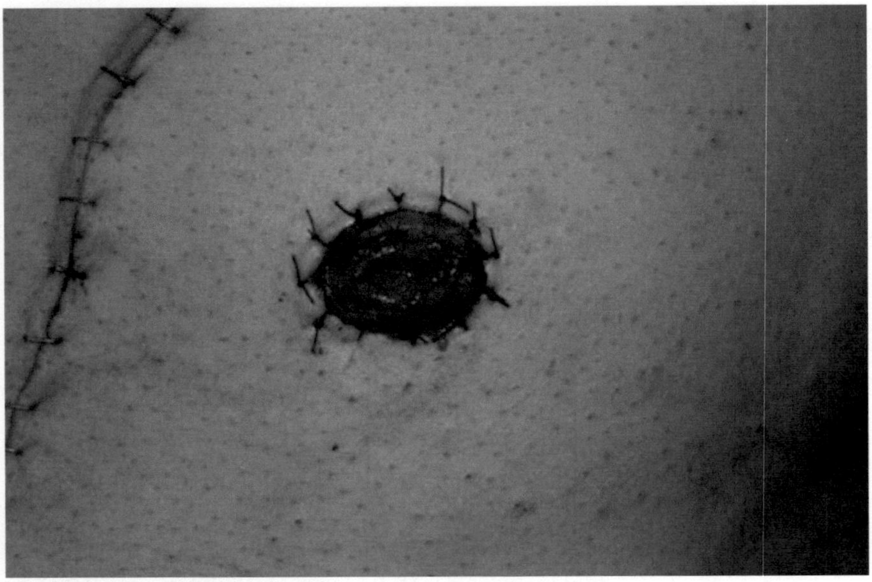

Fig. 8. End colostomy following APR.

A parastomal hernia is the commonest complication following stoma formation. Predisposing factors are obesity, chronic respiratory disease and a predisposition to other abdominal hernias. Ideally, the colostomy should be sited over the rectus muscle and brought out through the split thickness of the muscle. Parastomal herniation is less likely to occur if the stoma is fashioned through the muscle rather than at the side of the rectus muscle. Furthermore, the stoma should ideally be situated below the belt-line at a distance from the bony promontories and the umbilicus. Local repair may involve suture approximation of the defect with or without mesh reinforcement and if this fails, reciting of the stoma may become necessary.
Colostomy prolapse is usually associated with a parastomal hernia, and is more common in obese patients. The prolapse, which is an intussusception of the proximal bowel, is easily reducible even by the patients themselves. Elective surgical treatment consists of excision of the redundant colon followed by local repair of the parastomal hernia (Boulos & O'Bichere as cited in Hakim & Papalois, 2007).

7.5 Oncologic outcomes: Local recurrence & survival following APR

Recent literature has shown that the local recurrence (LR) of lower rectal cancers is higher, compared to the middle and upper ones (Daniels et al., 2006). This may be due to a lack of mesorectum below the levator sling, which increases the chance of tumor spread to the perirectal tissues, increasing the risk of the surgical resection margin being invaded by tumor. In addition to that, low rectal cancers present with more significant factors that predict recurrence, such as lymphatic and vascular invasion, perineural invasion and positive nodal disease. Other factors are involvement of the circumferential resection margin (CRM), tumor distance from the anal verge, tumor differentiation, nodal status, extent of extramural spread and peritoneal perforation by the tumor (Birbeck et al., 2002; Hermanek et al., 1989).
In Heald's series, 45% of patients had cancers in the lower rectum. Of the patients who had a curative LAR, the 5-year LR rate was 7% and systemic recurrence rate was 27%, compared

with 17% and 27% in patients who had curative APR. The LR rate after an APR tends to be higher than for LAR in most series comparing rectal cancers of all stages, with a range of 10–33% (Dehni et al., 2003). This comes in contrast with a LR rate of 4–8% for anterior resection with TME for all stages of rectal cancer, as reproduced by Enker in the USA (Enker et al., 1995). Studies by Quirke have shown that an involved CRM and the depth of extramural invasion are independent markers of poor prognosis and correlate with high LR rates due to residual microscopic disease. In patients with an involved CRM, the LR rate was 64%, compared with 9% in patients with a clear CRM (Quirke et al., 1988). Recent data suggests that a CRM at risk of tumor involvement can be accurately predicted on preoperative MRI.

Marr et al examined the cause of LR and patient survival following APR and LAR for rectal carcinoma and the effect of TME (Marr et al., 2005). There was a significant difference in both LR rates (23.8% versus 13.5%, p=0.002) and cancer-specific 5-year survival (52.3% versus 65.8%, p=0.003) between the APR and LAR groups. The conclusion of the study was that patients treated by an APR have a higher rate of CRM involvement, a higher LR and poorer prognosis than LAR. The frequency of CRM involvement for an APR has not diminished with TME. CRM involvement in the APR specimens is related to the removal of less tissue at the level of the tumor. Where possible, a more radical operation should be considered for all low rectal cancer tumors. The high rates of LR following APR could be explained by a number of factors. APR may be associated with a different pattern of lymphatic spread, which is not included in the "tumor package" excised by TME, or inadequate surgical resection may occur in a higher proportion of patients (Marr et al., 2005). Lymphatic spread to the iliac or obturator nodes occurs and removal of these nodes is reported as a determinant of LR. Inadequate excision appears to be the major factor determining outcome.

In advanced extraperitoneal rectal cancer, Japanese surgeons perform a lateral pelvic nodal dissection with only partial pelvic autonomic nerve preservation. Most Western surgeons prefer the total mesorectal excision (TME) with complete pelvic nerve sparing except for the cases with evident neoplastic neural involvement. Another study was performed to identify long-term oncological results of the total nerve-sparing TME between LAR and APR. The 5-year overall and disease-free survival rates were 88.8% and 77.7%, 90% and 75.1% and 62.3% and 45% for stage I, II and III respectively. The 8-year overall and disease-free survival rates were 77.7% and 77.7%, 78.3% and 75.1% and 50.4% and 40% for stage I, II and III respectively (Peparini et al., 2006).

It has been shown that staging MRI can define the mesorectal fascia and its proximity to the tumor and thereby help identify the expected TME resection margin. This should be extended to early pT1/pT2 low rectal cancers with the possible addition of EUS. The identification of the proximity of the expected surgical CRM to the tumor in the low rectum is an important challenge to the radiologist in order to predict the likelihood of complete excision. pT3 low rectal cancers are unlikely to be completely excised by surgery, and either wider surgical excision with en bloc removal of the levators and anal sphincters or a reduction of the tumor size by preoperative radiochemotherapy is required. Over the last years, there is a trend towards accurate MRI staging and preoperative radio-chemotherapy. Adjustments to the treatment of low rectal cancer are urgently required to achieve the lower rates of involvement of the CRM that are now obtained following mesorectal excision for high and mid rectal excisions. This should greatly improve local recurrence rates and 5-year survival in patients with such disease (Christoforidis et al., 2004; Marr et al., 2005).

Another study was performed by den Dulk in order to identify tumor and patient related risk factors in patients with distal rectal cancer treated by an APR and associated with positive CRM, LR and overall survival. It is concluded that anterior tumor location, advanced T-stage, and higher N-stage were independent risk factors for positive CRM. Positive CRM, higher T-stage, and higher N-stage were risk factors for local recurrence. In addition to the risk factors for LR, distal tumor location and older age were associated with reduced overall survival (den Bulk et al., 2007).

Preoperative chemoradiotherapy (CRT) has contributed remarkably to the increase of sphincter-preserving procedures (SPP) for lower rectal cancer. Kim et al compared the outcomes between APR and SPP after preoperative CRT in patients with locally advanced lower rectal cancer. Patients who underwent APR had a higher 5-year local recurrence (22.0% vs 11.5%, p=0.028) and lower 5-year cancer-specific survival rate (52.9% vs 71.1%, p=0.03) compared to patients who underwent SPP. This study shows that APR following preoperative CRT exhibited more adverse oncologic outcomes compared to SPP. This result may be due to higher rates of CRM involvement in APR even following preoperative CRT. The authors suggest that sharp perineal dissection and wider cylindrical excision at the level of the anorectal junction are required to avoid CRM involvement and improve oncologic outcomes in patients who undergo APR following preoperative CRT (Kim et al., 2009).

With regards to whether specific histopathological parameters can predict local recurrence, Dresen et al studied $T_xN_xM_0$ patients treated for locally recurrent rectal cancer over a period of 12 years. These patients were matched with a control group of patients who did not develop LR after primary rectal cancer treatment for at least 2 years based on the type of neoadjuvant treatment in an 1:2 ratio. The pathology of all primary rectal cancers was reviewed. Patient, treatment and histopathological characteristics were studied in relationship with the development of LR. The results indicate that the presence of lymphovascular invasion (LVI), extramural venous invasion (EMVI), positive CRM, serosal involvement and poor differentiation are factors leading to an increased risk of LR. However, higher age was a protective factor. The study concluded that apart from a positive CRM and serosal involvement, LVI, EMVI and poor differentiation are important independent predictive factors for the development of LR. Adjuvant therapy may be considered in the presence of these features in order to decrease the risk of a local recurrence (Dresen et al., 2009).

Laparoscopic resection for rectal cancer is feasible and safe, with acceptable morbidity and long-term results in patients receiving neoadjuvant treatment. In a study by Pugliese et al, the 5-year survival rate was 74.6% after laparoscopic LAR and 53% after laparoscopic APR (Pugliese et al., 2009). Baek et al, in an effort to evaluate oncologic outcomes after robotic-assisted LAR and APR with TME, analyzed prospectively sixty-four consecutive rectal cancer patients with stage I-III disease. The study showed that the CRM was negative in all surgical specimens, no port-site recurrence occurred in any patient and 6 patients developed recurrence: 2 combined local and distant, and 4 distal alone (mean follow-up of 20.2 months). None of the patients developed isolated local recurrence. The mean time to local recurrence was 23 months and 3-year overall and disease-free survival rates were 96.2% and 73.7%, respectively (Baek et al., 2010; Kanellos D et al., 2010).

7.6 Functional outcomes and quality of life

Avoiding a permanent stoma following rectal cancer excision is believed to improve quality of life (QoL), but evidence from comparative studies is contradictory. The results of a meta-analysis comparing QoL following APR with that after LAR in patients with rectal cancer show that the argument for restorative resections for rectal cancer cannot hinge solely on the issue of a perception of superior QoL outcomes for patients. It is clear that the preconception of many surgeons and patients is that QoL will be better if a permanent stoma is avoided. To the contrary, patients undergoing APR experience postoperatively a global QoL - incorporating the physical and psychological effects of treatment with or without a permanent stoma - that appears to be equivalent to that after LAR. Overall measures of QoL, measured using a variety of validated tools, are not significantly different between APR and LAR patients, but further comparative studies with longer periods of follow-up are needed. Individual domains do highlight significant differences between the two surgical approaches which may help the preoperative decision making process, but individualisation of care incorporating QoL outcomes and functional, oncological and technical considerations is essential for rectal cancer patients (Cornish et al., 2007).

Emotional and cognitive scores from the QLQ C30 questionnaire were consistently shown to be better for APR patients, while physical function was shown to be better for LAR patients using both tools. The improved emotional scores for APR patients may represent the finality of the treatment, as a patient no longer needs to be concerned about invasive examinations of the lower GI tract or worry about future complications once healed adequately.

While some authors have reported that functional recovery following LAR is complete by the 6th postoperative month, others have suggested that at 1 year following LAR, stool frequency is still significantly higher than that preoperatively and that the so-called "anterior resection syndrome" lasts for at least 1 year (Kakodkar et al., 2006).

The decision of which operation to perform would depend on a number of variables, including the likely oncological outcome, the life expectancy of the individual patient and their attitude towards a permanent stoma. There is evidence to suggest that oncological outcomes such as circumferential resection margins and rates of local recurrence are less favourable following APR than LAR. Such results may reflect technical factors that render APR a more complex procedure or differences in anatomy and tumour biology that may negatively impact on lower rectal tumours, which are more likely to be treated with sphincter-sacrificing surgery. In some cases, however, the height of the lesion will necessitate APR, as even ultra-low LAR with inter-sphincteric dissection will be inadequate to permit a safe oncological excision (Tekkis et al., 2005).

The overall findings of the meta-analysis by Cornish et al, highlighting no overall difference in QoL between those patients with and without permanent stomas, challenge the conclusions that may be drawn from other reports which have highlighted rates of stoma-related complications of up to 34%, with deterioration in overall lifestyle and sexual activity by 80% and 43%, respectively. Meta-analyses of individual domains from the QoL instruments suggested improved cognitive, emotional and future perspective scores for those undergoing APR (Cornish et al., 2007).

8. Treatment algorithm for cancer of the rectum

Pramateftakis MG, Spanos K, Tepetes K

Treating rectal cancer certainly requires a multidisciplinary approach involving surgery, radiology, pathology and oncology. Even though chemoradiotherapy has made huge advances over the last years, especially in the form of neoadjuvant therapy, radical surgery and lymphatic clearance remain the key elements to treating rectal cancer. It is therefore

crucial to say that designing a treatment plan should be "individualised" to each patient, depending on location and stage of the disease (Kanellos et al., 2010).
Pre-operative tumor staging will determine the tumor stage. Depending on the T stage of the cancer, three treatment categories can be identified: The early stage, the intermediate stage and the advanced stage cancer. The treatment approach one should follow is shown in Table 3:

Cancer stage	Treatment
Early cancer (T1)	Local transanal resection / Radical resection
Intermediate cancer (T2)	Radical resection followed by adjuvant chemo-radiotherapy (depending on N status)
Advanced cancer (T3,T4)	Neo-adjuvant chemo-radiotherapy followed by major radical resection

Table 3. Treatment according to stage.

After the decision on the treatment plan has been made, the surgeon has to decide on his approach to the tumor. The position of the tumor with regards to the dentate line plays a significant role in the approach chosen by the surgeon, a fact that was analyzed in detail in the previous chapters. Therefore, depending on the tumor distance from the dentate line, four treatment categories can be identified. These are shown in Table 4:

Distance	*Stage*	*Approach*
≥4-5 cm from dentate line	T1-T4	Low anterior resection
<4 cm from dentate line	T1 (well-differentiated, <3 cm diameter)	Transanal resection
1-3 cm from dentate line	T1 or T2 with "un-favourable" characteristics	Intersphincteric resection
0-3 cm from dentate line	T3-T4	Abdominoperineal resection

Table 4. Treatment according to location.

9. Conclusion

Pramateftakis MG

In order to be successful in treating rectal cancer, good oncologic outcome is the first priority. Equally important is the achievement of an acceptable quality of life for the patient. The avoidance of a permanent stoma, with all of the concomitant morbidity associated with it, may be of greater importance to the patient.
Despite advances in surgical technique along with improvements in neoadjuvant and adjuvant therapy, the surgical treatment of rectal cancer involving the pelvic floor and sphincter complex remains complicated. The decision on the type of surgery to perform depends on a number of variables including stage of the disease, tumour characteristics, condition of the anal sphincter mechanism, bowel function, patient's age, concomitant diseases, life expectancy and capability of stoma self-care.

Why are survival rates worse after abdominoperineal resections compared to low anterior resections? Patients with very low rectal cancer treated by an APR have worse tumor characteristics and higher involved margin rates compared to patients treated by LAR. Furthermore, they have more locally extensive tumors despite a greater proportion undergoing neoadjuvant treatment. Patients with low rectal cancer pose difficulties with regards to optimal management. Targeted strategies are needed to improve outcome in this complex and common cancer.

Careful patient selection, high quality preoperative imaging and functional assessment, with emphasis on sound operative technique should lead to superior results.

10. References

Akasu T, Takawa M, Yamamoto S, et al. (2008). Intersphincteric resection for very low rectal adenocarcinoma: univariate and multivariate analysis of risk factors for recurrence. *Ann Surg Oncol*; 15(10): 2668-2676

Baek JH, McKenzie S, Garcia-Aguilar J & Pigazzi A. (2010). Oncologic outcomes of robotic-assisted total mesorectal excision for the treatment of rectal cancer. *Ann Surg*; 251(5): 882-886

Balch G, Ce Meo A & Guillem G. (2006). Modern management of rectal cancer: A 2006 update. *World J Gastroenterol*; 12(20): 3186-3195

Bayar S, Saxena R, Emir B, et al. (2002). Venous invasion may predict lymph node metastasis in early cancer. *Eur J Surg Oncol*; 28(4): 413-417

Bedrosian I, Rodrifuez-Bigas MA, Feig B, et al. (2004). Predicting the node-negative mesorectum after preoperative chemoderation for locally advanced rectal carcinoma. *J Gastrointest Surg*; 8: 56-62.

Bennet RC. (1986). Abdomino-anal pull-through resection of the rectum. *Ann Chir Gynaecol*; 75: 95-9

Birbeck KF, Macklin CP, Tiffin NJ, et al. (2002). Rates of circumferential resection margin involvement vary between surgeons and predict outcomes in rectal cancer surgery. *Ann Surg*; 235: 449–457.

Bittorf B, Stadelmaier U, Merkel S, et al. (2003). Does anastomotic leakage affect functional outcome after rectal resection for cancer? *Langenbecks Arch Surg*; 387: 406-410

Bleday R & Garcia-Aguilar J. (2007). Surgical Treatment of Rectal Cancer, In: *The ASCRS Textbook of Colon and Rectal Surgery*. Springer, XXIV, pp. 413-436

Bonnem M, Crane C, Vauthey JN, et al. (1999). Long-term results using local excision after preoperative chemoradiation among selected T3 rectal cancer patients. *Int J Radiat Oncol Biol Phys*; 44: 1027-1038

Boulos PB & O'Bichere A. (2007). Complications of colorectal surgery, In: *Surgical complications - Diagnosis and Treatment*, Hakim NS, Papalois VE, pp. 363-390, Imperial College Press

Bouvet M, Milas M, Giacco GG, et.al. (1999). Predictors of recurrence after local excision and postoperative chemoradiation therapy of adenocarcinoma of the rectum. *Ann Surg Oncol*; 6(1): 26-32

Branagan G & Finnis D. (2005). Wessex Colorectal Cancer Audit Working Group. Prognosis after anastomotic leakage in colorectal surgery. *Dis Colon Rectum*; 48(5): 1021–1026

Bretagnol F, Rullier E, Laurent C, et al. (2004). Comparison of functional results and quality of life between intersphincteric resection and conventional coloanal anastomosis for low rectal cancer. *Dis Colon Rectum*; 47: 832-838

Carlsen E, Schlichting E, Guldvog I, et al. (1998). Effect of the introduction of total mesorectal excision for the treatment of rectal cancer. *Br J Surg*; 85: 526-529.

Chamlou E, Parc Y, Simon T et al. (2007). Long term results of intersphincteric resection for low rectal cancer. *Ann Surg*; 246: 916-922

Chen CC, Lee RC, Lin JK, et al. (2005). How accurate is magnetic resonance imaging in restaging rectal cancer in patients receiving preoperative combined chemoradiotherapy; *Dis Colon Rectum*; 48: 722-728

Chen CC, Leu SY, Liu MC, et al. (2005). Transanal local wide excision for rectal adeonocarcinoma. *Hepatogastroenterology*; 52(62): 460-463

Chiappa A, Biffi R, Bertani E, et al. (2006). Surgical outcomes after total mesorectal excision for rectal cancer. *J Surg Oncol*; 94(3): 182-93

Christoforidis E, Kanellos I, Tsachalis T, et al. (2004). Locally recurrent rectal cancer after curative resection. Tech Coloproctol; 8: 132-134.

Compton CC, Fielding LP, Burgart LJ et al. (2000). Prognostic factors in colorectal cancer. College of American Pathologists Consensus Statement. *Arch Pathol Lab Med*; 124: 979–994

Cornish JA, Tilney HS, Heriot AG, et al. (2007). A Meta-Analysis of Quality of Life for Abdominoperineal Excision of Rectum versus Anterior Resection for Rectal Cancer. *Ann Surg Oncol*; 14(7): 2056–2068

Daniels IR, Strassburg J & Moran BJ. (2006). The need for future surgical low rectal cancer studies. *Colorectal Disease*; 8(3): 25-29

Dehni N, McFadden N, McNamara DA et al. (2003). Oncologic results following abdominoperineal resection for adenocarcinoma of the low rectum. *Dis Colon Rectum*; 46: 867–874.

Demetriades H, Kanellos I, Vasiliadis K et al. (2004). Age-associated prognosis following curative resection for colorectal cancer. *Tech Coloproctol*; 8(S1): 144-146

den Dulk M, Marijnen CAM, Putter H, et al. (2007). Risk factors for adverse outcome in patients with rectal cancer treated with an abdominoperineal resection in the total mesorectal excision trial. *Ann Surg*; 246: 83–90

Dresen RC, Peters EEM, Rutten HJT, et al. (2009). Local recurrence in rectal cancer can be predicted by histopathological factors. *Eur J Surg Oncol*; 35: 1071-1077

Eickenberg, HU, Amin M, Klompus W & Lich R. (1976). Urologic complications following abdominoperineal resection. *J Urol*; 115: 180

Endreseth BH, Myrvold HE, Rumundstand P, et al. (2005). Transanal excision vs. major surgery for T1 rectal cancer. *Dis Colon Rectum*; 48: 1380-1388

Enker WE, Thaler HT, Cranor ML & Polyak T. (1995). Total mesorectal excision in the operative treatment of carcinoma of the rectum. *J Am Coll Surg*; 181: 335–346

Fowler JW, Bremner DN & Moffat L. (1978). The incidence and consequences of damage to the parasympathetic nerve supply to the bladder after abdominoperineal resection of the rectum for carcinoma. *Br J Urol*; 50: 95

Garcia-Aguilar H, Mellgren A, Sirivongs P, et al. (2000). Local excision of rectal cancer without adjuvant therapy. *Ann Surg*; 231: 345-351

Harewood GC. (2005). Assessment of publication bias in the reporting of EUS performance in staging rectal cancer, *Am J Gastroenterol*; 100: 808-816

Heald RJ & Karanjia ND. (1992). Results of radical surgery for rectal cancer. *World J Surg*; 16: 848–857

Heald RJ, Husband E & Ryall R. (1982). The mesorectum in rectal cancer surgery – the clue to pelvic recurrence? *Br J Surg*; 69: 613-618

Heriot AG, Tekkis PP, Darzi A, et al. (2006). Surgery for local recurrence of rectal cancer. *Colorectal Dis*; 8: 733-747

Heriot AG, Hicks RJ, Drummond EG, et al. (2004). Does positron emission tomography change management in primary rectal cancer? A prospective assessment. *Dis Colon Rectum*; 47: 451-458

Hermanek P, Guggenmoos-Holzmann I & Gall FP. (1989). Prognostic factors in rectal carcinoma. A contribution to the further development of tumour classification. *Dis Colon Rectum*; 32: 593–599

Hohenberger P, Schlag P, Kretzschmar U, et al. (1991). Regional mesenteric recurrence of colorectal cancer after anterior resection or left hemicolectomy: inadequate primary resection demonstrated by angiography of the remaining arterial supply. *Int J Colorectal Dis*; 6: 17-23

Jeng-Kai J, Yang SH & Lin JK. (2005). Transabdominal anastomosis after low anterior resection: A prospective, randomized, controlled trial comparing long-term results between side-to-end anastomosis and colonic J-pouch. *Dis Colon Rectum*; 48: 2100-2108

Kakodkar R, Gupta S & Nundy S. (2006). Low anterior resection with total mesorectal excision for rectal cancer: functional assessment and factors affecting outcome. *Colorectal Dis*; 8: 650–656

Kanellos D, Pramateftakis MG & Kanellos I. (2010). Standardization and time trends in laparoscopic colorectal surgery. *Surg Endosc*; 24(3): 726-727

Kanellos D, Pramateftakis MG, Vrakas G et al. (2010). Anastomotic leakage following low anterior resection for rectal cancer. *Tech Coloproctol*; 14: 35-37

Kanellos I, Vasiliadis K, Angelopoulos S, et al. (2004). Anastomotic leakage following anterior resection for rectal cancer. *Tech Coloproctol*; 8: s79-81

Kim HJ & Wong WD. (2000). Role of endorectal ultrasound in the conservative management of rectal cancers. *Semin Surg Oncol*; 19: 358-366

Kim JS, Hur H, Kim NK, et al. (2009). Oncologic outcomes after radical surgery following preoperative chemoradiotherapy for locally advanced lower rectal cancer: abdominoperineal resection versus sphincter-preserving procedure. *Ann Surg Oncol*; 16(5): 1266-1273.

Kohler A, Athanasiadis S, Ommer A, et al. (2000). Long-term results of low anterior resection with intersphincteric anastomosis in carcinoma of the lower one-third of the rectum: analysis of 31 patients. *Dis Colon Rectum*; 43: 843-850

Kuhry E, Schwenk W, Gaupset R, et al. (2008). Long-term outcome of laparoscopic surgery for colorectal cancer: Cochrane systematic review of randomised controlled trials. *Cancer Treat Rev*; 34: 498-504

Kurt M, Ozkan L, Yilmazlar T, et al. (2005). Postoperative concomitant chemoradiotherapy in locally advanced rectal cancer. *Hepatogastroenterology*; 52(65): 1411-5

Kwok H, Bissett IP & Hill GL. (2000). Preoperative staging of rectal cancer. *Int J Colorectal Dis*; 15: 9-20

Law WL, Chu KW & Choi HK. (2002). Randomized clinical trial comparing loop ileostomy and loop transverse colostomy for faecal diversion following total mesorectal excision. *Br J Surg*; 89: 704–708

Marakis G, Demetriades H, Ziogas D & Kanellos I. (2009). Local excision for rectal cancer-safety and efficacy challenges. *Ann Surg Oncol*; 16: 2369-2370

Marr R, Birbeck K, Garvican J et al. (2005). The modern abdominoperienal excision: the next challenge after total mesorectal excision. *Ann Surg*; 242: 74–82

Matthiessen P, Hallbook O, Rutegard J, et al. (2007). Defunctioning stoma reduces symptomatic anastomotic leakage after low anterior resection of the rectum for cancer. A randomized multicenter trial. *Ann Surg*; 246(2): 207-214

Matzel KE, Bittorf B, Gunther K, et al. (2003). Rectal resection with low anastomosis: functional outcome. *Colorectal Dis*; 5: 458-464

Mellegren A, Sirivongs P, Rothenberg DA, et al. (2000). Is local excision adequate therapy for early rectal cancer? Dis Colon Rectum; 43: 1064-1071

Meyerhardt JA, Tepper JE, Niedzwiecki D, et al. (2004). Impact of hospital procedure volume on surgical operation and long-term outcomes in high-risk curatively resected rectal cancer: findings from the Intergroup 0114 Study. *J Clin Oncol*; 22(1): 166-174

Miles WE. A method of performing abdomino-perineal excision for carcinoma of the rectum and of the terminal portion of the pelvic colon. (1971). *Ca Cancer J Clin*; 21: 361-364

Mohiuddin M, Hayne M, Regine WF et al. (2000). Prognostic significance of postchemoradation stage following preoperative chemotherapy and radiation for advanced/recurrent rectal cancers. *Int J Radiat Oncol Biol Phys*; 45: 1075-1080.

Nesbakken A, Nygaard K, Westerheim O, et al. (2002). Audit of intraoperative and early postoperative complications after introduction of mesorectal excision for rectal cancer. *Eur J Surg*; 168: 229-235

Ng SM, Leung KL, Lee JFY, et al. (2008). Laparoscopic-Assisted Versus Open Abdominoperineal Resection for Low Rectal Cancer: A Prospective Randomized Trial. *Ann Surg Oncol*; 15(9): 2418–2425

Nicholls RJ & Tekkis PP. (2008). Multidisciplinary treatment of cancer of the rectum: a European approach. *Surg Oncol Clin N Am*; 17: 533-551.

Nicholls RJ. (1991). Surgical treatment of adenomas. *World J Surg*; 15: 20-24

Nissan A, Guillem JG, Paty PB et al. (2001). Abdominoperineal resection for rectal cancer at a specialty center. *Dis Colon Rectum*; 44: 27–36.

Nugent KP, Daniels P, Stewart B, et al. (1999). Quality of life in stoma patients. *Dis Colon Rectum*; 42: 1569–1574

Otchy D, Hyman NH, Simmang C, et al. (2004). Practice Parameters for Colon Cancer. The American Society of Colon and Rectal Surgeons. *Dis Colon Rectum*; 47: 1269–1284

Peparini N, Maturo A, Di Matteo FM, et al. (2006). Long-term survival and recurrences after total nerve-sparing surgery for rectal cancer. *Hepatogastroenterology*; 53(72): 850-853

Piso P, Dahlke MH, Mirena P, et al. (2004). Total mesorectal excision for middle and lower rectal cancer: a single institution experience with 337 consecutive patients. *J Surg Oncol*; 86: 115–121.

Pramateftakis MG, Kanellos D & Kanellos I. (2010). Progress in rectal cancer staging and treatment. *Tech Coloproctol;* 14(1): 29-31

Pramateftakis MG, Vrakas G, Hatzigianni P, et al. (2010). The handsewn anastomosis after colon resection due to colonic cancer. *Tech Coloproctol;* 14(1): 57-59

Ptok H, Marusch F, Meyer F, et al. (2007). Impact of anastomotic leakage on oncological outcome after rectal cancer resection. *Br J Surg;* 94: 1548–1554

Pugliese R, Di Lernia S, Sansonna F, et al. (2009). Laparoscopic resection for rectal adenocarcinoma. *Eur J Surg Oncol;* 35(5): 497-503

Quirke P & Dixon MF. (1988). The prediction of local recurrence in rectal adenocarcinoma by histopathological examination. *Int J Colorectal Dis;* 3: 127–131

Rasmussen OO, Petersen IK & Christiansen J. (2003). Anorectal function following low anterior resection. *Colorectal Dis;* 5: 258-261

Rees JR, Carney L, Gill TS, et al. (2004). Management of recurrent anastomotic stricture and iatrogenic stenosis by circular stapler. *Dis Colon Rectum;* 47: 944-947

Rothenberger DA & Wong WD. (1992). Abdominoperineal resection for adenocarcinoma of the low rectum. *World J Surg;* 16: 478-485

Rullier E, Laurent C, Bretagnol, et al. (2005). Sphincter-saving resection for all rectal carcinomas: the end of the 2-cm distal rule. *Ann Surg;* 241(3): 465-469

Rullier E, Cunha AS, Coudere P, et al. (2003). Laparoscopic intersphincteric resection with coloplasty and coloanal anastomosis for mid and low rectal cancer. *Br J Surg;* 90: 445–451

Rullier E, Cunha AS, Coudere P, et al. (1999). Intersphincteric resection with excision of internal anal sphincter for conservative treatment of very low rectal cancer. *Dis Colon Rectum;* 42: 1168-1175

Rullier E, Laurent C, Garrelson JL, et al. (1998). Risk factors for anastomotic leakage after resection of rectal cancer. *Br J Surg;* 85: 355-358

Saito N, Sugito M, Ito M, et al. (2009). Oncologic outcome of intersphincteric resection for very low rectal cancer. *World J Surg;* 33: 1750-1756

Sangwan YP & Solla JA. (1998). Internal anal sphincter: advances and insights. *Dis Colon Rectum;* 41: 1297-1311

Schwenk W, Neudecker J, Raue W, et al. (2006). "Fast-track" rehabilitation after rectal cancer resection. *Int J Colorectal Dis;* 21: 547–553

Staudacher C, Vignali A, Di Palo S, et al. (2007). Laparoscopic vs Open Total Mesorectal Excision in unselected patients with rectal cancer: Impact on early outcome. *Dis Colon Rectum;* 50: 1324-1331

Sugarbaker PH. (1996). Rectovaginal fistula following low circular stapled anastomosis in women with rectal cancer. *J Surg Oncol;* 61: 155-158

Taflampas P, Christodoulakis M & Tsiftsis D. (2009). Anastomotic leakage after low anterior resection for rectal cancer: Facts, Obscurity, and Fiction. *Surg Today;* 39: 183–188.

Tekkis PP, Heriot AG, Smith J, et al. (2005). Comparison of circumferential margin involvement between restorative and nonrestorative resections for rectal cancer. *Colorectal Dis;* 7: 369–374

Tilney HS & Tekkis PP. (2007). Extending the horizons of restorative rectal surgery: intersphincteric resection for low rectal cancer. *Colorectal Dis;* 10: 3-16

Tsarkov P. (2005). Abdominoperineal resection. In: *Rectal Cancer: New frontiers in diagnosis, treatment and rehabilitation*, Dilaini G.G., 157-165, Springer

Vordermark D, Sailer M, Flentje M, et al. (1999). Curative-intent radiation therapy in anal carcinoma: quality of life and sphincter function. *Radiother Oncol*;52: 239-243

Vrakas G, Pramateftakis MG, Kanellos D, et al. (2010). Defunctioning ileostomy closure following low anterior resection by chemotherapy. *Tech Coloproctol*; 14(S1): 77-78

Wagman R, Minsky BD, Cohen AM, et al. (1999). Conservative management of rectal cancer with local excision and postoperative adjuvant therapy. *Int J Radiat Oncol Biol Phys*; 44: 841-846.

Wibe A, Rendedal PR, Svenson E, et al. (2002). Prognostic significance of circumference resection margin following total mesorectal excision for rectal cancer. *Br J Surg*; 89: 327-334

Wiggers T, Jeekel J, Arends JW, et al. (1988). No-touch isolation technique in colon cancer: a controlled prospective trial. *Br J Surg*; 75: 409-415

Williams NS, Dixon MF & Johnston D. (1983). Reappraisal of the 5-cm rule of distal excision for carcinoma of the rectum: a study of distal intramural spread and of patients' survival. *Br J Surg*; 70: 150-154

Yamada K, Ogata S, Saiki Y, et al. (2009). Long-term results of intersphincteric resection for low rectal cancer. *Dis Colon Rectum*; 52: 1065-1071

Young-Fadok TM, Wolff BG, Nivatrongs S, et al. (1998). Prophylactic oophorectomy in colorectal carcinoma: preliminary results of a randomized, prospective trial. *Dis Colon Rectum*; 41: 277–285

4

Helping Patients Make Treatment Choices for Localized Prostate Cancer

Ravinder Mohan, Hind Beydoun and Paul Schellhammer
Eastern Virginia Medical School, Norfolk, Virginia
USA

1. Introduction

One in six men in the U.S. will be diagnosed with prostate cancer in his lifetime; however, only one in 35 men will die from the cancer.[1] As prostate-specific antigen (PSA) screening has become widespread, about 90 percent of patients are diagnosed with localized prostate cancer which will not lead to death in the majority of patients.[2] As a result, over treatment of localized prostate cancer (LPC) has been an increasing concern. [3] However, prostate cancer is the second most common cause of cancer-related death in U.S. men, after lung cancer. Therefore not treating aggressive cancers which are detected early carries a grave risk.

Treatment of localized cancer by surgery or radiotherapy can be curative; however, in about one-half to three-fourths of patients, the risk of death from screening-detected prostate cancer is very low, even if they choose observation. [4,5] A large U.S. retrospective study found that about 20 percent of low-risk patients who chose observation died from prostate cancer over 20 years of follow-up.[6] A Swedish randomized controlled trial also found a survival benefit after eight years of treatment in low-risk patients.[7] However, patients in both of these studies had higher-stage cancer at diagnosis (i.e., their cancer was clinically diagnosed and was not detected by PSA screening). The Swedish trial also found that prostate cancer–specific mortality was only 2.4 percent at 10 years in low-risk patients who were randomized to active surveillance.[8] A large study of 44,630 low-risk U.S. patients found a survival benefit of treatment, [9] but only 2.1% of the patient sample had died because of prostate cancer.

Treatment is associated with urinary, sexual, and bowel dysfunction, and enhances the quality-adjusted survival of low-risk patients by only 1.2 months. [10] Five years after treatment in 3,533 patients, 79.3% of surgery patients and 63.5% of radiotherapy patients had erectile dysfunction, 15% of surgery patients and 4% of radiotherapy patients had at least frequent urinary leakage, and 19% of surgery patients and 29% of radiotherapy patients had bowel urgency.[11] Side effects are unpredictable and vary very widely,[12] and decisional regret is common.[13] In addition, the cost of each potentially unnecessary prostatectomy or radiation treatment was about $10,000 to $25,000 in 2000 dollars. [14] Despite these concerns, about 94 percent of patients with localized prostate cancer choose treatment.[15] In patients treated from 2000 to 2002, the rate of overtreatment (i.e., treatment in low-risk patients) was estimated to be about 55 percent.[16]

Under-treatment of localized prostate cancer has also been a concern for over two decades. The incidence and mortality of the cancer are two to three times higher in black men.[17]

However, black and Hispanic men are more likely to be monitored instead of receiving treatment, possibly because they are more likely to present late, have poorer access to care, and sometimes a cultural preference for conservative treatment but many of these factors are not well evidenced.[18]

Few randomized controlled trials have compared outcomes of different treatments for localized prostate cancer. A survey of 504 urologists and 559 radiation oncologists found that for the same hypothetical patient, 93 percent of urologists would recommend surgery, and 72 percent of radiation oncologists would recommend radiotherapy. [19] Although treatment of localized prostate cancer is unlikely to improve the survival of low-risk patients and has potentially negative effects on health-related quality of life, about 70 to 90 percent of patients choose a treatment during the first visit to a urologist after a positive biopsy.[20]

In our survey of 184 men with newly diagnosed prostate cancer, more than one-half significantly overestimated the survival benefit of treatment. [21] Education, income, and health literacy did not affect the results; 60 percent of the survey respondents were college educated and had an annual income more than $50,000, and more than 90 percent had at least a ninth-grade health literacy. [22] Although these patients had been counseled by their urologists and had already elected treatment or observation, more than 50 percent incorrectly answered more than one-half of the 18 items in a questionnaire designed to test their knowledge, understanding, and judgment about the advantages and disadvantages of treatment options for prostate cancer. This questionnaire[22] can be used to identify patients who need further counseling about treatment choices.

Over-, and Under-treatment occur because without the use of guidelines, it is extremely difficult for even the most intelligent LPC patient to make a good decision. Patients must choose from treatments with marginally different HRQOL outcomes, and without clear numerical probabilities of the frequency, severity, and duration of side effects. Finding the HRQOL outcome that can best match the patient's preference can eclipse the bigger question of whether any treatment will enhance survival. Urologists are unsure too, which is reflected in their need to develop newer nomograms to predict survival even though 40 nomograms already exist. [23] Most urologists recommend definitive treatment for low risk young patients. [24] Observation is inappropriate in many patients, and until better evidence is obtained, a balanced decision-aid with numerical probabilities is recommended. [25] This could be very difficult, given that for LPC patients, urologists have more than 69 tools to predict prognosis, [26] and more than 800 articles [27] about HRQOL outcomes have been reported.

Dahm et al [83] have suggested that such a complex decision should not be left to expert opinion alone, and that national guidelines can help in preventing over-, or under-treatment because guidelines are developed by panels of individuals who have the access and time to understanding and balance the available evidence. Guidelines aim to maximize both survival and HRQOL, are freely available on the Internet, are likely without much bias, and can give a point of reference from where patients may deviate by personal preference. However, in the literature, we found 160 articles with combinations of search terms and Medical Subject Headings including "prostate cancer, practice guidelines, NCCN, medical oncology/standards, evidence-based practice, urology/standards, and neoplasms/ therapy". Except for a Japanese study on the outcomes of brachytherapy, [29] and a case report by Walsh [30] suggested that any named guideline was used in choosing a treatment for LPC. Our publication in 2010 was the first to show the use of guidelines; we have described a new method to estimate co-morbidity adjusted life expectancy that makes the use of guidelines feasible.[31]

Among ten guidelines published for choosing a treatment for LPC, the guideline by the National Comprehensive Cancer Network (NCCN)[32] was rated as the most evidenced-based. [28] NCCN risk categories use the D'Amico criteria for survival prediction in LPC patients, [33] all NCCN guidelines require continuous review, and their recommendations are level 2A or better (either high level evidence or uniform consensus). The goal of NCCN guidelines is "to extend life expectancy while minimizing excess morbidity," and the guidelines are based on the thinking that "despite differences in values, most patients would make the same choice." An algorithm based on the NCCN guideline is presented in Figure 1. Four factors are used in determining the recommended treatment. These are: the cancer's stage, its grade i.e, the Gleason score, the PSA level, and the estimated baseline co-morbidity adjusted life expectancy of the patient.

Stages T1 (not palpable) and T2 (palpable but limited to the prostate) are considered localized if there are no lymph nodes involved and no distant metastasis.

The Gleason score is determined by adding the grades of the two most common histologic patterns seen in each biopsy core. Each pattern is scored from 1 to 5, with 5 being most poorly differentiated. For example, if grade 3 is the most common pattern and grade 4 is the

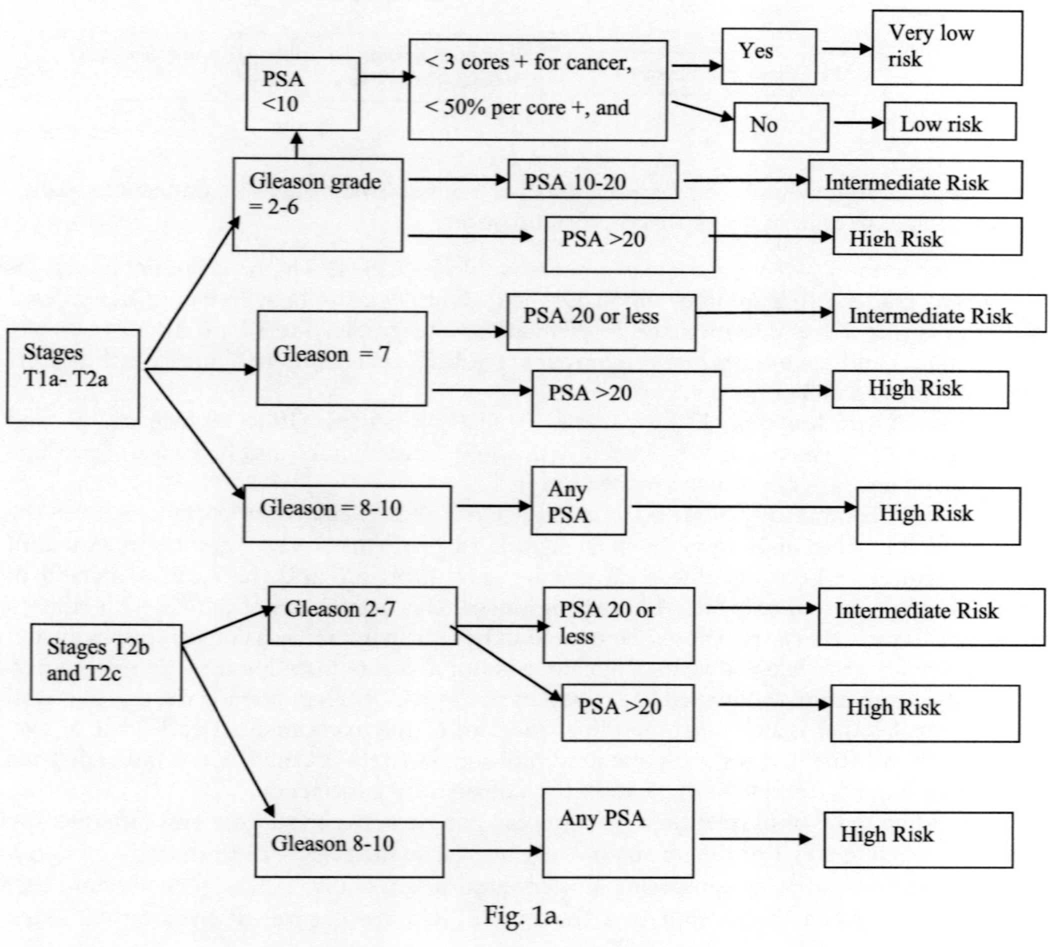

Fig. 1a.

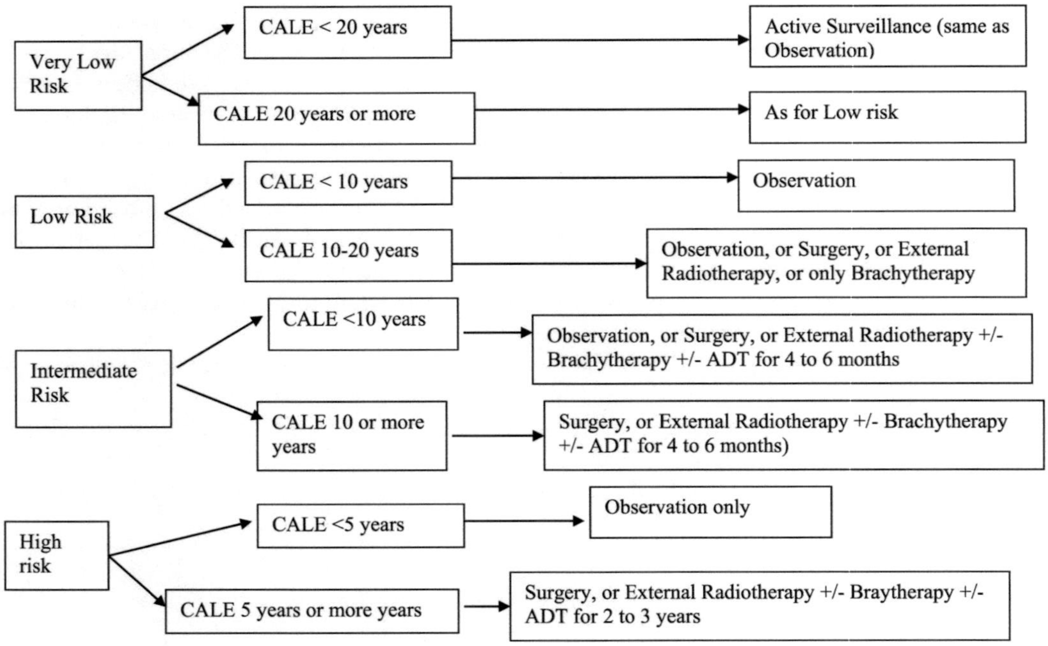

Fig. 1b.

Fig. 1a and 1b. Algorithm based on guideline by National Comprehensive Cancer Network for selection of treatment for localized prostate cancer.

next most common pattern, the Gleason score would be 7 (3+4). The most common grade is 6, whereas grades 2 to 5 are uncommon. Grade 6 identifies a tumor with well-differentiated histology; grade 7 has intermediate differentiation; and grades 8 to 10 are the most poorly differentiated and have the worst prognosis. A grade 7 cancer is more aggressive if its scoring is 4+3 instead of 3+4.

PSA levels of 4 to less than 10 ng per mL, 10 to20 ng per mL (10 to 20 mcg per L), and greater than 20 ng per mL are associated with a low, intermediate, and high risk of prostate cancer recurrence after treatment, respectively.

The factor of Comorbidity-adjusted Life Expectancy is particularly important because the number of comorbid diseases is the most significant predictor of survival after treatment of prostate cancer. [34] Prostate cancer is usually slow growing, and the survival benefit of treatment may present only after 10 years or longer. This is the basis of the "10-year rule": a patient with prostate cancer should be treated only if the patient has a comorbidity-adjusted life expectancy of at least 10 years. Age alone is not accurate in estimating life expectancy. To estimate comorbidity-adjusted life expectancy, the NCCN recommends the use of health status quartiles that match corresponding quartiles of life expectancy at each year of age. Tables 1a [35] and 1b [31] give a short patient-administered Charlson Comorbidity Index that can be used for a quick estimation of comorbidity-adjusted life expectancy.

After deciding in favor of treatment, patients can choose between surgery and radiotherapy based on the side-effect profile of treatments. A systematic review did not find any good-quality head-to-head trials comparing surgery and radiotherapy. [36] The review found that surgery and external beam radiation therapy (EBRT) are equivalent in controlling the cancer, especially if the baseline PSA level is greater than 10 ng per mL.[36] Many trials studied biochemical progression but not long-term survival, and some trials were conducted before the advent of PSA testing. No trial has compared treatment outcomes by race or ethnicity, and most trials do not provide baseline racial characteristics. Among patients in whom cancer was detected clinically (not by PSA screening), those who underwent radical prostatectomy (RP) had fewer prostate cancer-related deaths than patients who chose watchful waiting, although this benefit was limited to patients younger than 65 years. [36] Patients who were operated on by surgeons who performed more than 40 RPs per year had fewer urinary adverse effects. Laparoscopic RP performed with or without the use of robotic technology is associated with less blood loss and shorter hospital stays, but all long-term outcomes are similar to open RP. In robotic laparoscopic RP, surgeons with more experience were more likely to achieve complete resection of the cancer.[36]

Which medical problems have you had?		Has this condition limited your activities, or do you need to take prescription medicine?	
		Yes	No
Inflammatory bowel disease	O	O	O
Liver disease	O	O	O
Stroke	O	O	O
Ulcer	O	O	O
Arthritis	O	O	O
Chest pain	O	O	O
Chronic lung disease	O	O	O
Depression	O	O	O
Diabetes mellitus	O	O	O
Heart attack	O	O	O
Heart failure	O	O	O
High blood pressure	O	O	O

Note: Inflammatory bowel disease, liver disease, stroke, and ulcers are scored as one disease each, regardless of severity. The remaining eight conditions are scored as one disease each only if the conditions limit the patient's activity or require prescription medications.

Table 1a. Patient-Administered 12-item Charlson Comorbidity Index

EBRT is given over eight to nine weeks and is associated with more bowel adverse effects than surgery. Surgery is more difficult if cancer recurs after EBRT. The review found one trial in which proton therapy was more effective than EBRT. [36] In patients with low-risk cancer, brachytherapy using iodine-125 or palladium-103 pellet implantation is recommended as monotherapy.[32] It is a preferred option in these patients because it controls the cancer as effectively as surgery or EBRT, and patients experience much less urinary incontinence and erectile dysfunction. Implantation may be difficult in patients who have bladder outlet obstruction or a very large or very small prostate, and in those who have had previous prostate surgery.

Hormone therapy (also known as androgen deprivation therapy) as an adjunct to surgical treatment is discouraged in low-risk patients because it does not increase treatment effectiveness and is associated with gynecomastia and erectile dysfunction. [32, 36] Cryotherapy and high-frequency ultrasound are not recommended as routine monotherapies.

Age (years)	Life expectancy (years)		
	Top percentile of health (no disease)*	Middle two percentiles of health (1 or 2 diseases)*	Bottom percentile of health (3 or more diseases)*
50	42.69	28.46	14.23
51	41.43	27.62	13.81
52	40.18	26.79	13.39
53	38.94	25.96	12.98
54	37.71	25.14	12.57
55	36.49	24.33	12.16
56	35.28	23.52	11.76
57	34.06	22.71	11.35
58	32.88	21.92	10.96
59	31.69	21.13	10.56
60	30.54	20.36	10.18
61	29.4	19.6	9.8
62	28.27	18.85	9.42
63	27.16	18.11	9.05
64	26.07	17.38	8.69
65	25.00	16.67	8.33
66	23.94	15.96	7.98
67	22.90	15.27	7.63
68	21.88	14.59	7.29
69	20.89	13.93	6.96
70	19.90	13.27	6.63
71	18.96	12.64	6.32
72	18.01	12.01	6.00
73	17.11	11.41	5.70
74	16.21	10.81	5.40
75	15.36	10.24	5.12
76	14.52	9.68	4.84
77	13.71	9.14	4.57
78	12.93	8.62	4.31
79	12.16	8.11	4.05
80	11.43	7.62	3.81

*—Number of diseases refers to the conditions listed in the Charlson Comorbidity Index.

Table 1b. Comorbidity-Adjusted Life Expectancy in U.S. Men

Adverse effects vary depending on the treatment modality used; the specialist's experience; the criteria used to assess the frequency, severity, and duration of symptoms and their baseline status; and the medications or devices used to treat the symptoms. Table 2 shows the incidence of adverse effects two years after surgery and EBRT. [37] Adverse effects noted five years after treatment include no urinary control or frequent urinary leakage (14 percent after surgery versus 5 percent after EBRT, with pad use in 29 percent of surgical patients and 4 percent of EBRT patients). [36] After adjusting for baseline factors, dripping or leaking urine was noted six times more often after surgery than after EBRT.[36] Erections insufficient for intercourse occurred in approximately three-fourths of patients after surgery or EBRT.[36] Despite these adverse effects, less than 5 percent of patients reported dissatisfaction with treatment, and more than 90 percent of patients said they would make the same decision again.[36] Patients who underwent surgery were most satisfied. Patient satisfaction was highly related with adverse effects, but also with the perception of freedom from prostate cancer.

Adverse effect	Watchful waiting (%)	Surgery (%)	External beam radiation (%)	Hormone therapy (%)
Bowel problems (urgency)	16	14	29	16
Erectile dysfunction (no erections at all)	33	58	43	86
Urinary problems (leaking)	7	35	12	11

Adapted from Agency for Healthcare Research and Quality. Treating prostate cancer. A guide for men with localized prostate cancer.
http://www.effectivehealthcare.ahrq.gov/ehc/products/9/98/ProstateCancerConsumer.pdf
Accessed June 4, 2010.

Table 2. Adverse Effects Two Years After Prostate Cancer Treatment

Compared with observation and watchful waiting, active surveillance is a more structured program to track the progression of prostate cancer, allowing for earlier intervention if the patient's risk is found to increase on follow-up. A protocol used in Canada is shown in Table 3 [10]; with the use of this protocol, patient survival is similar to that after treatment (99.2 percent at eight years in 299 patients).[10] About 25 percent of patients in this protocol proceed to intervention.9 Patient survival in a European study was 100 percent at 10 years in 616 patients. [38] In this ongoing study, patients continue with active surveillance only if their PSA level (checked every three months) doubles in more than three years; if cancer is present in only one or two biopsy cores; and if their Gleason score remains 6 (3+3) or lower (biopsy is done if the PSA doubling time is three to 10 years, and routinely at one, three, five, and seven years, then every five years thereafter). Active surveillance is recommended for low- and very low-risk patients. Drawbacks include the potentially increased difficulty of curative or nerve-sparing surgery in patients for whom intervention is delayed despite increasing risk, and mild anxiety. However, men following this protocol have been found to have favorable levels of anxiety and distress.[39]

In summary, with the use a new, easy and quick method that we have described to estimate a newly-diagnosed patient's co-morbidity adjusted life expectancy, physicians can help patients in choosing treatment or observation according to evidence-based national guidelines. This may reduce reluctance among patients and physicians in getting PSA screening and may reduce worry regarding over-diagnosis of low-risk cancers and the potential damage to the patient's health-related quality of life through unnecessary treatment of such cancers. We have recently published our algorithm in the journal American Family Physician, [40] which is the most widely read journal in primary care; this may help primary care physicians in counseling newly-diagnosed patients; until now patients return to primary care physicians after they have chosen a course of treatment as recommended by the urologist who had done the biopsy. [41] Although in October 2011 the United States Preventive Services Task Force has recommended against PSA testing,[42] this recommendation is based on the potential harms that can result from treatment of low-risk cancers. However, to not screen for prostate cancer- which is the second most common cause of cancer death in American men, will inevitably lead to even more deaths from untreated advanced cancer. A more prudent approach might be to screen for the cancer, but to use the approach in this article to convince low-risk patients to choose active surveillance instead of immediate treatment.

Eligibility criteria
• PSA level ≤ 10 ng per mL (10 μg per L), Gleason score of 6 or lower, and stage T1c or T2a cancer • For men with more than 15-year life expectancy: fewer than three cores and less than 50 percent of any one core involved
Follow-up schedule
• PSA testing and digital rectal examination every three months for two years, then every six months as long as PSA level is stable • 10 to 12 core biopsies at one year, then every three years until 80 years of age • Optional: transrectal ultrasonography on alternate visits
Indications for intervention
• PSA doubling time less than three years (based on at least eight determinations; required in about 20 percent of patients) • Progression to Gleason score of 7 (4+3) or higher (required in about 5 percent of patients)

PSA = prostate-specific antigen. Adapted with permission from Klotz L. Active Surveillance for prostate cancer: for whom? J Clin Oncol 2005; 23(32): 8167

Table 3. Canadian Protocol for Active Surveillance of Prostate Cancer

2. References

[1] American Cancer Society. What are the key statistics about prostate cancer? http://www.cancer.org/Cancer/ProstateCancer/DetailedGuide/prostate-cancer-key-statistics. Accessed June 4, 2010.

[2] National Cancer Institute. Cancer advances in focus: prostate cancer. http://www.cancer.gov/cancertopics/factsheet/cancer-advances-in-focus/FS12_7.pdf. Accessed July 9, 2011.

[3] Miller D, Gruber S, Hollenbeck B, Montie J, Wei J. Incidence of initial local therapy among men with lower-risk prostate cancer in the United States. J Natl Cancer Inst 2006; 98(16):1134-1141.

[4] Cooperberg MR, Broering JM, Kantoff PW, Carroll PR. Contemporary trends in low risk prostate cancer: risk assessment and treatment. J Urol. 2007;178 (3 pt 2):S14-S19.

[5] Parker C, Muston D, Melia J, Moss S, Dearnaley D. A model of the natural history of screen-detected prostate cancer, and the effect of radical treatment on overall survival. Br J Cancer. 2006; 94(10):1361-1368.

[6] lbertsen PC, Hanley JA, Fine J. 20-year outcomes following conservative management of clinically localized prostate cancer. JAMA. 2005;293(17):2095-2101.
[7] Bill-Axelson A, Holmberg L, Ruutu M, et al.: Scandinavian Prostate Cancer Group Study No. Four. Radical prostatectomy versus watchful waiting in early prostate cancer. N Engl J Med. 2005;352(19):1977-1984.
[8] Stattin P, Holmberg E, Johansson JE, Holmberg L, Adolfsson J, Hugosson J. Outcomes in localized prostate cancer: National Prostate Cancer Register of Sweden follow-up study. J Natl Cancer Inst. 2010;102(13):950-958.
[9] Wong YN, Mitra N, Hudes G, et al: Survival associated with treatment versus observation of localized prostate cancer in elderly men. JAMA 296:2683-93, 2006
[10] Klotz L. Active surveillance for prostate cancer: for whom? J Clin Oncol. 2005;23(32):8165-8169.
[11] Potosky AL, Davis WW, Hoffman RM et al. Five-year outcomes after prostatectomy or radiotherapy for prostate cancer: the prostate cancer outcomes study J Natl Cancer Inst. 96:1358-67, 2004.
[12] Thompson I, Thrasher JB, Aus G, et al. Guideline for the management of clinically localized prostate cancer: 2007 update. http://www.usrf.org/CaP%20Guidelines,%20AUA,%202007.pdf
[13] Hu JC, Kwan L, Saigal CS et al. Regret in men treated for localized prostate cancer J Urol. 169:2279-83, 2003
[14] Ruchlin HS, Pellisier JM. An economic overview of prostate carcinoma. Cancer 92: 2796-810, 2001
[15] Harlan SR, Cooperberg MR, Elkin EP, et al. Time trends and characteristics of men choosing watchful waiting for initial treatment of localized prostate cancer: results from CaPSURE. J Urol. 2003; 170(5):1804-1807.
[16] Miller DC, Gruber SB, Hollenbeck BK, Montie JE, Wei JT. Incidence of initial local therapy among men with lower-risk prostate cancer in the United States. J Natl Cancer Inst. 2006; 98(16):1134-1141.
[17] Jemal A, Siegel R, Xu J, Ward E. Cancer statistics, 2010. CA Cancer J Clin. 2010;60(5): 277-300.
[18] Shavers VL, Brown ML, Potosky AL, et al. Race/ethnicity and the receipt of watchful waiting for the initial management of prostate cancer. J Gen Intern Med. 2004; 19(2):146-155.
[19] Fowler FJ Jr, McNaughton Collins M, Albertsen PC, Zietman A, Elliott DB, Barry MJ. Comparison of recommendations by urologists and radiation oncologists for treatment of clinically localized prostate cancer. JAMA. 2000; 283(24):3217-3222.
[20] Cohen H, Britten N. Who decides about prostate cancer treatment? A qualitative study. Fam Pract. 2003; 20(6):724-729.
[21] Mohan R, Beydoun H, Barnes-Ely ML, et al. Patients' survival expectations before localized prostate cancer treatment by treatment status. J Am Board Fam Med. 2009; 22(3):247-256.
[22] Beydoun HA, Mohan R, Beydoun MA, Davis J, Lance R, Schellhammer P. Development of a scale to assess patient misperceptions about treatment choices for localized prostate cancer. BJU Int. 2010;106 (3):334-341.
[23] Ross RW, Kantoff PW: Predicting outcomes in prostate cancer: How many more nomograms do we need? J Clin Oncol 25:3563-3564, 2007

[24] Jang TL, Yossepowitch O, Bianco FJ et al. Low risk prostate cancer in men under age 65: the case for definitive treatment. Urol Oncol: seminars and original investigations 25:510-514, 2007
[25] Feldman-Stewart D, Brennenstuhl S, McIssac K et al. A systematic review of information in decision aids. Health Expect. 10:46-61, 2007
[26] Shariat SF, Karakiewicz PI, Margulis V et al. Inventory of prostate cancer predictive tools. Curr Opin Urol. 18:279-296, 2008.
[27] Visser A, van Andel G. Psychosocial and educational aspects in prostate cancer patients. Patient Educ Couns. 49:203-206, 2003
[28] Dahm P, Kunz R, Schünemann H: Evidence-based clinical practice guidelines for prostate cancer: the need for a unified approach. Curr Opin Urol.17:200-7, 2007
[29]Ebara S, Katayama N, Tanimoto R et al. Iodine-125 seed implantation (permanent brachytherapy) for clinically localized prostate cancer Acta Med Okayama.62:9-13, 2008
[30] Walsh PC., DeWeese TL, Eisenberger M. Localized Prostate Cancer N Engl J Med 357: 2696-2705, 2007
[31] Mohan R, Beydoun H, Davis J, Lance R, Schellhammer P. Feasibility of using guidelines to choose treatment for prostate cancer. Can J Urol. 2010 17:4975-84
[32] National Comprehensive Cancer Network. Prostate cancer.2010 Practice guidelines in oncology v.2. http://www.nccn.org/professionals/physician_gls/f_guidelines.asp (registration required). Accessed June 4, 2010.
[33] D'Amico AV, Whittington R, Malkowicz SB et al. Pretreatment nomogram for prostate-specific antigen recurrence after radical prostatectomy or external beam radiation therapy for clinically localized prostate cancer. J Clin Oncol 17:168-172, 1999
[34] Post PN, Hansen BE, Kil PJ, Janssen-Heijnen ML, Coebergh JW. The independent prognostic value of comorbidity among men aged < 75 years with localized prostate cancer: a population-based study. BJU Int. 2001; 87(9):821-826.
[35] Hoffman RM, Stone SN, Espey D, Potosky AL. Differences between men with screening-detected versus clinically diagnosed prostate cancers in the USA. BMC Cancer. 2005;5:27.
[36] Agency for Healthcare Research and Quality. Comparative effectiveness of therapies for clinically localized prostate cancer. Executive summary. http://www.effectivehealthcare.ahrq.gov/ehc/products/9/79/2008_0204ProstateCancerExecSum.pdf. Accessed June 4, 2010.
[37] Agency for Healthcare Research and Quality. Treating prostate cancer. A guide for men with localized prostate cancer. http://www.effectivehealthcare.ahrq.gov/ehc/products/9/98/ProstateCancerConsumer.pdf. Accessed June 4, 2010.
[38] van den Bergh RC, Roemeling S, Roobol MJ, et al. Outcomes of men with screen-detected prostate cancer eligible for active surveillance who were managed expectantly. Eur Urol. 2009;55 (1):1-8.
[39] van den Bergh RC, Essink-Bot ML, Roobol MJ, et al. Anxiety and distress during active surveillance for early prostate cancer. Cancer. 2009; 115(17):3868-3878.
[40] Mohan R, Schellhammer P. Treatment options in Localized Prostate Cancer. American Family Physician, August 15th, 2011. 84(4):413-20.
[41] Mohan R . Family physicians could help in predicting life expectancy without prostate cancer. Journal Clin Oncol. 26:690-1, 2008.
[42] Screening for prostate cancer: draft recommendation statement. Rockville, MD: U.S. Preventive Services Task Force, October 7, 2011

5

Automatic Diagnosis of Breast Tissue

Atef Boujelben[1], Hedi Tmar[2], Mohamed Abid[2] and Jameleddine Mnif[1]
University of Sfax
[1]*ANIM "Departement of Radiology and Medical Imaging- Habib Bourguiba Hospital-Sfax. Faculty of Medicine",*
[2]*CES "National Engineers School of Sfax"*
Tunisia

1. Introduction

The Breast cancer whose region is difficult to be visually detected is a major cause of death among women (Nishikawa, 2007). So, the quality of radiologist judgment of whether the suspected region is malignant or benign will not be guaranteed. So far, screening mammography has been the best available radiological technique for an early detection of breast cancer (Siddiqui et al., 2005). However, because of the large number of mammograms to be analysed, radiologists can make false detections. Thus, there are new solutions of automatic detection pertaining to the problems of analysis that can be explored. In this context, Computer Aided Diagnosis (CADi) and Computer Aided Detection (CADe) are two systems that can solve these problems (Rangayyan et al., 2007). In fact, CADe System is based on the detection of Region Of Interest (ROI) and decision. As for, CADi build on good isolation of ROI, analysis and classification to have a decision and/or aid for decision.

This paper proposes a CADi System based on Texture/Shape characterization to reduce the load of radiologists work. In fact, in the past several years the mammography process has seen tremendous evolution. In processing and analysis techniques, many methods based on shape characterization are adopted. So, breast tumours and masses appear in mammograms with different shapes and characteristics. There are two kinds of tumours: malignant ones which usually have rough, microlobulated, or spiculated contours, and benign tumours that have commonly smooth, round, macrolobulated, or oval contours (Reston, 1998). It is true that this type of characterization is efficient and allows good mammogram exploration, but the quality of results is women-old dependent: if the woman is younger, it is too hard to analyse his mammogram. For this reason, we include a texture description of the region to cope with this problem. So, the density of the region can discriminate the malignity or benignity of ROI by analysing the texture. Thus, the technique adopted in this work takes into consideration both texture and shape characterisation. In general, the quality of analysis is dependent on the quality of segmentation. However, current approaches do not guarantee a good quality of segmentation. The majority of segmentation-methods take only edge (inter-area) aspects into account to delimit the ROI. In this context, the manual segmentation and semi-automatic method are widely used. In (Boujelben et al., 2009a) (Boujelben et al., 2009b), the threshold-based segmentation is carried out by fixing a rectangular box around the suspicious tumour area and then using Sobel filter in order to avoid noise. However, this can affect noise and discontinuities in the border of ROI. In addition, active contours, depending on edge criterion, solve the problems of segmentation as noise and discontinuities (Osher & Fedkiw, 2002). However, breast quality makes segmentation effective only by taking both intra-area and inter-area aspects into account. To attain our objective which is the ROI segmentation in mammographic images, we apply the Level Set method based on external function (convergence function) that represents area and contour criteria as much as possible. In this paper, we include the texture/shape detection in the process of mammograms diagnosis. The main purpose of this work is the elaboration of a CADi to reach a good identification of ROI and contribute to a better quality of analysis. This work, is integrate within the MIPAX (Medical Image Processing and Analysis eXchange) project which was defined as the object of CES (Computer, Electronic And Smart engineering systems design Laboratory in National School of Engineers of Sfax) and ANIM(Numeric Archiving and Medical Imaging in National School of Medicine) collaboration. So, this project was split in three parts; Numeric Archiving PACS (Picture Archiving and Communication System), Data Base of User Environment and Automatic Analysis of Medical Images. This present work articulate around the last part. To attain our objective (CADi), we firstly show why and how to adapt Level Set-based approach in case of pseudo-detection, which is a semi-automatic detection by using level-set technique; and secondly, we study the performance of boundary, region and texture features in a mammogram diagnosis process. The remainder of this paper is organised as follows. Section 2 presents the state of the art of shape/texture analysis; without loss of generality, we outline the most original and important work addressing mammogram analysis. Section 3 describes the proposed block diagram for mass diagnosis. Section 4 illustrates the deformable model, namely, Level Set approach adopted in segmentation and its adaptation in case of breast cancer detection. Afterwards, section 5 presents the adopted method for analysis and shows how a combination of shape and texture features could be advantageous for a good diagnosis. As for section 6, it presents the results obtained by the proposed scheme. Lastly, section 7 gives some concluding remarks and draws some future work.

2. Context of state of the art

The medical imaging is an active domain that embraces various topics like image processing, mass segmentation or detection, mass analysis and decision or aid for decision. The results of our research can be viewed in the context of two areas of related work: the detection of breast cancers, and the analysis of detected breast cancers. The purpose of this paper is to examine how to differentiate the malignant tumours from the benign ones. So, the analysis steps are related to pseudo-detection results. In this context, we attempt to present an adaptation of Level Set technique for pseudo-detection and investigate two approaches for shape and texture analysis. Therefore, the analysis of texture is used to qualify the density of ROI or to have an idea about the space distribution of micro-calcification (Dheeba & Wiselin, 2010) (Wiesmiller & Chandy, 2010)(Boujelben et al., 2011). Generally, texture feature extraction methods can be classified into three major categories; namely statistical, structural and spectral. In a biomedical image like mammogram, the characteristics of the pixels in the texture pattern are not similar everywhere. To cope with this specificity, statistical approaches for texture analysis such as the moments of gray-level histogram, based on a Gray-Level Co-occurrence Matrix (GLCM), is used. It is computed to discriminate different textures in mammographic images (Oliver et al., 2007) (Zwiggelaar & .R.Denton, 2004) (Lambrou et al., 2002) (Masala et al., 2007) (Ahirwar & Jadon, 2011). In this context, Zwiggelaar et *al.*(Zwiggelaar & .R.Denton, 2004) include some mathematic operators like translation and transportation in order to select a sub-set of features from GLCM to have a decision about tumour characterisation. Quite close from ours, Lambrou et *al.* (Lambrou et al., 2002) studied the effectiveness of GLCM and the higher-order-statistic based on twenty features. In (Masala et al., 2007), ROI is characterised by eight features extracted from GLCM. Thereafter, four classifiers were evaluated: Multilayer Perception (MLP), Probabilistic Neural Network (PNN), Radial Basis Function Network (RBF) and k-Nearest Neighbours (KNN). In opposition to (Masala et al., 2007), we evaluate the effectiveness of two classifiers: MLP and KNN classifiers. Using statistical approaches, we extract six characteristics from Co-occurrence matrix. Therefore, we compute the average value of each characteristic over each orientation(0, 45, 90 and 135). The second criterion in medical image analysis process is the analysis of shape which is built over two phases, namely boundary and region analysis. In case of boundary, many work focused on the Radial Distance Measure (RDM)(Rangayyan et al., 2006)Boujelben et al. (2009a)(Alvarenga et al., 2006), Convexity (CVX), Fourier Fraction (FF) (Rangayyan et al., 1997), Fractal Dimension (FD) (Nguyen & Rangayyan, 2005) (Nguyen & Rangayyan, 2006) and the angular measure (Yang et al., 2005) (Denise et al., 2008) (Rangayyan et al., 2006). However, methods defined in the context of angular measures provides so far either of the two categories: Radial Angle (RA) (Yang et al., 2005) or Turning Angle(TA) (Denise et al., 2008) (Rangayyan et al., 2006). In this context, Sheng Chih et *al.* (Yang et al., 2005) used the RA, which is the smallest angle included between the gradient direction and the radial direction of the edge. The RA forms a good feature for a malignant/benign discrimination. In fact, if the angle increases towards 180 degree, then it is a benign mass. In contrast, if the angle decreases towards zero degree, then it is a malignant mass. Nevertheless, the computation of RA takes many times. His temporel complexity increases because alarge number of points in the perimeter of the region are taken into account through the calculus. Unlike RA, TA tackle the problem of temporel complexity. However, the calculus is limited to the convex points that forms the perimeter of the region(Rangayyan et al., 2006) with preserving the result quality. Quite close from (Rangayyan et al., 2006), we propose a novel measure denoted Index Angle (IA)(Boujelben et al., 2009b). Its based on the external and internal angle concepts. We will show in section 5 the technical details of the IA calculus. We will also show how the IA can be efficient to differentiate malignant mass from benign ones. On the other hand, the RDM descriptor (Alvarenga et al., 2006) (Delogu et al., 2008) was taken a great importance in medical imaging litterature. It is based on the computation of the distances between contour points and gravity center of the region. However, it provides a complete knowledge concerning circularity of the region. The RDM technique presents any advantages like normalized computation and insensibility to affine transformations. From the RDM, Alvarenga et *al.*(Alvarenga et al., 2006) and Delogu et *al.* (Delogu et al., 2008) extracted many features like Roughness (R), Standard DEViation (SDEV), etc. They combined the RDM and the region features to improve mass description. In (Alvarenga et al., 2006), the performance and relevance of a set of shape features extracted from the RDM method and the Convex-Hull are evaluated. In contrast, Delogu et *al.* (Delogu et al., 2008) evaluated the combination of some features extracted from RDM and others like Convexity and Circularity. The RDM is a method that can differentiate between the malignant and benign cases, but, it can cause noise in the calculation of each boundary point. Furthermore, it can also cause a long time of calculation. To deal with these problems, we propose to calculate the features only in the concave and convex points. In fact, the extended RDM that we propose, XRDM (Boujelben et al., 2009a), is shown in section 5. Like contour descriptor explained above, region descriptor was taken a great importance in image description. It is used to describe the regularity of the mammogram masses. However, simple morphologic features like Circularity and Eccentricity are extracted through this descriptor (Yang et al., 2005)(Boujelben et al., 2009b)(Delogu et al., 2008). Alvarenga et *al.* (Alvarenga et al., 2006) evaluated the performance and relevance of seven shape features; namely Perimeter (P), Normalized Radial Length (NRL), SDEV, Area Ratio (AR), contour roughness (R), Circularity and Mshape. These characteristics are enriched by adding some other ones in (Retico et al., 2007). The most important added characteristics are Zero Crossing (ZC) (i.e. a count of the number of times the radial distance plot crosses the average radial distance) and Convexity, which allows the representation of the studied shape better than the characteristics cited above. In this chapter, we present an approach of shape analysis in our diagnosis process of mammograms. From region criteria we use characteristics like Circularity, which can be useful in this direction and can give an indication on the regularity of a given mammogram mass, Internal/External Circle (IEC), which can be used to measure the elongation of shape, and NRV. Added to that, the features combination based on shape and texture is used in the CADi systems. In (Maglogiannis et al., 2007), Maglogiannis et *al.* proposed an intelligent system for automatic breast cancer diagnosis using Support-Vector-Machines based classifiers (SVM). The features used are based on texture and shape criteria like radius (means of distances from centre to points on the perimeter), SDEV of grey-scale values, Perimeter, Area, Smoothness (local variation in radius lengths), Compactness, Concavity (severity of concave portions of the contour), concaves points (number of concave portions of the contour), symmetry and FD. Furthermore, 22 features based on edge-sharpness, shape and texture are extracted by Nandi et *al.* (Nandi et al., 2006). They adopted Genetic Programming (GP) for features classification. This method handles implicit feature selection. The GP is also used in (Zadeh et al., 2001) to compare the performance of four different texture and shape feature extraction methods which are conventional shape quantifiers, co-occurrence-based method of Haralick, wavelet transformations and multi-wavelet transformations. Zadeh et *al.* (Zadeh et al., 2004) began again their work done in (Zadeh et al., 2001) by considering 17 shape and 44 texture features. They selected the best feature using Genetic Algorithm (GA).

In summary, the medical imaging literature is splited so far either of two orientations: many methods independently process on contour, region and texture indexes while others attempt a combination of all these indexes and a selection of the more important features with GA. Yet, it is clear that the characteristic of masses has information based on these proprieties (region, contour and texture). The subject matter is that the combination of the characteristics of different properties can lead or not to a good quality of diagnosis.

However, the identification of breast region is important to improve the analysis process. So, breast tumours and masses appear in mammograms with different shape characteristics. Detecting the region can give an idea about the nature of diagnosis. However, in the past several years there has been tremendous evolution in mammography process. In this context, two approaches are used in the literature: automatic detection and region segmentation. Concerning detection, Torrent et *al.* (Torrent et al., 2008) presents a comparison of two clustering based algorithms and one region based algorithm for segmenting fatty and dense tissue in mammographic images. The first algorithm is a multiple thresholding algorithm based on the excess entropy, the second one is based on the Fuzzy C-Means clustering algorithm, and the third one is based on a statistical analysis of the breast. In addition, method based on multiresolution approach to the computer aided detection of clustered micro-calcifications in digitized mammograms based on Gabor elementary functions is illustrated in (Catanzariti et al., 2003). So, a bank of Gabor functions with varying spatial extent and tuned to different spatial frequencies is used for the extraction of micro-calcifications characteristics. Firstly, results show that most micro-calcifications, isolated or clustered, are detected and secondly the classification is illustrated by an Artificial Neural Network with supervised learning. On the other hand, Thangavel et *al.* (Thangavel

& Karnan, 2005) present an Ant Colony Optimization (ACO) and Genetic Algorithm (GA) for the identification of suspicious regions in mammograms. The proposed method uses the asymmetry principle (bilateral subtraction): strong structural asymmetries between the corresponding regions in the left and right breasts are taken as evidence for the possible presence of micro-calcifications in that region. Bilateral subtraction is achieved in two steps. First, the mammogram images are enhanced using median filter, then pectoral muscle region is removed and the border of the mammogram is detected for both left and right images from the binary image. Further GA is applied to enhance the detected border. So, the nipple position is identified for both left and right images using GA and ACO, and their performance is studied. Second, using the border points and nipple position as the reference of mammogram images are aligned and subtracted to extract the suspicious region. In the context of detection ROI, Schiabel et *al.* (Schiabel et al., 2008) proposed a methodology based on the Watershed transformation, which is combined with two other procedures; histogram equalization, working as pre-processing for enhancing images contrast, and a labelling procedure intended to reduce noise. But, Jadhav et *al.* (Jadhav & Thorat, 2009) used statistical feature extraction method by using a sliding window analysis, for detecting circumscribed masses in mammograms. This procedure is implemented by taking into account the multi-scale statistical properties of the breast tissue, and succeeds in finding the exact tumour position by performing the mammographic analysis using first few moments of each window. We have demonstrated that fast implementation in both feature extraction and neural classification module can be achieved. Nevertheless, a system processes for the mammograms in several steps is adopted in (Arodz et al., 2006). First, we filter the original picture with a filter that is sensitive to micro-calcification contrast shape. Then, authors enhance the mammogram contrast by using wavelet-based sharpening algorithm. Afterwards, present to radiologist, for visual analysis, such a contrast-enhanced mammogram with suggested positions of micro-calcification clusters. However, a multi-resolution representation of the original mammogram is obtained using a linear phase non-separable 2-D wavelet transform which is adopted in (Liu & Delp, 1997). This is chosen for two reasons. First, it does not introduce phase distortions in the decomposed images. Second, no bias is introduced in the horizontal and vertical directions as a separable transform would. Authors used coefficients of the analysis low pass filter. A set of features are then extracted at each resolution for every pixel. Detection is performed from the coarsest resolution using binary tree classifiers. This top-down approach requires less computation by starting with the least amount of data and propagating detection results to finer resolutions. In addition, wavelet coefficients describe the local geometry of an image in terms of scale and orientation apart from being flexible and robust with respect to image resolution and quality (Oliver et al., 2007). In addition, Marti et *al.* (Marti et al., 2003) propose a supervised method for the segmentation of masses in mammographic images. Based on the active region approach, an energy function which integrates texture, contour and shape information is defined. Then, pixels are aggregated or eliminated to the region by optimizing this function allowing the obtention of an accurate segmentation. The algorithm starts with a selected pixel inside the mass, which has been manually selected by an expert radiologist. Recently, explicit and implicit methods of deformable model are used in different applications (Brox et al., 2009). In this context, for breast cancer detection, Ferrari et *al.* (Ferrari et al., 2004) used a traditional active deformable contour model (Snake) to limit the breast in the image. To injure the problem of initialisation, they used an adaptative thresholding. For the elimination of the pectoral muscle, Boucher et *al.* (Boucher et al., 2009) used the snake and Ball et *al.* (Ball & Bruce, 2007) used the Narrow Band level set methodology with an adaptative segmentation threshold controlled by a border complexity term. An overview of the literature shows that many methods of segmentation and identification are used to detect ROI. In this paper, we propose method based on Level Set approach which includes edge and region proprieties. So, in the Level Set approach, two major problems are usually discussed in the bibliographies: initialisation and evolution function which is the point of interest in section 4. In the next section, we describe the proposed block diagram for mass diagnosis.

3. Overview

The proposed approach consists of three subtasks. Firstly, the identification of ROI is done using a level-set-based approach which includes edge and region criteria. Secondly, features are extracted, using shape/texture descriptors. Finally, in order to take decision about diagnosis, we are interested in MLP and KNN classifiers. Figure 1 shows the bloc diagram of the proposed scheme. The first point of this workflow is the segmentation which will be detailed in details in next section.

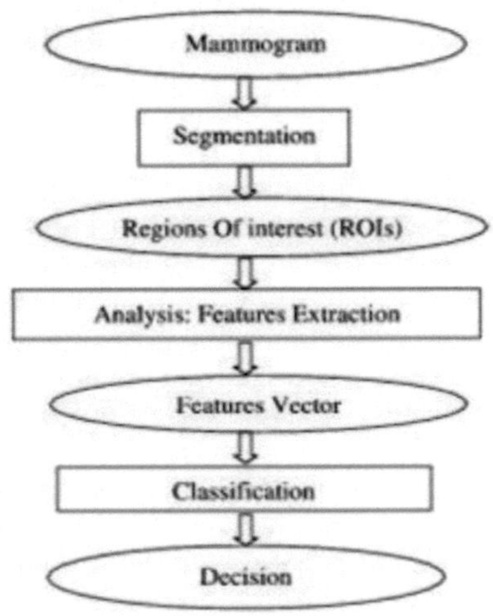

Fig. 1. Proposed Flow

4. Segmentation with deformable models

Image Segmentation is an important step to handle a good analysis. However, it is based on homogeneity and/or edge criteria of the region. It consists of ROI extraction. So, the choice of a segmentation technique depends on regularity/irregularity of the edge of the ROI. In addition, the noise can affect the segmentation quality. However, we are interested in noise avoiding. Generally, to tackle this problem in medical imaging, explicit and implicit methods of deformable model are used.

4.1 Explicit deformable models

The active contour model, or snake, is used to detect region of interest (ROI) or contour in image. It is an energy-minimising-spline technique. The result of this minimisation is guided by two terms; the first term controls the aspect of the curve: it is often called internal energy. The second term attracts the curve C towards object which one seeks the borders: it is often called external energy. The detail of this method is illustrated in (Kass et al., 1988). The main concepts are:

- The snake is parametrically defined as:

$v(s) = (x(s), y(s))$, with $s \in [0, 1]$

- The energy is defined by:

$$E = \int_0^1 \alpha \| \acute{V(s)} \| + \beta \| \acute{\acute{V(s)}} \|^2) ds - \lambda \int_0^1 (\| \nabla I(V(s)) \|^2) ds \tag{1}$$

Where:

- α, β and λ are real constants, respectively coefficients of elasticity, rigidity and contraction (or dilation) from the curve.

- $\nabla I(V(s))$: is the gradient of image in s.

4.2 Implicit deformable models

Contrary to the explicit models, the implicit deformable models or Level Set approach (Casselles et al., 1997) uses a dense contour in which the implicit evolution avoids the needs to track surface markers in relation to each other. So, the Level Set is a method which studies the evolution of the curve and surfaces (Osher & Fedkiw, 2002). The points defining this interface will move towards the normal at a speed F according to the following equation:

$$\frac{\partial C(t)}{\partial t} = F \vec{N} \tag{2}$$

$\vec{N}$: Normal with the curve.

F: speed term depends on the curve.

The parametric curve C(t) is improved by the detection of the level zero and the function F evolves and moves according to:

$$\frac{\partial \phi}{\partial t} = F \| \nabla \Phi \| \tag{3}$$

The Evolution of this function depends on an initial curve $\Phi 0$. In this case, there are two aspects of research which are the initialization and the function F. The former is adopted in the present paper with a special focus on the region to be detected. In general (Sethian, 1998), speed F depends on three terms: first, on the local curve in each point (pondered with ϵ), second, on the term which is dependent on the image (pondered with β), and third, on a constant term (pondered with ν). The evolution of the interface is given by the following equation:

$$\frac{\partial \phi}{\partial t} = \epsilon * g(I) \| \nabla \Phi \| * div(\frac{\nabla \phi}{|\nabla \phi|}) - \beta * \nabla g(I) \| \nabla \Phi \| + \nu * g(I) \| \nabla \Phi \| \tag{4}$$

where: I is the point (i,j) of image matrix

$\epsilon, \beta, \nu \in [0, 1]$
$g(I) = \frac{1}{1 + \| \nabla \Phi \|}$

To minimize the temporal complexity of this equation, we adopt the Narrow Band and Fast Marching method in the implementation algorithm of Level Set. Narrow band consists of computing Level Set on evolution from contour for early inside and outside near the Level Set zero (Osher & Fedkiw, 2002). The reasons for using this approach are twofold. The first reason is to optimize time computation efficiency for a numerical calculation Level set method. The second one is the fact that, in general, regions in breast are difficult to be detected. In fact, we should focus locally near to the zero Level Set and its neighbouring Level Set because the local contour has more information significance than distant ones. Still, to accelerate the convergence of Level Set approach, we adopt a monotonically advancing front based on Fast Marching approach (Osher & Fedkiw, 2002). Its idea is that if T(x,y) is the time at which the curve crosses the point (x,y) then the surface T(x,y) satisfies the equation:

$$\|\nabla T\|.F = 1 \tag{5}$$

where:

$$F = \frac{1}{\exp(-\alpha \nabla I)} \tag{6}$$

This equation allows us to make a good implementation of deformable contours. Indeed, the changes of topology are automatically managed. Thus, if the image contains several objects, the contour is divided during its evolution including each object separately. Contour can also become deformed in order to be adjusted with complex forms, which cannot do explicit active contours (Snakes). Another positive point is that this method does not depend on initialization. Nevertheless, in the case of textured images, the criteria of gradient (edge properties) on which depends this equation (uniformity inter-region) affected a over-segmentation. So, the presence of textures in a mammographic image generates bad results because the small areas are privileged. But one can resort to a measurement of containing area in order to improve the quality of detection.

4.3 Adaptation of a Level Set approach

To solve the problem of mammographic images, which also depends on the information of the intra-region included in the information of inter-region, we added the criterion of the area. So, the region property is adopted firstly with the notion of image and secondly with the notion of propagation (addition of a fourth term). The evolution of the interface which has indeed ameliorated eq 4 is given by the following equation:

$$\frac{\partial C(t)}{\partial t} = \epsilon * g(I)\|\nabla\Phi\| * div(\frac{\nabla\phi}{|\nabla\phi|} - \beta * (\nabla g(I)\|\nabla\Phi\| + \frac{Moy(I)}{Max(I)}) - \nu * g(I)\|\nabla\Phi\| - \Theta * SkewCN(I) \tag{7}$$

where: $\Theta \in [0,1]$
Max(I)=maximum of gray-level in image.
Moy(I)=average of gray-level 3*3 centred in (x,y)
SkewCN(I)=$\frac{SkewnessCentred}{Max(Skewness)}$

The SkewnessCentred corresponds to the moment around the average. It measures the deviation of the distribution of the gray-level compared to a symmetrical distribution. For a deviation towards raised values, the Skewness-Centred is positive; whereas for a deviation towards low values, it is negative. Then SkewCentred can be calculated as follows:

$$SkewnessCentred = \frac{1}{9}\sum_{x}\sum_{y}(I(x,y) - MoY(x,y)) \tag{8}$$

Figure 2 show the result of segmentation in the proposed scheme. In the first line, the first

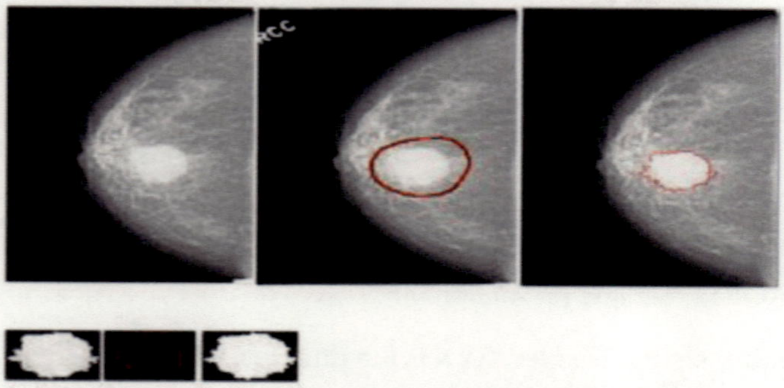

Fig. 2. ROI segmentation with mammogram; The first line showing from left to right: 1- the original image without contour, 2- the original image in DDSM database detoured by an experimented radiologic (red line), 3-the image segmented in this approach (red line). The second line showing the ROI isolated region in three cases: texture, boundary and area.

image is the original image without contour, the second image is the original image in DDSM database detoured by a radiologic (red line), and the third image is segmented in the context of this approach (red line) and in the second line, in every raw, we have region isolated ROI in the original texture, boundary and region, respectively. These three sub-images will be like entries for the vector which is based on texture, boundary and region. Likewise, it is clear that our results about segmentation are quite close to the manual segmentation results obtained by the radiologist. So, what remains is to see the quality of the segmentation that can be proven by the analysis step. Moreover, breast tumours and masses appear in mammograms with different shape characteristics. In this context, the method can reflect the irregularity or regularity of region and more precisely if compared to the manual process. Hence, the performance is illustrated according to two standpoints: precision of ROI segmentation in diagnostic relevance and computation time of optimization. After the ROI segmentation, the extraction of features is adopted in ROI: this is the point of interest that we will focus on, in the next section of the paper.

5. Analysis: Features extraction

In the ROI segmentation, we use an adaptation of a Level Set Approach with an edge and a region criterion. In this section, the features extraction is illustrated on any ROI. The mass have different shape characteristics, particularly, in breast cancer. In this framework, we can introduce a method based on shape analysis, basically, boundary analysis. Figure 3 shows the overall shape of benign and malignant mass. Firstly, we start with boundary information.

5.1 Boundary descriptor

Boundary analysis is often referred to in order to help to define regions according to any criteria. To differentiate between microlobulated region from macrolobulated ones, we can measure the convexity which is based on boundary. In fact, Retico et *al.* (Retico et al., 2007) used CVX in which feature depends on region (ratio of region-air detected by perimeter/or Air for his Convex envelop). In this subsection, we attempt to improve the importance of the

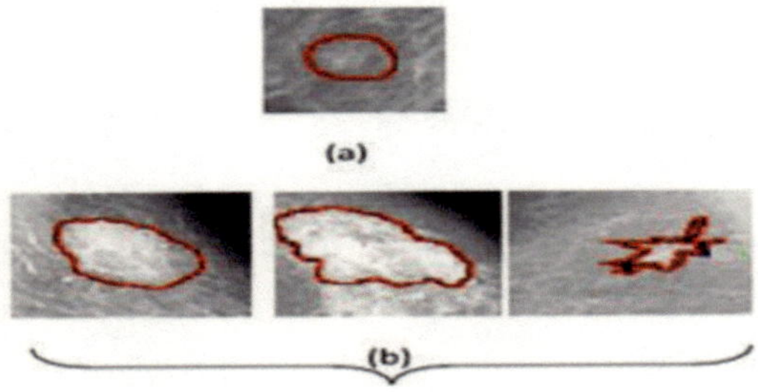

Fig. 3. Types of ROI: (a) benign, (b) malignant

analysis of boundary shape. Besides, CVX is the ratio of Convex envelop by perimeter for its perimeter of the region detected. When the mass tends to be round, its CVX tend to be near the 1. Conversely, a mass with speculated edge will have a CVX smaller than 0.5. Then, the CVX can be calculated as follows:

$$CVX = \frac{Perimeter(ConvexEnvelop)}{Perimeter(region)} \tag{9}$$

The advantage of this feature is that it is standardized and it is invariant with any affine transformation. After that we can differentiate between the macrolobulated and microlobulated region. Subsequently, to describe the rough ones, any researchers use RDM (Boujelben et al., 2009a) and Turning angle (Denise et al., 2008) (Rangayyan et al., 2006). In fact, RDM is a well-known method used in shape analysis. However, Euclidian distances d(i) are calculated between the gravity centre in the region and all the points in boundary region (Figure 4). where:

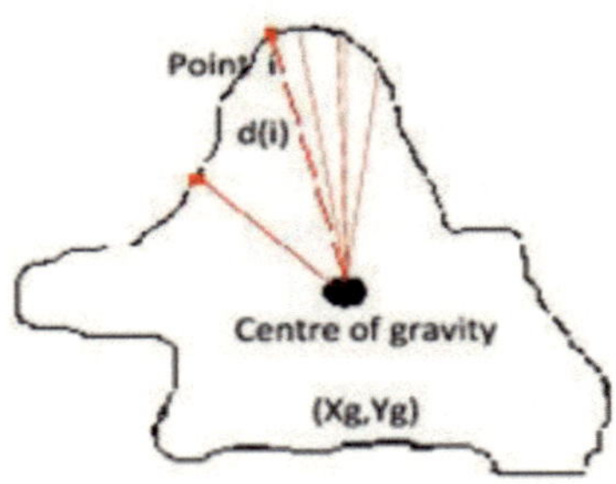

Fig. 4. Illustrative figure of RDM

$$d(i) = \sqrt{(Xi - Xg)^2 + (Yi - Yg)^2} \tag{10}$$

To eliminate large calculations from characteristics, all radial distances were normalized by using the maximum value of the radial distances.

$$dn(i) = \frac{d(i)}{max[d(i)]} \tag{11}$$

where n: is the number of points (pixels) of the region boundary (the perimeter of region).

$$Xg = \frac{\sum_N X}{N} \tag{12}$$

$$Yg = \frac{\sum_N Y}{N} \tag{13}$$

where N: is the number of points (pixels) in the region area.

$$dmoy = \frac{1}{n}\sum_N dn(i) \tag{14}$$

The features extracted in the RDM are cited below. We will only give the expressions of the RDM features related to this work.

- The Standard Deviation of the Normalized Radial Distance Measure (SDEV) is defined as the variance of the distances around the ray (the average distance dmoy previously defined) of a circle. This characteristic gives a good quality of information concerning the irregularity of contour. Indeed, when it is about a malignant tumour, the value of SDEV tends to move towards 0.5, and when it is in the case of benign tumour, the SDEV tends to move towards 0.

$$SDEV = \sqrt{\frac{1}{N}\sum_N (dn(i) - dmoy)^2} \tag{15}$$

- Rugosity (R): treats angular contours (contours which contain concave segments). It is given by the following equation:

$$R = \frac{1}{N}\sum_N \|dn(i) - dn(i+1)\| \tag{16}$$

- Area ratio (Ar): this characteristic differentiates between stellar contours and smooth contours. It is illustrated in the following equation:

$$Ar = \frac{1}{N * dmoy} * \sum_N (dn(i) - dmoy) \tag{17}$$

where Ar=0, if(dn(i)$\leq dmoy$)

In practice, the computation of these features increases the complexity of calculation. To deal with the problem of complexity, we propose to calculate the features only in the concave and convex points. The RDM is a method that can differentiate between the malignant and benign cases, but, it can cause noise in the computation of each point of boundary. Furthermore, it can also cause a long-time calculation. To solve the problem of noise and computing time, one can improve the method of RDM. This can be done by implementing the idea of the eXtended Radial Distance Measure (for more details see (Boujelben et al., 2009a)). In fact, the eXtended RDM "XRDM" is adopted. So, to solve the problem of complexity, we propose to calculate the features only in the local concave and convex points as in Figure 5. These points are defined as follows:

- The concave point (Pconcave (i)) of the contour is a point which have a radial distance d(i) lower than the radial distance d(i-1) and the radial distance d(i+1).

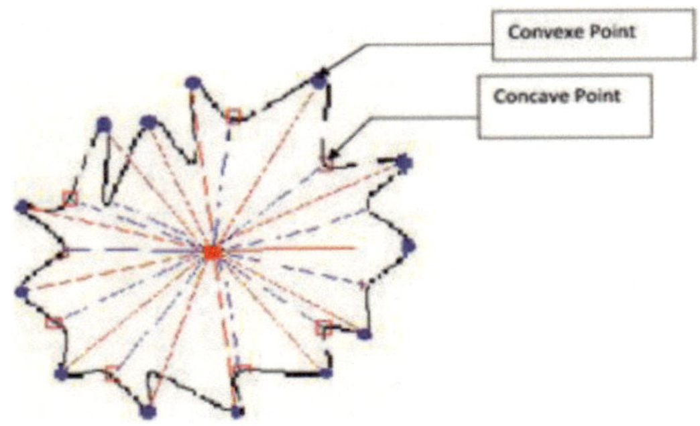

Fig. 5. Illustrative figure of eXtended RDM

- The convex point (Pconvexe (i)) of the contour is a point whose radial distance d(i) is higher than the radial distance d(i-1) and the radial distance d(i+1).

More formally:
Pconcave (i) = (i; $d(i) \leq d(i-1)$ et $d(i) \leq d(i+1)$)
Pconvexe (i) = (i; $d(i) \geq d(i-1)$ et $d(i) \geq d(i+1)$)

In the speculated region, the feature like turning angle cannot be applied because of the problem of segment tangents (Figure 5). However, RDM and XRDM can be used with regions that have an elliptic shape. In fact the major problem is when there is a speculated region.

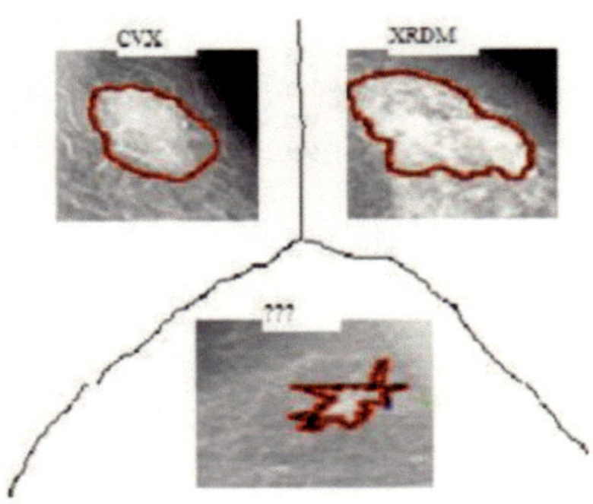

Fig. 6. Problem space convergence in malignant boundary

To solve this problem, we introduce a new angular characteristic named Index Angle (IA).

- The IA is the ratio of all the internal angles by external ones: the external angle is the angle between central convex points (Convex point pi) and their "next-least" convexes points (Convex point pi-1, p+1). In fact, the internal angle is the angle between a central convex point and its "next-least" concave points (Figure 7). The IA is applied to make a distinction between the edge shapes of the mass as being speculated or as being round. When the mass tends to be round, its IA tends to be near the 1. In opposition, a mass with speculated edge will have an IA smaller than 0.5. Then, the IA can be calculated as follows:

$$IA = \frac{\sum_i \phi(i)}{\sum_i \theta(i)} \tag{18}$$

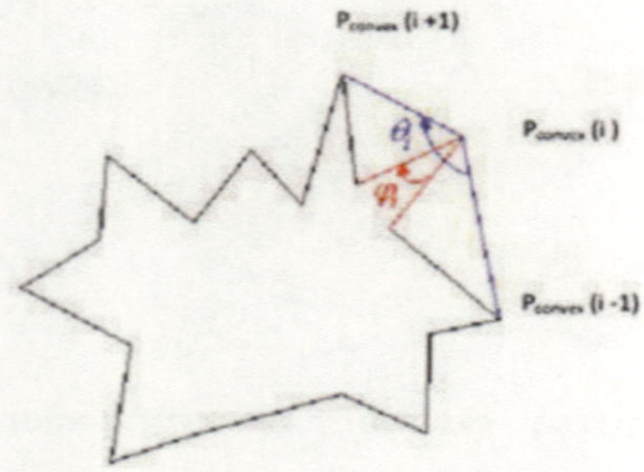

Fig. 7. An example of Index Angle computation

So, the IA is used only in the concave and convex points and not to any other points. Our objective is to minimize the temporal complexity differently from the radial angle used in (Rangayyan et al., 2006). Added to that, the advantage of this characteristic is that it is standardized and invariant with any affine transformation. In this subsection, we discussed boundary information of opacity (boundary vector) composing on CVX, XRDM and IA, in the next subsection, we will put our interest on the region criteria.

5.2 Region descriptor

We use Region Features to describe the mammographic masses through features extracted region. For this reason, we illustrate a method based on Circularity (C), Internal/External Circle (IEC) and Normalized Residual Value (NRV)

- Circularity (C): it describes the areas that can be circular. It can be useful in this direction and can give an indication of the regularity of a given mammogram mass. This feature is given by the following equation:

$$C = \frac{4 * Pi * Aire}{Perimeter * Perimeter} \tag{19}$$

where: P is the perimeter and A is the area of the segmented mass.

- Internal External Circle (IEC): This feature can be used to measure the shape elongation used by Chettaoui et *al.* (Chettaoui et al., 2005). In our work, we exploit this feature to describe mass region. The IEC feature is given by the following equation:

$$IEC = \frac{Inf - Radius}{Sup - Radius} \tag{20}$$

where: Sup-Radius represents the largest internal circle and Inf-Radius represents the smallest external circle(Figure 8).

For a round mass, the value of IEC is close to 1 since the value of Inf-Radius is very close to the value of Sup-Radius, whereas for a lengthened mass the value of IEC becomes close to 0 since the value of Inf-Radius is far from the value of Sup-Radius.

The advantage of this characteristic is that it is invariant with affine transformation and it is adequate to our work. In fact, its calculation is slow, since for each form, we should pass through all the points to determine the circle inscribed in the object which contains this point.

- Normalized Residual Value (NRV): This feature is extracted from the convex-hull by using the residual region. NRV gives best performances compared to the characteristics that can

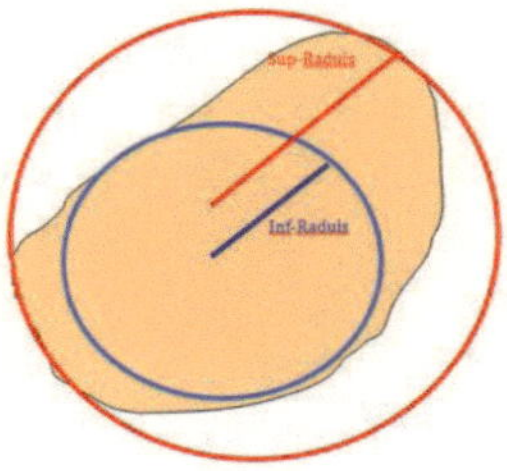

Fig. 8. Illustrative figure of internal/external circle computation

be extracted from the convex-hull, and can be useful in the distinction between the regular and irregular area. It is given by the following equation:

$$NRV = \frac{Aire(Resudial - Region)}{Perimeter(Convex - Envelop)} \tag{21}$$

where: Perimeter is the perimeter of the convex-hull and Aire is the area of the residual region(Figure 9).

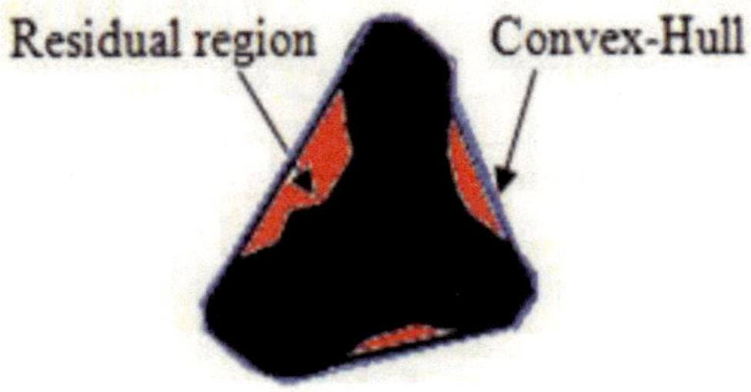

Fig. 9. Example of breast tumour and its respective Convex-Hull

In the two last subsections, we focused on shape features which are boundary and region. In the next subsection we will put emphasis on texture criteria.

5.3 Texture descriptor

The density (Figure 10) of breast region is an important property in ROI. To determine this quality, we adopt the texture method. In approach to texture feature extraction, which is frequently cited in the literature, is based on the use of CGLM. Co-occurrence matrix is a second-order statistical measure of image variation. In this subsection, we detail the feature of co-occurrence approach.

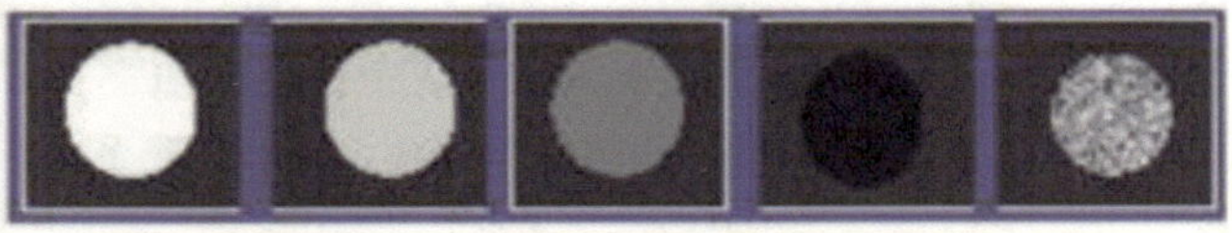

Fig. 10. The density of ROI opacity

We represent our analysis by texture statistical. From this approach, we extract six characteristics which are defined as follows:

$$mean = \frac{1}{N^2} \sum_x \sum_y p(x,y) \tag{22}$$

where: p(x,y) denotes the gray-level in the co-occurrences matrix.

N: denote the width and the height of co-occurrences matrix. In order to reduce calcul of co-occurrence characteristics we adopted the original matrix of region, where Gray Level value are between 0 and maximum of Gray Level value, to adopt a region with size 32X32(i.e. Gray Level value between 0 and 31)

$$Variance = \sum_x \sum_y (x - moy)^2 p(x,y) \tag{23}$$

$$Energy = \sum_x \sum_y p(x,y)^2 \tag{24}$$

$$Contrast = \sum_x \sum_y (x - y)^2 p(x,y) \tag{25}$$

$$Entropy = -\sum_x \sum_y p(x,y) \log p(x,y) \tag{26}$$

$$Homogenety = \sum_x \sum_y \frac{1}{1 + (x - y)^2} p(x,y) \tag{27}$$

The algorithm evaluates the properties of the region of the mammographic image. We investigate the performance of feature in texture from GLCM in diagnosis by using four orientations 0, 45, 90, 135. From each one, we inspect six features (then we take the average of one feature of the four orientations). In the next section, we will show the performance of the textural and shape vector in analyzing ROI in terms of diagnosis relevance by using kNN and MLP classifier.

6. Results and discussion

The terminology which is used to determine the performance of a CADi System is defined as follows:

- Sensitivity: percentage of pathological ROIs which is correctly classified.
- Specificity: percentage of non-pathological ROIs which is correctly classified.
- Accuracy: percentage of correctly classified pathological and non-pathological cases.

Because of the variation in the types of breast cancer, a large number of cases can reduce the dependency of analysis techniques versus image sets. The performance of an algorithm is affected by the characteristics of a database like the digitization techniques which are namely pixel size, subtlety of cases, choice of training/testing subsets, etc.

6.1 The DDSM dataset

The establishment of the DDSM allows the possibility of the common training and testing Dataset. The DDSM is the largest publicly available database of mammographic data. It contains approximately 2620 screening mammography cases. From the total number of mammographic images included in the DDSM database, we use 200 malignant images and 200 benign ones. To make a good evaluation, we use the remaining 400 images which are divided into 200 ground malignant regions together with 200 entirely benign ones. To classify the area segmented with Level Set Approach using DDSM dataset with vector illustrated in the least section, one will use two classifiers which are kNN (K=7) and MLP. In the next subsection, we illustrate the results of sensibility and specificity adopted with an analysis method.

6.2 Experimental results: Performance in terms of diagnosis quality

The basic classification is based on two methods of classification KNN (K=7) and MLP as shown in Table 1, Table 2 and Table 3. It represents the results from different analysis in boundary, region and texture vector respectively.

classifier	Kppv	MLP
Sensitivity	87 %	92%
Specificity	88%	90%
Exactitude	88%	91%

Table 1. Results from analysis based on boundary description vector

classifier	Kppv	MLP
Sensitivity	92%	89%
Specificity	89%	90%
Exactitude	90%	89%

Table 2. Results from analysis based on region description vector

classifier	Kppv	MLP
Sensitivity	93%	90%
Specificity	87%	87%
Exactitude	89%	89%

Table 3. Results from analysis based on texture description vector

The sensitivity result varies between 87% in boundary vector and 93% in texture feature using KNN (K=7) classifier. But the result of specificity varies between 87% using KNN classifier in texture vector and 90% in both MLP classifier region and boundary classifier. These results seem to be variable because of a variation of result: 6% in pertaining to sensibility and 3% relating to specificity. In fact, breast tumour sometimes depends on the region, or/and contour or/and texture criteria. To solve this problem, we propose to combine features vectors. The results are shown on Table 4, Table 5 and Table 6.

classifier	Kppv	MLP
Sensitivity	90%	89%
Specificity	86%	89%
Exactitude	88%	89%

Table 4. Results from the analysis based on shape (boundary and region) description vector

classifier	Kppv	MLP
Sensitivity	92%	87%
Specificity	92%	88%
Exactitude	92%	88%

Table 5. Results from analysis based on boundary-texture description vector

classifier	Kppv	MLP
Sensitivity	89%	89%
Specificity	93%	93%
Exactitude	91%	91%

Table 6. Results from the analysis based on region-texture description vector

Table 4, Table 5 and Table 6 show the results of combination of region/boundary features, region/texture feature and boundary/texture feature, respectively. Table 4 illustrates the importance of shape information in this analysis. The result in terms of sensitivity tends to move towards 90% in KNN classifier. The result in terms of specificity tends to move towards 89% using MLP classifier. So, we can assume that shape vector is a good feature in differentiating the benign from the malignant mass. In boundary texture-combination, we find a good result in terms of sensibility and specificity by using KNN classifier differently from MLP classifier. Table 6 shows the result of features region-texture. In this approach we can assume good specificity using both MLP and KNN classifiers differently from sensibility. So, the majority of classifications that are obtained are favourable, but, the problem is in the stability of result in terms of sensibility, specificity and accuracy. This is conducted by the combination of all features in Table 7. However, all result are about 90% of sensibility, specificity and accuracy. This result seems to be logical: ROIs in mammographic image depends on taking account of region, boundary and texture properties.

classifier	Kppv	MLP
Sensitivity	90%	89%
Specificity	90%	90%
Exactitude	90%	89%

Table 7. Results from the analysis based on texture-shape description vector

These results are not the best result compared to local works (Boujelben et al., 2009a) (Boujelben et al., 2009b). However, in (Boujelben et al., 2009b) the result is about 94% in boundary information; and in (Boujelben et al., 2009a) the result is between 90% and 92% using XRDM method. In such work, we used DDSM database but the ROI is selected from the image by fixing a rectangular box around the suspicious lesion area and the classical method of segmentation based on Sobel filter and thresholding. But, in this approach, we note the stability of result which is an important quality in analysis of medical imaging. Comparing these results with other related work, we notice important ameliorations. In fact, Alvarenga et *al.* (Alvarenga et al., 2006) obtained 88% of sensitivity and 90% of specificity. In their experiments, they used a local images dataset and LDA (Linear Discriminant Analysis) method for classification. Additionally, Rangayyan et *al.*(Rangayyan et al., 1997) have used the LDA classifier and their result reaches 95% in terms of classification accuracy. Conversely, the result of Retico et *al.*(Retico et al., 2007) using a MLP classifier can reach 78.1% and 79.1% in sensitivity and specificity, respectively. Using a SVM classifier, Chang et *al.* (Chang et al., 2005) obtained 88.89% and 92.5% in terms of sensitivity and specificity, respectively. Yet, the characterization of mammographic masses and tumours and their classification as being benign or malignant is difficult. In spite of acceptable results found by our proposed features, we should not make an assumption that it is the best or the worst because we did not use the same Database. In fact, the digitization can reflect the final result. However, we can assume that by combining feature vector based on shape/texture, we attempt to have good stability of results in differentiating between the benign and the malignant masses.

7. Conclusion

In this work, we attempted to improve the classification performance of shape and texture in analyzing ROI in case of mammographic images. We introduced the adaptation of Level Set approach to detect ROI by combining edge and region criteria. We also presented cooperation of features to have stability of results because the ROI depends on both shape and texture properties. The results in terms of sensitivity and specificity tend to reach 90%. The results have been validated via two algorithms of classification: kNN (K=7) and MLP. These results seem to be sufficient and an automatic method of detection based on a Level Set Approach can ameliorate the CADi system to have a CADe one.

8. References

Ahirwar, A. & Jadon, R. (2011). Characterization of tumor region using som and neuro fuzzy techniques in digital mammography, *International Journal of Computer Science and Information Technology* 3(1): 199–211.

Alvarenga, A., Fernando, A. & Albuquerque, C. W. C. (2006). Assessing the performance of the normalised radial length and convex polygons in distinguishing breast tumours on ultrasound images, *Pereira Revista Brasileira de Engenharia Biomédica* 22: 181–189.

Arodz, T., Kurdziel, M., Popiela, T. J., Sevre, E. & Yuen, D. (2006). Detection of clustered microcalcifications in small field digital mammography, *computer methods and programs in biomedicine* 81: 56–65.

Ball, J. & Bruce, L. (2007). Digital mammogram spiculated mass detection and spicule segmentation using level set, *Conference of the IEEE EMBS* pp. 23–26.

Boucher, A., Jouve, P., F.Cloppet & Vincent, N. (2009). Pectoral muscle segmentation on a mammogram, *ORASIS* .

Boujelben, A., Chaabani, A., Tmar, H. & Abid, M. (2009a). An approach based on rdm for analysis in breast cancer detection, *International Conference on Applied Informatics*, Bordj Bou Arerig Algeria.

Boujelben, A., Chaabani, A., Tmar, H. & Abid, M. (2009b). Feature extraction from contours shape for tumor analyzing in mammographic, *IEEE Digital Image Computing: Techniques and Applications*, Melbourne, pp. 395–399.

Boujelben, A., Tmar, H., Mnif, J. & Abid, M. (2011). Automatic application level set approach in detection calcifications in mammographic image, *International Journal of Computer Science and Information Technology* 3(4): 1–14.

Brox, T., Rousson, M., Deriche, R. & Weickert, J. (2009). Colour, texture, and motion in level set based segmentation and tracking, *Image and Vision Computing: Elsevier* .

Casselles, V., Kimmel, R. & Sapiro, G. (1997). Geodesic active contours, *International Journal of Computer Vision* (22): 61Ű79.

Catanzariti, E., Ciminello, M. & Prevete, R. (2003). Computer aided detection of clustered microcalcifications in digitized mammograms using gabor functions, *IEEE Image Analysis and Processing* pp. 266–270.

Chang, R., W.Wu, Moon, W. & D.R.Chen (2005). Automatic ultrasound segmentation and morphology based diagnosis of solid breast tumors, *Springer* 89: 179–185.

Chettaoui, C., Djamel, K., Djouak, A. & Maaref, H. (2005). Etude de formes des globules drépanocytaires par traitement numérique des images, *International Conferance SETIT Tunisia* .

Delogu, P., Fantacci, M., Kasae, P. & Retico, A. (2008). Characterization of mammographic masses using a gradient-based segmentation algorithm and a neural classifier, *Computer Biologie Medecal* .

Denise, G., Rangayyan, R., Carvalho, D. & Santiago, S. (2008). Polygonal modeling of contours of breast tumors with the preservation of spicules, *IEEE Transations In Biomedical Engineering* 55.

Dheeba, J. & Wiselin, G. (2010). Detection of microcalcification clusters in mammograms using neural network, *International Journal of Advanced Science and Technology* 19.

Ferrari, R., Frere, A., R.M.Rangayyan, desautels, J. & Borges, R. (2004). Identification of the breast boundary in mammograms using active contour models, *Medical Biological Engineering and Computing* 42.

Jadhav, R. & Thorat, R. (2009). Computer aided breast cancer analysis and detection using statistical features and neural networks, *International Conference on Advances in Computing, Communication and Control* (23-24): 283–290.

Kass, M., Witkin, A. & Terzopoulos., D. (1988). Snakes: Active contour models, *International Journal of Computer Vision*, 1: 321–332.

Lambrou, T., Linney, A. D., Speller, R. D. & Todd-Pokropek, A. (2002). Statistical classification of digital mammograms using features from the spatial and wavelet domains, *Medical Image Understanding and Analysis* 3.

Liu, S. & Delp, E. (1997). Multiresolution detection of stellate lesions in mammograms, *IEEE International Conference on Image Processing* pp. 109–112.

Maglogiannis, I., Zafiropoulos, E. & Anagnostopoulos, I. (2007). An intelligent system for automated breast cancer diagnosis and prognosis using svm based classifiers, *Springer Science Business* .

Marti, J., Freixenet, J., Munoz, X. & Arnau, A. (2003). Active region segmentation of mammographic masses based on texture contour and shape features, *A Pattern Recognition and Image Analysis Springer* 2652: 478–485.

Masala, G., Tangaro, S., Golosio, B., Oliva, P., Stumbo, S., Bellotti, R., Carlo, F. D., Gargano, G., Cascio, D., Fauci, F., Magro, R., Raso, G., Bottigli, U., Chincarini, A., Mitri, I. D., Nunzio, G. D., Gori, I., Retico, A., Cerello, P., Cheran, S. C., Fulcheri, C. & Torres, E. L. (2007). Comparative study of feature classification methods for mass lesion recognition in digitized mammograms, *Maggio-Giugno nuovo cimento* 30(3).

Nandi, R., Nandi, A., Rangayyan, R. & Scutt, D. (2006). Classification of breast masses in mammograms using genetic programming and feature selection, *International Federation for Medical and Biological Engineering* .

Nguyen, T. & Rangayyan, R. (2005). Fractal analysis of contours of mammographic masses, *International Conference on Biomedical Engineering Innsbruck Austria* pp. 186–191.

Nguyen, T. & Rangayyan, R. (2006). Shape analysis of breast masses in mammograms via the fractal dimension, *In Proceedings of the 27th Annual International Conference of the IEEE Engineering in Medicine and Biology Society Shanghai China* pp. 3210–3213.

Nishikawa, R. (2007). Current status and future directions of computer-aided diagnosis in mammography, *Computerized Medical Imaging and Graphics* 31: 224–235.

Oliver, A., Llado, X., Marti, R., Freixenet, J. & Zwiggelaar, R. (2007). Classifying mammograms using texture information, *Medical Image Understanding and Analysis*, Aberystwyth and Wales and UK, pp. 223–227.

Osher, S. & Fedkiw, R. (2002). Level set methods and dynamic implicit surfaces, *Springer-Verlag New York, Applied Mathematical Sciences* .

Rangayyan, R., Ayres, F. & Desautels, J. (2007). A review of computer-aided diagnosis of breast cancer: Toward the detection of subtle signs, *Journal of the Franklin Institute* 344(3-4): 312–348.

Rangayyan, R., Faramawy, N., Desautels, J. & Alim, O. (1997). Measures of acutance and shape for classification of breast tumors, *IEEE Transactions on Medical Imaging* 16: 799–810.

Rangayyan, R., Guliato, D., Carvalho, J. & Santiago, S. (2006). Feature extraction from the turning angle function for the classification of contours of breast tumors, *IEEE-The International Special Topics Conference on Information Technology in Biomedicine* pp. 1–6.

Reston, V. (1998). Illustrated breast imaging reporting and data system (bi-radstm), *American College of Radiology* 3.

Retico, A., Delogu, P., Fantacci, M. & Kasae, P. (2007). An automatic system to discriminate malignant from benign massive lesions on mammograms, *Medical Physics* 14: 596–600.

Schiabel, H., Santos, V. & Angel, M. (2008). Segmentation technique for detecting suspect masses in dense breast digitized images as a tool for mammography cad schemes, *ACM Special Interest Group on Applied Computing* 20(16): 1333–1337.

Sethian, J. (1998). Adaptive fast marching and level set methods for propagating interfaces, *Cambridge Univ Press* pp. 3–15.

Siddiqui, M., Anand, M., mehrotra, P., Sarangi, R. & Muthur, N. (2005). Biomonitoring of organochlorines in women with benign an malignant breast disease, *Technical report*, 250-257, Environmental Research.

Thangavel, K. & Karnan, M. (2005). Computer aided diagnosis in digital mammograms: Detection of micro-calcifications by meta heuristic algorithms, *GVIP Journal* 7(5): 41–55.

Torrent, A., Oliver, A., Freixenet, J., Boada, I., Feixes, M., Marti, R., Llado, X., Pont, J., Perez, E., Pedraza, S., Marti, J., & Krupinski, E. (2008). Breast density segmenattion: A comparaison of clustering and region based techniques, *Springer-Verlag Berlin Heidelberg IWDM* pp. 9–16.

Wiesmiller, S. & Chandy, D. A. (2010). Content based mammogram retrieval using gray level aura matrix, *International Joint Journal Conference on Engineering and Technology* pp. 217–221.

Yang, S. C., Wang, C., Chung, Y., Hsu, G., Lee, S., Chung, P. & Chang, C. (2005). A computer-aided system for mass detection and classification in digitized mammograms, *In Biomed Eng Appl Basis Comm* pp. 215–228.

Zadeh, H., Radc, F. & Nejad, S. (2001). Shape-based and texture-based feature extraction for classification of microcalcification in mammograms, *Medical Imaging: Image Processing* pp. 301–310.

Zadeh, H., Radc, F. & S.P.Nejad (2004). Comparison of multiwavelet, wavelet, haralick, and shape features for micro-calcification classification in mammograms, *Pattern Recognition* pp. 1973–1986.

Zwiggelaar, R. & .R.Denton, E. (2004). Optimal segmentation of mammographic images, *International Workshop on Digital Mammography*, Norwich, UK.

6

Testosterone for the Treatment of Mammary and Prostate Cancers: Historical Perspectives and New Directions

Moshe Rogosnitzky and Rachel Danks
MedInsight Research Institute
Israel

1. Introduction

After lung cancer, breast cancer and prostate cancer are the two most common forms of cancer. Approximately 209,060 women were thought to have been diagnosed with breast cancer in the US in 2010, and 217,730 men with prostate cancer (National Cancer Institute, 2007). Furthermore, a total of 39,840 women and 32,050 men were expected to have died of breast or prostate cancer during this year (National Cancer Institute, 2007).

It has been known for some time that the sex hormones, estrogen and testosterone, play a major role in the etiology of breast and prostate cancer (Bonkhoff & Berges, 2009; Carruba, 2007; Dimitrakakis & Bondy, 2009; Folkerd & Dowsett, 2010; Ho, 2004; Mcleod, 2003; Meyer, 1955; Suzuki et al., 2010). However, determining their precise impact in these cancers has proved controversial, and theories of their involvement have been repeatedly revised with the emergence of new scientific evidence (Drewa & Chlosta, 2010; Jensen et al., 2010; Margo & Winn, 2006; Morgentaler, 2006). Because causation has often been assumed where in fact mere association exists, ineffective treatment strategies have frequently been adopted while potentially successful avenues have been neglected.

A key insight that was missing for many years was that testosterone and estrogen can be considered as two sides of a see-saw. In other words, manipulation of one has a direct effect upon the other (Ellem & Risbridger, 2010). This connection was realized with the discovery of aromatization (Santen et al., 2009), but unfortunately did not lead to the necessary re-examination of previous findings in the treatment of hormone-related cancers.

Despite enormous clinical and research efforts, hormonal treatments for advanced breast cancer and prostate cancer have not resulted in significant prolongation of survival over the last few decades. A comprehensive reassessment of prevailing hormonal treatment strategies and the scientific logic behind them is therefore long overdue.

The following chapter examines the role of testosterone and estrogen in breast and prostate cancer from an historical perspective, and suggests that a revised approach of combined therapies targeting multiple pathways in the hormonal cascade is required in order to lead to the meaningful hormonal manipulation of these cancers.

2. Estrogen and testosterone: a biological balancing act

Although people have been aware of the sex hormones since ancient times (Freeman et al., 2001), estrogen and testosterone were only isolated and fully characterized in the 1920s and

1930s. The structure of estrogen was the first to be determined when Adolf Butenandt and Edward Adelbert Doisy independently identified the chemical configuration in 1929 (Tata, 2005). Isolation of testosterone quickly followed in 1935 (David et al., 1935), and this was characterized and named once again by Butenandt (Butenandt & Hanisch, 1935).
New organic synthetic methods emerging during and after the 1930s created ready access to testosterone and estrogen and their derivatives, allowing a period of prolific research into the sex hormones in what has been termed 'The Golden Age of Steroid Chemistry' from the 1930s until the 1950s (Schwarz et al., 1999).
The studies conducted during this time began to reveal similarities between the androgens and estrogens, and it was speculated that it might be possible to convert the C19 androgens directly into C18 estrogens (Santen et al., 2009). Indeed, in 1934, the German-Jewish gynecologist Bernhard Zondek demonstrated remarkable early insight when he stated, '*the female hormone which is regularly present in the male organism represents a normal physiological product of the metabolism of the sex hormones, especially since – due to our present chemical knowledge – a conversion of the male hormone into the female one appears to be quite possible*' (Zondek et al., 1934). This speculation was further supported when the Austrian endocrinology pioneer Steinach and his colleague Kun showed enhanced estrogenic activity in the urine of men administered testosterone propionate (Steinach & Kun, 1937).
The crucial biochemical step in the conversion of testosterone to estradiol, the major estrogen present in humans, is the formation of an aromatic ring from the only unsaturated ring of testosterone (ring 'A', Figure 1). This process is known as 'aromatization'.

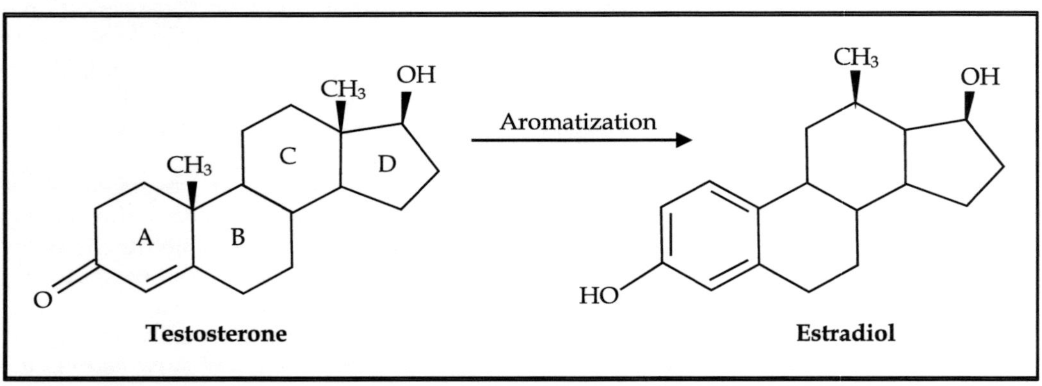

Fig. 1. Aromatization of testosterone to estradiol.

In 1955, a Swiss chemist named Meyer achieved this aromatization using bovine adrenal extracts (Meyer, 1955; Meyer et al., 1955). He recognized that this transformation was likely to be enzyme catalyzed, but the specific enzyme involved was not purified until the 1980s. The enzyme responsible for the aromatization of testosterone was ultimately found to be a member of the P450 cytochrome family of enzymes, and was named aromatase. Eventually, the full mechanism for the conversion of testosterone to estradiol was established (Figure 2).

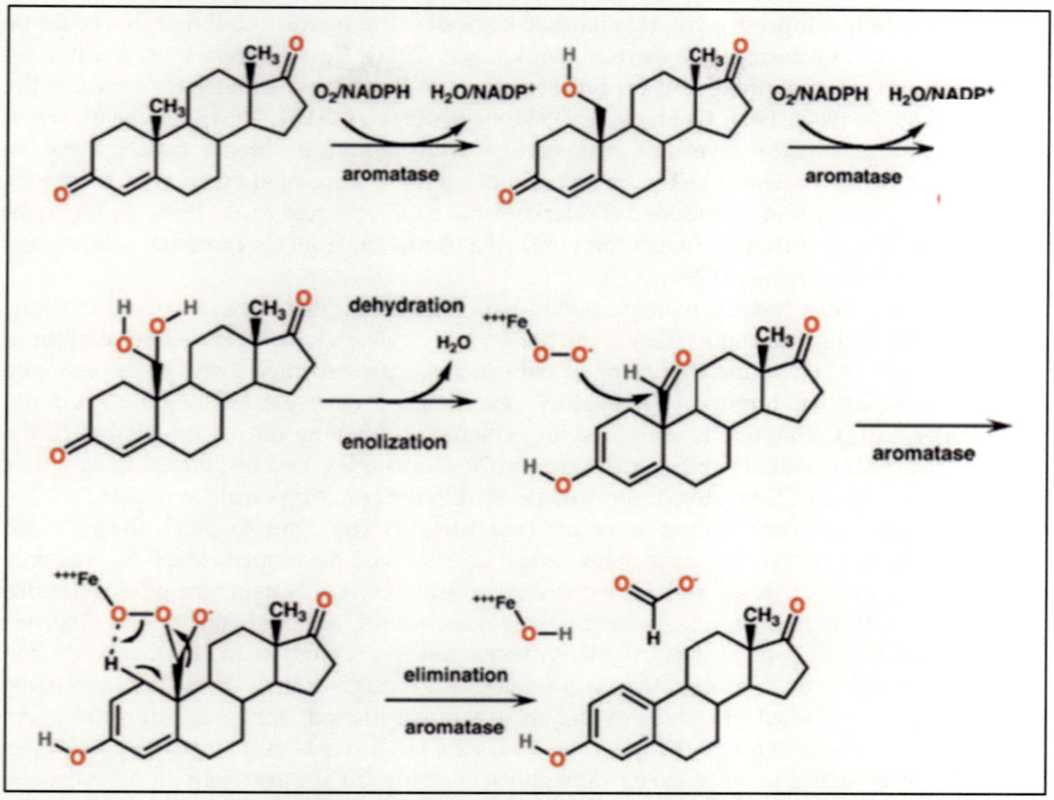

Fig. 2. Mechanism of action of aromatase in the conversion of testosterone to estradiol.

3. Hormonal manipulation in breast and prostate cancer: the controversy begins

3.1 Breast cancer

The first link between estrogen and breast cancer was observed in the late 1890s by a Scottish surgeon by the name of George Beatson (Mukherjee, 2011). Beatson had noticed that removal of the ovaries altered the capacity of cows to lactate, establishing for the first time a connection between breast and ovary. From this, he made the leap to speculate that removal of the ovaries in women with breast cancer may prove therapeutic. He successfully demonstrated the benefit of this intervention in a small group of his breast cancer patients when the tumors of three of his patients shrank dramatically following ovary removal (Beatson, 1896). Butenandt and Doisy's discovery of estrogen was still decades away and Beatson had no understanding of any mechanism for this effect. However, Beatson was convinced he had found a route to control breast cancer. When Beatson's experiments were repeated by others, around two thirds of breast cancer patients were found to benefit (Mukherjee, 2011). This was an important observation, the relevance of which would not become apparent for many years.

Despite its apparent success, removal of the ovaries was not considered a practical or viable treatment for breast cancer as it caused many side effects, including osteoporosis. The alternative was to suppress estrogen pharmacologically, and it was found that this could be achieved by administering testosterone (Mukherjee, 2011). Testosterone soon became an important and effective treatment for breast cancer, and was used extensively between the 1930s and 1960s (Fels, 1944; Goldenberg, 1964; Segaloff et al., 1951, 1964). However, when raised blood and urine levels of testosterone were found in breast cancer patients, testosterone was assumed to be the cause and not a simple associated factor, and successful testosterone therapy was abandoned (Malarkey et al., 1977; Secreto et al., 1983). Subsequent discovery of the confusion between total and free testosterone levels came too late redress the error (Vitola & Zeĭkate, 1976).

In 1968, an American chemist named Elwood Jensen made an important discovery when he identified the estrogen receptor (ER) in the breast, and began to look for the same receptor in breast cancer cells. He found that some breast cancers expressed high levels of the estrogen receptor (ER-positive tumors), while others expressed low levels (ER-negative tumors) (Mukherjee, 2011). This finally provided an explanation for why only a proportion of the early breast cancer patients investigated around 70 years earlier had responded to complete ovary removal. Only ER-positive tumors responded to the resulting estrogen deprivation.

Following this discovery, efforts were directed towards strategies to block the estrogen receptor in breast cancer. The first nonsteroidal antiestrogen developed, MER-25, was only weakly active in large doses and caused severe central nervous system side effects (Gajdos & Jordan, 2002). However, an alternative was soon found, although through an indirect route. Tamoxifen (Figure 3) was originally developed in an attempt to create an estrogen stimulator which would be effective as a female contraceptive drug. However, tamoxifen was very quickly shown to induce ovulation in women instead, acting as a fertility agent rather than a contraceptive (Klopper & Hall, 1971). Instead of stimulating estrogen, tamoxifen was acting as an estrogen antagonist, turning off the estrogen signal in many tissues. As an estrogen antagonist was thought to have no possible clinical benefit, clinical development of tamoxifen was very nearly abandoned.

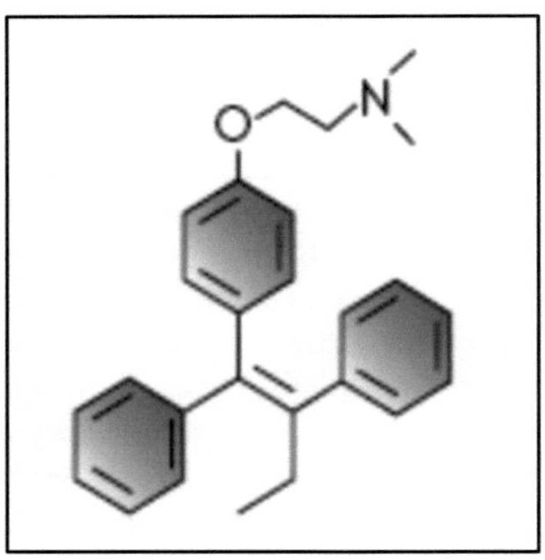

Fig. 3. Chemical structure of tamoxifen.

However, one chemist at ICI where tamoxifen had first been synthesized saw a possible connection between fertility drugs and cancer. Arthur Walpole had been intimately involved in the development of tamoxifen and knew of previous experiments of the sex hormones in prostate and breast cancer. Walpole wondered whether an estrogen antagonist could have a role in ER-positive breast cancer (Furr & Jordan, 1984). Unlike MER-25, tamoxifen is a selective estrogen receptor modulator (SERM), which means it is a partial antagonist effective in only a number of sites, and has relatively low toxicity (Cole et al., 1971; Furr & Jordan, 1984). Tamoxifen therefore appeared to have the attributes of a potential chemotherapeutic candidate for breast cancer.

In collaboration with an oncologist from Manchester, a clinical trial of tamoxifen in 46 women with breast cancer was quickly designed. The results were astonishing. An almost immediate response was observed in ten patients in the trial, with tumors visibly shrinking in the breast, reductions in lung metastases, and a dramatic reduction in bone pain.

Tamoxifen was quickly discovered to improve survival of ER-positive breast cancer patients (Early Breast Cancer Trialists' Collaborative Group, 1998) and soon became a standard adjunctive therapy (Lerner & Jordan, 1990). Tamoxifen held the dominant position for treatment of ER-positive breast cancer for nearly three decades, although numerous other SERMs were also developed (Gajdos & Jordan, 2002). The reduction in the number of deaths from breast cancer in the Western world over recent decades can largely be attributed to tamoxifen therapy (Gajdos & Jordan, 2002; Gradishar, 2010; Hackshaw et al., 2011).

For many years, tamoxifen was considered to act exclusively through its anti-estrogen activity. However, recent evidence has emerged to suggest that its benefit in breast cancer may be due to the up-regulation of androgen receptors (Labrie et al., 2003; Somboonporn & Davis, 2004; Wierman et al., 2006; Zhou et al., 2000). Thus tamoxifen therapy represents an indirect return to the testosterone therapy which was abandoned during the 1950s.

To complete the circle, a review of studies of androgen therapy has recently suggested testosterone itself has a protective effect against breast cancer (Dimitrakakis & Bondy, 2009), while the role of estrogen in the development of breast cancer is now firmly established (Ekmektzoglou et al., 2009; Rana et al., 2010; Sonne-Hansen & Lykkesfeldt, 2005; Thijssen & Blankenstein, 1989).

3.2 Prostate cancer

Just as female hormones were known to control the growth of breast tissue, so it was speculated around the same time that the androgens were responsible for the control of prostate growth. In the 1920s and 1930s, experiments conducted by the urologist Charles Huggins working at the University of Chicago showed that surgical removal of dog testicles led to a dramatic reduction in prostate size, an effect that could be ameliorated by injecting purified exogenous testosterone (Mukherjee, 2011). Soon, Huggins and his colleague, Hodges, published a paper reporting that reducing testosterone levels through castration or estrogen therapy achieved regression of metastatic prostate cancer, while administration of exogenous testosterone resulted in growth of prostate cancer (Huggins & Hodges, 1941). This paper marked the beginning of the long association of testosterone with increased prostate cancer risk and progression, establishing the enduring perception of testosterone as 'food for a hungry cancer' (Morgentaler, 2006). From this time onwards, the presence of prostate cancer, or any prior history of prostate cancer, became an absolute contraindication for use of testosterone therapy.

In an attempt to achieve medical, rather than surgical, castration, estrogens began to be routinely administered to prostate cancer patients in an attempt to halt the production of testosterone. The first results with diethylstilbestrol (DES), a xenoestrogen, appeared extremely encouraging. Patients with aggressive prostate cancer treated with estrogen derivatives responded rapidly and markedly (Mukherjee, 2011).

Estrogen therapy was soon hailed as the salvation for prostate cancer. The reduced side effects achieved were considered particularly important as the current pharmaceutical model of cancer management involved increasingly aggressive cytotoxic drugs which took patients to the very limits of their tolerance. Although patients frequently relapsed, remission could often be achieved for several months. It seemed that prostate cancer would finally be beaten by hormonal manipulation through estrogen therapy.

Over time, new methods for restricting testosterone levels became common place, notably novel phytoestrogens (Castle & Thrasher, 2002; Morrissey & Watson, 2003) and synthetic estrogens (Kim et al., 2002). Yet decades of estrogen-based therapies and testosterone deprivation have failed to make a significant impact on survival and have resulted in significant toxicities.

Despite numerous studies investigating the proposed link between testosterone and prostate cancer, no direct correlation has in fact been found (Jannini et al., 2011; Morgentaler, 2006). Equally, low testosterone levels have not conclusively been linked with the absence of prostate cancer (Jannini et al., 2011; Morgentaler, 2006). For example, prostate biopsies in a study of hypogonadal men revealed prostate cancer in 14.3% of men (Morgentaler et al., 1996), comparable with the 15.2% found in the placebo arm of the Prostate Cancer Prevention Trial (Thompson et al., 2004). Of even greater concern, neither prostate specific antigen (PSA), prostate volume, nor cancer progression has been found to increase with increasing testosterone levels in men with untreated prostate cancer (Morgentaler et al., 2011). Interestingly, evidence is even emerging to show that patients with a lower serum testosterone level may have a higher risk of prostate cancer than patients with high serum testosterone (Shin et al., 2010).

Recent scrutiny of the seminal work conducted by Huggins and Hodges has revealed some fundamental flaws and methodological failings (Morgentaler, 2006). Perhaps the most damning criticism of the causative link between testosterone and prostate cancer comes from the observation that prostate cancer rates are lowest during the late teens and early 20s when testosterone levels are highest, and highest in old age when testosterone levels are at their lowest (Figure 4). If testosterone truly was a cause of prostate cancer, the reverse relationship would be expected.

Not only does it appear that testosterone should be exonerated from its role in causing prostate cancer, but evidence is emerging to suggest that it may actually be beneficial in managing the condition (Gardiner et al., 2009; Dorff & Vogelzang, 2011; Algarté-Génin et al., 2004). For example, two preliminary phase I studies have shown that high-dose exogenous testosterone therapy can safely be administered in patients with castrate-resistant metastatic prostate cancer (Szmulewitz et al., 2009; Morris et al., 2009). Some response in terms of PSA reduction was noted in these trials, but neither study was designed to investigate efficacy of this regimen. A larger, randomized trial is under way to further characterize efficacy and impact on quality of life measures more fully.

To complete the absolute reversal of the conventional dogma regarding the role of estrogen and testosterone in prostate cancer, there is also now considerable evidence to suggest that estrogens, once used to treat prostate cancer, actually contribute to the genesis of the disease (Bonkhoff & Berges, 2009; Carruba, 2007; Jensen et al., 2010; Prins & Korach, 2008; M Singh et al., 2008; P Singh et al., 2008; Wibowo et al., 2011)

In summary, after decades of research and contradictory claims it now seems that, contrary to the received wisdom, estrogen is a causative factor in breast and prostate cancer while

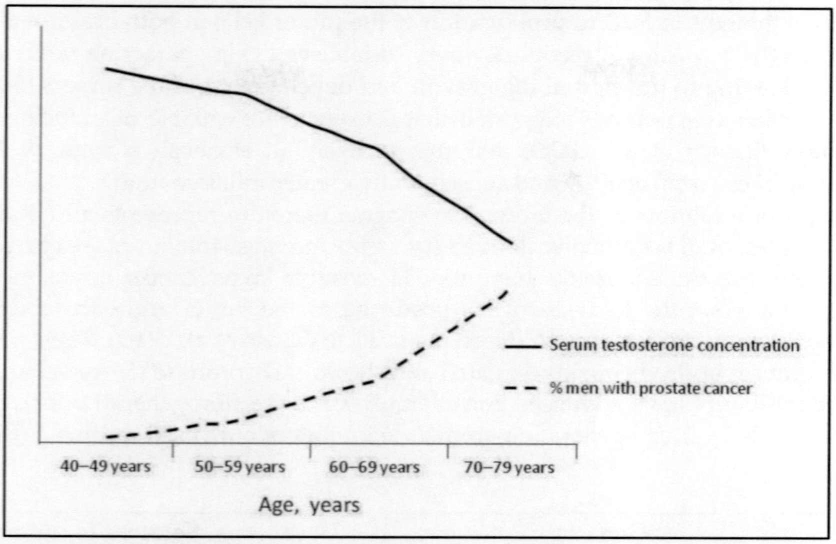

Fig. 4. Prostate cancer prevalence and testosterone levels with ageing. pCA: prostate cancer, T: testosterone. Reproduced from Morgentaler, 2006 with permission.

	Prostate cancer	**Breast cancer**
Estrogen	Causative	Causative
Testosterone	Protective	Protective

Table 1. Current understanding of the relationship between estrogen/testosterone and prostate/breast cancer.

testosterone actually offers protection against the conditions (Table 1). The concept of aromatization is the key to understanding the conflicting findings.

3.3 The importance of aromatization

From the earliest studies of the sex hormones, it was widely believed that estrogen was only formed in the ovaries and testosterone in the testes. However, research conducted during the 1970s demonstrated that aromatase was abundant in the adipose tissue of both men and women, demonstrating that the peripheral tissue is the major source of estrogen synthesis in men and postmenopausal women (Grodin et al., 1973; MacDonald et al., 1967; Santen et al., 2009).

The close connection between estrogen and testosterone in both men and women presented the possibility of fine-tuning the balance of the two hormones in the body. Scientists began to recognize the therapeutic potential of targeting aromatase to control the biosynthesis of estrogen, and started to develop selective aromatase inhibitors for therapeutic purposes (Barone et al., 1979; Santen et al., 2009; Thompson & Siiteri 1973, 1974).

Research conducted over recent years suggests that aromatase expression and activity in the breast and prostate may be up-regulated at the tumour site, resulting in an altered local hormonal environment and an increased estrogen/testosterone ratio (Ellem & Risbridger,

2010). This is thought to lead to proliferation of the tumor cells in both breast and prostate cancer through a positive feedback loop, established via paracrine and autocrine mechanisms leading to the continuing growth and development of the tumors (Simpson et al., 1997). Further research has suggested that estrogens are capable of inducing prostatic inflammation (Bianco et al., 2006), and this is likely to establish a cycle of increased aromatase, local estrogen activity and subsequently greater inflammation.

Development of inhibitors of the aromatase enzyme therefore represents a logical strategy for the management of hormonally-derived tumors. Aromatase inhibitors are currently used with great effect in the endocrine therapy of ER-positive breast cancer in postmenopausal women to counteract the local estrogens produced in the tumor and surrounding tissue which act as a stimulant for growth (Eisen et al., 2008; Ghosh et al., 2009). Their potential in male breast cancer is also being investigated and shows early promise (Doyen et al., 2010).

Aromatase inhibitors have advanced considerably since the first generation of agents was developed (Table 2). Third-generation aromatase inhibitors now used routinely (Bhatnagar, 2007).

Type	Generic	Dose	Selected brand names
First generation (non-selective)	Aminoglutethimide	250 mg	Cytadren®, Orimeten®
	Testolactone	50 mg	Fudestrin®, Teslac®
Second generation (selective)	Formestane	250 mg	Lentaron®
	Fadrozole	1 mg	Afema®
Third generation (selective)	Exemestane	25 mg	Aromasin®
	Anastrozole	1 mg	Arimidex®
	Letrozole	2.5 mg	Femara®
	Vorozole	2.5 mg	Rivizor®

Table 2. Aromatase inhibitors.

4. Applying current knowledge in future directions

After more than a century of research and controversy surrounding the hormonal treatment of breast and prostate cancer, some conclusions can finally be drawn. First, excessive estrogen levels can be implicated in both breast and prostate cancer, while testosterone appears to offer a protective effect. Second, aromatase inhibitors reduce the conversion of testosterone to estrogen, thus lowering levels of estrogen and increasing testosterone activity. Third, the SERM tamoxifen blocks estrogen activity and both directly and indirectly increases testosterone activity by up-regulating androgen receptors.

In view of these findings, the most rational approach to treatment of breast and prostate cancer would be to administer a combination of three drugs - tamoxifen, an aromatase inhibitor and testosterone. The combination of these three drugs would allow patients to greatly benefit from their synergistic effects in maintaining a desirable hormonal balance in the following way:

1. **Aromatase inhibitor** would allow both endogenous and exogenous testosterone levels to be maintained and estrogen levels to be reduced;

2. **Tamoxifen** would allow upregulation of androgen receptors and downregulation of estrogen receptors, thereby both increasing testosterone's action and ensuring further suppression of estrogen activity;
3. **Exogenous testosterone** in the presence of the aromatase inhibitor would allow increased testosterone levels whilst halting its aromatization to estrogen.

These effects are summarized in Figure 5.

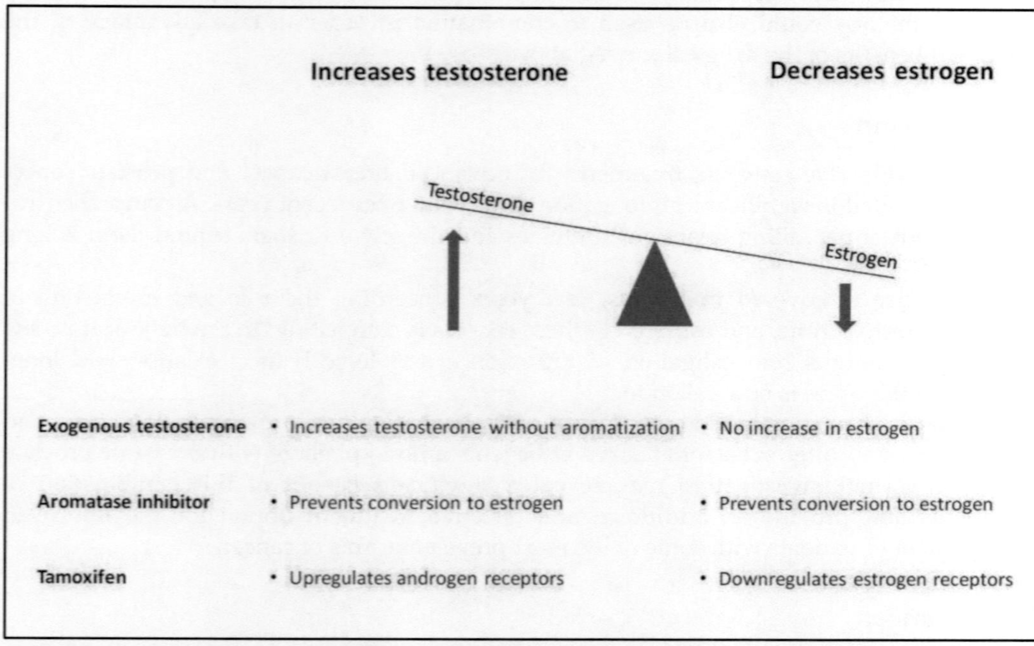

Fig. 5. Rationale for the combination of exogenous testosterone, an aromatase inhibitor, and tamoxifen for the treatment of breast or prostate cancer through elevation of testosterone and reduction of estrogen levels.

Considerable research efforts continue to be devoted to the development of new SERMs to improve upon tamoxifen (Clarke & Khosla, 2009; Silverman 2010). However, the now off-patent tamoxifen confers a significant advantage over newer drugs in being inexpensive and well-tolerated with a known side-effect profile. As well as an established role in the treatment and chemoprevention of hormone-related breast cancer, tamoxifen is also cardioprotective and increases bone mineral density, and appears to have other beneficial physiological effects (M Singh et al., 2008). Although usually prescribed at 20 mg daily, studies have revealed that tamoxifen may be as effective, and perhaps even more effective, at one-tenth the dose (Tormey et al., 1983). This is highly desirable as the risks associated with high dose tamoxifen include thrombo-embolism and uterine cancer.

Testosterone has been safely used for decades and its use does not require any regulatory approval. When used in combination with other drugs, it may have beneficial effects at much lower doses than usual. Ideally it would be possible to use at physiologic doses that would mean customizing the dose to each patient's individual requirement. This could be determined with comprehensive individual hormonal assessments.

There have been several clinical trials in the past 30 years demonstrating superior effects of combining a synthetic androgen with tamoxifen in treating advanced breast cancer over using tamoxifen alone (Ingle et al., 1991; Swain et al., 1988; Tormey et al., 1983), as well as preliminary research into thecombination of tamoxifen with an aromatase inhibitor (Coombes et al., 1982).

Combination therapy has been a common practice in the treatment of cancer for many years, and new combinations continue to be investigated (Lin et al., 2010). It is proposed here that hormonal therapy could also be used in combination in order to take advantage of the combined benefits of the drugs discussed above.

5. Conclusion

Despite considerable research, treatments for advanced breast cancer and prostate cancer have not resulted in significant prolongation of survival over recent years. A comprehensive reassessment of prevailing treatment strategies and the scientific logic behind them is long overdue.

New evidence discovered in the last few years concerning the role and interaction of tamoxifen, testosterone, and estrogen in these cancers is compelling. In the light of this new evidence a rigorous reinvestigation of the science and logic behind existing and long-abandoned therapies is now called for.

We propose that combination treatment with tamoxifen, an aromatase inhibitor, and testosterone may offer substantial survival benefits among patients with breast or prostate cancer. A formal investigation may reveal a significant benefit of this combination of treatments and provide an additional and effective treatment option for the improved management of patients with some of the most prevalent forms of cancer.

6. References

National Cancer Institute. (2007). United States Cancer Statistics (USCS): 1999-2007, In *Incidence and Mortality Web-based ReportExternal Web Site Policy.* 28.02.2011, Available from: http://seer.cancer.gov/csr/1975_2007/results_single/sect_01_table.01.pdf

Early Breast Cancer Trialists' Collaborative Group. (1998). Tamoxifen for early breast cancer: an overview of the randomised trials. *Lancet*, Vol.351, No.9114, pp. 1451-1467

Algarté-Génin, M.; Cussenot, O. & Costa, P. (2004). Prevention of prostate cancer by androgens: experimental paradox or clinical reality. *European Urology*, Vol.46, No.3, pp. 285-294

Barone, R.; Shamonki, I.; Siiteri, P. & Judd, H. (1979). Inhibition of peripheral aromatization of androstenedione to estrone in postmenopausal women with breast cancer using delta 1-testololactone. *The Journal of Clinical Endocrinology and Metabolism*, Vol.49, No.5, pp. 672-676.

Beatson, G. (1896). On the treatment of inoperable cases of carcinoma of hemamma. Suggestions for a new method of treatment with illustrative cases. *Lancet II*, 104-107

Bhatnagar, A. (2007). The early days of letrozole. *Breast Cancer Research and Treatment*, Vol.105, Suppl 1, pp. 3-5

Bianco, J.; McPherson, S.; Wang, H.; Prins, G. & Risbridger, G. (2006). Transient neonatal estrogen exposure to estrogen-deficient mice (aromatase knockout) reduces prostate weight and induces inflammation in late life. *The American Journal of Pathology*, Vol.168, No.6, pp. 1869-1878

Bonkhoff, H. & Berges, R. (2009). The evolving role of oestrogens and their receptors in the development and progression of prostate cancer. *European Urology*, Vol.55, No. 3, pp. 533-542

Butenandt, A. & Hanisch, G. (1935). Umwandlung des Dehydroandrosterons in Androstendiol und Testosterone; ein Weg zur Darstellung des Testosterons aus Cholestrin [About Testosterone. Conversion of Dehydro-androsterons into androstendiol and testosterone; a way for the structure assignment of testosterone from cholestrol]. *Hoppe Seylers Z Physiol Chem*, Vol.237, No. 2, pp. 89

Carruba, G. (2007). Estrogen and prostate cancer: an eclipsed truth in an androgen-dominated scenario. *Journal of Cellular Biochemistry*, Vol.102, No. 4, pp. 899-911

Castle, E. & Thrasher, J. (2002). The role of soy phytoestrogens in prostate cancer. *The Urologic Clinics of North America*, Vol.29, No.1, pp. 71-81

Clarke, B. & Khosla, S. (2009). New selective estrogen and androgen receptor modulators. *Current Opinion in Rheumatology*, Vol.21, No.4, pp. 374-379

Cole, M.; Jones, C. & Todd, I. (1971). A new anti-oestrogenic agent in late breast cancer. An early clinical appraisal of ICI46474. *British Journal of Cancer*, Vol.25, No.2, pp. 270-275

Coombes, R.; Powles, T.; Rees, L.; Ratcliffe, W.; Nash, A.; Henk, M.; Ford, H.; Gazet, J. & Neville, A. (1982). Tamoxifen, aminoglutethimide and danazol: effect of therapy on hormones in post-menopausal patients with breast cancer. *British Journal of Cancer*, Vol.46, No.1, pp. 30-34

David, K.; Dingemanse, E.; Freud, J. & Laqueur, E. (1935). Über krystallinisches mannliches Hormon aus Hoden (Testosteron) wirksamer als aus harn oder aus Cholesterin bereitetes Androsteron [On crystalline male hormone from testicles (testosterone) effective as from urine or from cholesterol]. *Hoppe Seylers Z Physiol Chem*, Vol.233, pp. 281

Dimitrakakis, C. & Bondy, C. (2009). Androgens and the breast. *Breast Cancer Research: BCR*, Vol.11, No.5, pp. 212

Dorff, T. & Vogelzang, N. (2011). Use of Testosterone Replacement Therapy in Patients with Prostate Cancer. *Current Urology Reports* (March 2).

Doyen, J.; Italiano, A.; Largillier, R.; Ferrero, J-M.; Fontana, X. & Thyss, A. (2010). Aromatase inhibition in male breast cancer patients: biological and clinical implications. *Annals of Oncology: Official Journal of the European Society for Medical Oncology*, Vol.21, No.6, pp. 1243-1245

Drewa, T. & Chłosta, P. (2010). Testosterone supplementation and prostate cancer, controversies still exist. *Acta Poloniae Pharmaceutica* Vol.67, No.5, pp. 543-546

Eisen, A.; Trudeau, M.; Shelley, W.; Messersmith, H. & Pritchard, K. (2008). Aromatase inhibitors in adjuvant therapy for hormone receptor positive breast cancer: a systematic review. *Cancer Treatment Reviews*, Vol.34, No.2, pp. 157-174

Ekmektzoglou, K.; Xanthos, T.; German, V. & Zografos, G. (2009). Breast cancer: from the earliest times through to the end of the 20th century. *European Journal of Obstetrics, Gynecology, and Reproductive Biology*, Vol.145, No.1, pp. 3-8

Ellem, S. & Risbridger, G. (2010). Aromatase and regulating the estrogen:androgen ratio in the prostate gland. *The Journal of Steroid Biochemistry and Molecular Biology*, Vol.118, No.4, pp. 246-251

Fels, E. (1944). Treatment of breast cancer with testosterone propionate.A preliminary report. *J Clin Endocrinol* 4: 121-125.

Folkerd, E. & Dowsett, M. (2010). Influence of sex hormones on cancer progression. *Journal of Clinical Oncology: Official Journal of the American Society of Clinical Oncology*, Vol.28, No.26, pp. 4038-4044

Freeman, E.; Bloom, D. & Mcguire, E. (2001). A brief history of testosterone. *The Journal of Urology*, Vol.165, No.2, pp. 371-373

Furr, B. & Jordan, V. (1984). The pharmacology and clinical uses of tamoxifen. *Pharmacology & Therapeutics*, Vol.25, No. 2, pp. 127-205

Gajdos, C. & Jordan V. (2002). Selective estrogen receptor modulators as a new therapeutic drug group: concept to reality in a decade. *Clinical Breast Cancer*, Vol.2, No.4, pp. 272-281

Gardiner, R.; Sweeney, C. & Tilley, W. (2009). Testosterone therapy in castrate-resistant prostate cancer: a possible new approach. *European Urology*, Vol.56, No.2, pp. 245-246

Ghosh, D.; Griswold, J.; Erman, M. & Pangborn, W. (2009). Structural basis for androgen specificity and oestrogen synthesis in human aromatase. *Nature*,Vol.457, No.7226, pp. 219-223

Goldenberg, I. (1964). Testosterone propionate therapy in breast cancer. *The Journal of the American Medical Association*, Vol.188, pp. 1069-1072

Gradishar, W. (2010). Adjuvant endocrine therapy for early breast cancer: the story so far. *Cancer Investigation*, Vol.28, No.4, pp. 433-442

Grodin, J.; Siiteri, P. & MacDonald, P. (1973). Source of estrogen production in postmenopausal women. *The Journal of Clinical Endocrinology and Metabolism*, Vol.36, No.2, pp. 207-214

Hackshaw, A.; Roughton, M.; Forsyth, S.; Monson, K.; Reczko, K.; Sainsbury, R. & Baum, M. (2011). Long-Term Benefits of 5 Years of Tamoxifen: 10-Year Follow-Up of a Large Randomized Trial in Women at Least 50 Years of Age With Early Breast Cancer. *Journal of Clinical Oncology*, doi:10.1200/JCO.2010.32.2933. http://www.ncbi.nlm.nih.gov/pubmed/21422412.

Ho, S-M. (2004). Estrogens and anti-estrogens: key mediators of prostate carcinogenesis and new therapeutic candidates. *Journal of Cellular Biochemistry*, Vol.91, No.3, pp. 491-503

Huggins, C. & Hodges, C. (1941). Studies on prostatic cancer, I: the effect of castration, of estrogen and of androgen injection on serum phosphatases in metastatic carcinoma of the prostate. *Cancer Res*, Vol.1, pp. 293-7

Ingle, J.; Twito, D.; Schaid, D.; Cullinan, S.; Krook, J.; Mailliard, J.; Tschetter, L.; Long, H.; Gerstner, J. & Windschitl, H. (1991). Combination hormonal therapy with tamoxifen plus fluoxymesterone versus tamoxifen alone in postmenopausal women with metastatic breast cancer. An updated analysis. *Cancer*, Vol.67, No.4, pp. 886-891

Jannini, E.; Gravina, G.; Mortengaler, A.; Morales. A.; Incrocci, L. & Hellstrom, W. (2011). Is testosterone a friend or a foe of the prostate? *The Journal of Sexual Medicine*, Vol.8, No.4, pp. 946-955

Jensen, E.; Jacobson, H.; Walf, A. & Frye, C. (2010). Estrogen action: a historic perspective on the implications of considering alternative approaches. *Physiology & Behavior*, Vol.99, No. 2, pp. 151-162

Kim, I.; Kim, B-C.; Seong, D.; Lee, D.; Seo, J-M.; Hong, Y.; Kim, H-T.; Morton, R. & Kim, S-J. (2002). Raloxifene, a mixed estrogen agonist/antagonist, induces apoptosis in androgen-independent human prostate cancer cell lines. *Cancer Research*, Vol.62, No.18, pp. 5365-5369

Klopper, A. & Hall, M. (1971). New Synthetic Agent for the Induction of Ovulation: Preliminary Trials in Women. *BMJ*, Vol.1, pp. 152-154

Labrie, F.; Luu-The, V.; Labrie, C.; Belanger, A.; Simard, J.; Lin, S-X. & Pelletier, G. (2003). Endocrine and Intracrine Sources of Androgens in Women: Inhibition of Breast Cancer and Other Roles of Androgens and Their Precursor Dehydroepiandrosterone. *Endocrinology Reviews*, Vol.24, No.2, pp. 152-182

Lerner, L. & Jordan, V. (1990). Development of antiestrogens and their use in breast cancer: eighth Cain memorial award lecture. *Cancer Research*, Vol.50, No.14, pp. 4177-4189

Lin, S-X.; Chen, J.; Mazumdar, M.; Poirier, D.; Wang, C.; Azzi, A. & Zhou, M. (2010). Molecular therapy of breast cancer: progress and future directions. *Nature Reviews. Endocrinology*, Vol.6, No.9, pp. 485-493

MacDonald, P.; Rombaut, R. & Siiteri, P. (1967). Plasma precursors of estrogen. I. Extent of conversion of plasma delta-4-androstenedione to estrone in normal males and nonpregnant normal, castrate and adrenalectomized females. *The Journal of Clinical Endocrinology and Metabolism*, Vol.27, No.8, pp. 1103-1111

Malarkey, W.; Schroeder, L.; Stevens, V.; James, A. & Lanese, R. (1977). Twenty-four-hour preoperative endocrine profiles in women with benign and malignant breast disease. *Cancer Research*, Vol.37, No.12, pp. 4655-4659

Margo, K.; & Winn, R. (2006). Testosterone treatments: why, when, and how? *American Family Physician*, Vol.73, No.9, pp. 1591-1598

Mcleod, D. (2003). Hormonal therapy: historical perspective to future directions. *Urology*, Vol.61, No.2, pp. 3-7

Meyer, A. (1955). Conversion of 19-hydroxy-delta 4-androstene-3,17-dione to estrone by endocrine tissue. *Biochimica Et Biophysica Acta*, Vol.17, No.3, pp. 441-442

Meyer, A.; Hayano, M.; Lindberg, M.; Gut, M. & Rodgers, O. (1955). The conversion of delta 4-androstene-3,17-dione-4-C14 and dehydroepiandrosterone by bovine adrenal homogenate preparations. *Acta Endocrinologica*, Vol.18, No.2, pp. 148-168

Morgentaler, A.; Bruning, C. & DeWolf, W. (1996). Occult prostate cancer in men with low serum testosterone levels. *The Journal of the American Medical Association*, Vol.276, No.23, pp. 1904-1906

Morgentaler, A. (2006). Testosterone and prostate cancer: an historical perspective on a modern myth. *European Urology*, Vol.50, No.5, pp. 935-939

Morgentaler, A.; Lipshultz, L.; Bennett, R.; Sweeney, M.; Avila, D. & Khera, M. (2011). Testosterone Therapy in Men With Untreated Prostate Cancer. *The Journal of Urology*. doi:10.1016/j.juro.2010.11.084. http://www.ncbi.nlm.nih.gov/pubmed/21334649.

Morris, M.; Huang, D.; Kelly, W.; Slovin, S.; Stephenson, R.; Eicher, C.; Delacruz, A.; Curley, T.; Schwartz, L. & Scher, H. (2009). Phase 1 trial of high-dose exogenous testosterone in patients with castration-resistant metastatic prostate cancer. *European Urology*, Vol.56, No. 2, pp. 237-244

Morrissey, C. & Watson, W. (2003). Phytoestrogens and prostate cancer. *Current Drug Targets*, Vol.4, No.3, pp. 231-241

Mukherjee, S. (2011). *The emperor of all maladies. A biography of cancer* (1st ed). HarperCollins Publishers. ISBN 978-0-00-725091-2, London, UK

Prins, G. & Korach, K. (2008). The role of estrogens and estrogen receptors in normal prostate growth and disease. *Steroids*, Vol.73, No.3, pp. 233-244

Rana, A.; Rangasamy, V. & Mishra, R. (2010). How estrogen fuels breast cancer. *Future Oncology*, Vol.6, No.9, pp. 1369-1371

Santen, R.; Brodie, H.; Simpson, E.; Siiteri, P. & Brodie, A. (2009). History of Aromatase: Saga of an Important Biological Mediator and Therapeutic Target. *Endocrinology Review* Vol.30,No.4, pp. 343-375

Schwarz, S.; Onken, D. & Schubert, A. (1999). The steroid story of Jenapharm: From the late 1940s to the early 1970s. *Steroids*, Vol.64, No.7, pp. 439-445

Secreto, G.; Recchione, C.; Grignolio, E. & Cavalleri, A. (1983). Increased urinary androgen excretion is a hormonal abnormality detectable before the clinical onset of breast cancer. *Cancer Detection and Prevention*, Vol.6, No.4, pp. 435-438

Segaloff, A.; Gordon, D.; Horwitt, B.; Schlosser, J. & Murison, P. (1951). Hormonal therapy in cancer of the breast. I. The effect of testosterone propionate therapy on clinical course and hormonal excretion. *Cancer*, Vol.4, No.2, pp. 319-323

Segaloff, A.; Weeth, J.; Cuningham, M. & Meyer, K. (1964). Hormonal therapy in cancer of the breast. 23. Effect of 7-alpha-methyl-19-nortestosterone acetate and testosterone propionate on clinical course and hormonal excretion. *Cancer*, Vol.17, pp. 1248-1253

Shin, B.; Hwang, E.; Im, C.; Kim, S-O.; Jung, S.; Kang, T.; Kwon, D.; Park, K. & Ryu, S. (2010). Is a decreased serum testosterone level a risk factor for prostate cancer? A cohort study of korean men. *Korean Journal of Urology*, Vol.51, No.12, pp. 819-823

Silverman, S. (2010). New selective estrogen receptor modulators (SERMs) in development. *Current Osteoporosis Reports*, Vol.8, No.3, pp. 151-153

Simpson, E.; Zhao, Y.; Agarwal, V.; Michael, M.; Bulun, S.; Hinshelwood, M. & Graham-Lorence, S. (1997). Aromatase expression in health and disease. *Recent Progress in Hormone Research*, Vol.52: 185-213

Singh, M.; Martin-Hirsch, P. & Martin, F. (2008). The multiple applications of tamoxifen: an example pointing to SERM modulation being the aspirin of the 21st century. *Medical Science Monitor: International Medical Journal of Experimental and Clinical Research*, Vol.14, No.9, pp. RA144-148

Singh, P.; Matanhelia, S. & Martin, F. (2008). A potential paradox in prostate adenocarcinoma progression: oestrogen as the initiating driver. *European Journal of* Cancer, Vol.44, No.7, pp. 928-936

Somboonporn, W. & Davis, S. (2004). Testosterone Effects on the Breast: Implications for Testosterone Therapy for Women. *Endocrinology Review*, Vol.25, No.3, pp. 374-388

Sonne-Hansen, K. & Lykkesfeldt, A. (2005). Endogenous aromatization of testosterone results in growth stimulation of the human MCF-7 breast cancer cell line. *The Journal of Steroid Biochemistry and Molecular Biology*,Vol.93, No.1, pp. 25-34

Steinach, E. & Kun, H. (1937). Transformation of male sex hormones into a substance with the action of a female hormone. *Lancet* Vol.133, pp. 845

Suzuki, T.; Miki, Y.; Takagi, K.; Hirakawa, H.; Moriya, T.; Ohuchi, N. & Sasano, H. (2010). Androgens in human breast carcinoma. *Medical Molecular Morphology* Vol.43, No.2, pp. 75-81

Swain, S.; Steinberg, S.; Bagley, C. & Lippman, M. (1988). Tamoxifen and fluoxymesterone versus tamoxifen and danazol in metastatic breast cancer-a randomized study. *Breast Cancer Research and Treatment*, Vol.12, No.1, pp. 51-57

Szmulewitz, R.; Mohile, S.; Posadas, E.; Kunnavakkam, R.; Karrison, T.; Manchen, E. & Stadler, W. (2009). A randomized phase 1 study of testosterone replacement for patients with low-risk castration-resistant prostate cancer. *European Urology* Vol.56, No.1, pp. 97-103

Tata, J. (2005). One hundred years of hormones. *EMBO reports*, Vol.6, No.6, pp. 490-496

Thijssen, J. & Blankenstein, M. (1989). Endogenous oestrogens and androgens in normal and malignant endometrial and mammary tissues. *European Journal of Cancer & Clinical Oncology*, Vol.25, No.12, pp. 1953-1959

Thompson, E. & Siiteri, P. (1973). Studies on the aromatization of C-19 androgens. *Annals of the New York Academy of Sciences*, Vol.212, pp. 378-391

Thompson, E. & Siiteri, P. (1974). The involvement of human placental microsomal cytochrome P-450 in aromatization. *The Journal of Biological Chemistry*, Vol.249, No.17, pp. 5373-5378

Thompson, I.; Pauler, D.; Goodman, P.; Tangen, C.; Lucia, M.; Parnes, H. & Minasian, L. (2004). Prevalence of prostate cancer among men with a prostate-specific antigen level < or =4.0 ng per milliliter. *The New England Journal of Medicine*, Vol.350, No.22, pp. 2239-2246

Tormey, D.; Lippman, M.; Edwards, B. & Cassidy, J. (1983). Evaluation of tamoxifen doses with and without fluoxymesterone in advanced breast cancer. *Annals of Internal Medicine*, Vol.98, No.2, pp. 139-144

Vitola, G. & Zeĭkate, G. (1976). Blood levels of testosterone and dihydrotestosterone in breast cancer. *Voprosy Onkologii* Vol.22, No.8, pp. 26-30

Wibowo, E.; Schellhammer, P. & Wassersug, R. (2011). Role of estrogen in normal male function: clinical implications for patients with prostate cancer on androgen deprivation therapy. *The Journal of Urology*, Vol.185, No.1, pp. 17-23

Wierman, M.; Basson, R.; Davis, S.; Khosla, S.; Miller, K.; Rosner, W. & Santoro, N. (2006). Androgen Therapy in Women: An Endocrine Society Clinical Practice Guideline. *J Clin Endocrinol Metab*, Vol.91, No.10, pp. 3697-3710

Zhou, J.; Ng, S.; Adesanya-Famuiya, O.; Anderson, K. & Bondy, C. (2000). Testosterone inhibits estrogen-induced mammary epithelial proliferation and suppresses estrogen receptor expression. *FASEB J.* Vol.14, pp. 1725-1730

Zondek, B. (1934). Oestrogenic hormone in the urine of the stallion. *Nature*, 133, pp. 494

7

Emerging Imaging and Operative Techniques for Glioma Surgery

Claude-Edouard Chatillon and Kevin Petrecca
Montreal Neurological Institute and Hospital, McGill University
Canada

1. Introduction

Malignant gliomas are the most common adult primary brain cancers and are amongst the most devastating of human malignancies. These cancers are characterized by high proliferation and invasion into normal brain. Treatment consists of a combination of surgery, radiotherapy, and chemotherapy. Despite years of experience and refinement of these treatments, patients suffering from World Health Organization grade four gliomas have a mean survival of 14 months (Stupp et al., 2005).

The goal of surgery is to remove the entirety of the tumor as strong emerging evidence suggests that completeness of resection improves cancer control and lengthens survival. Extent of resection, for malignant gliomas, is based on gadolinium-enhanced magnetic resonance imaging (MRI). In cases of complete resection, radiotherapy is then delivered to a 2 cm border along the resection cavity. In cases of incomplete resection, radiotherapy is delivered to the residual tumor and a 2 cm border along the residual tumor and resection cavity. The rational for this radiotherapy strategy is that invasive cancer cells can be found up to 2 cm distant from the main tumor mass.

Studies examining the location of malignant glioma recurrence following surgery and adjuvant radiotherapy and chemotherapy have found that most cancers recur within a 1 cm border along the surgical resection cavity, even in cases in which no residual gadolinium-enhancing tumor was evident on immediate post-operative MRI. This suggests that gadolinium-enhanced MRI does not sufficiently reveal the entire tumor resulting in residual tumor post-operatively. Other common MRI sequences, including FLAIR and T2, do not adequately distinguish non-gadolinium enhancing cancer cells from peritumoral edema. The inability to accurately visualize the whole tumor, including invasive cells, on imaging decreases the likelihood of complete resection. Recently, attempts to visualize malignant gliomas with newer imaging techniques, including metabolic labeled positron emission tomography (PET), have identified tumor borders beyond those seen with gadolinium-enhanced MRI. These technologies may have profound implications regarding surgical planning in malignant glioma surgery.

Historically, extent of tumor resection has been determined by the surgeon's qualitative assessment at the time of operation, often reporting a gross total resection. More recently, the use of immediate post-operative MRI has revealed that complete resection of the gadolinium-enhancing portion of the tumor is achieved at a much lower rate. This overestimation by surgeons is, in part, owing to the difficulty distinguishing cancer cells from normal brain. Since malignant gliomas are highly invasive tumors, the margin between tumor and normal brain is typically not obvious. Reluctant to cause an irreversible neurological deficit, surgeons will error on the side of caution. The downside is that malignant cancer cells will remain. Since adjuvant radiation and chemotherapies are only modestly effective (Stupp et al., 2005), these cancer cells that remain along the border of the original tumor mass will recur. Intraoperative tools designed to help surgeons distinguish cancer cells from normal brain include ultrasound and fluorescence guided surgical resection. Comparative studies using these tools have shown higher rates of complete resection compared to standard operating techniques.

Here we review current and emerging imaging technologies designed to better visualize the tumor on preoperative imaging. We also review developing surgical technologies to help surgeons distinguish cancer cells from normal brain intraoperatively. The development of these technologies will lead to an increased rate of complete resection and thus improved cancer control.

2. Preoperative glioma imaging

2.1 Tumour delineation in glioma

The accurate characterisation of tumour size and location is crucial to decisions in diagnosis, presurgical planning and adjuvant therapy, as well as assessment of treatment response or failure in patients with a glioma. The diagnostic and tumour delineation gold standard remains the MRI using T1 with and without gadolinium-enhancement, T2 and fluid attenuation inversion recovery (FLAIR) sequences. However, classical MRI sequences provide an indirect assessment of tumour grade by relying on tissue density, fluid content and blood-brain barrier breakdown patterns. Advanced MRI techniques aim to measure water molecule diffusion patterns (diffusion weighted imaging), cerebral blood volume (perfusion-weighted MRI) and metabolic tissue composition (magnetic resonance spectroscopy), which are more direct measures of tumour metabolism. Furthermore, PET using the classical metabolic tracer fluorodeoxyglucose (FDG) or novel amino acid tracers have been shown to provide complimentary information to MRI in presurgical planning and improve outcome in low and high grade gliomas.

2.2 Conventional MRI

Since its first clinical use in the 1980s, MRI rapidly became the imaging modality of choice in cerebral tumors, owing to its resolution, grey-white matter distinction and radiation sparing advantages over computed tomography (CT). To image glioma invasion, changes in tissue density, fluid content and blood brain barrier breakdown underlie the abnormalities seen on classical MRI sequences. Tumour delineation in low grade gliomas (LGG) is usually determined by the extent of hyperintense signal on a T2 sequence. Edema is usually absent in LGGs and should therefore not be a confounder of T2 hyperintensity. Areas of enhancement after gadolinium enhancement are typically not seen in LGG and are, in fact, a marker of anaplastic transformation. In contrast, tumour delineation in high grade gliomas (HGG) cannot rely on the T2 sequence, due to the often significant edema surrounding the lesion. The area of enhancement on the gadolinium-enhanced T1 sequence is usually used for pre-operative planning, post-operative extent of resection assessment and evaluation of progression, treatment response or recurrence.

The reliability of classical MRI to fully delineate the tumour has been questioned in low and high grade tumours. In particular, the absence of enhancement after gadolinium injection does not exclude the presence of high grade cancer cells. This has been shown within non-enhancing, T2 hyperintense lesions suspected of being LGG (Kunz et al., 2011) and outside the enhancement perimeter in HGG (Pauleit et al., 2005). Furthermore, the effects of various treatments on the blood-brain barrier, at times independent of their anti-tumoural effects, have highlighted the need for imaging modalities more directly linked to metabolic tumoural activity. For example, radiation alone or combined with chemotherapy can lead to a regional blood-brain barrier breakdown in 20 to 50% of treated patients, leading to new or increase in size of exisiting areas of enhancement on gadolinium-injected T1 sequences in treated patients, an entity known as pseudoprogression (de Wit et al., 2004; Brandsma et al., 2008; Taal et al., 2008; Brandsma et al., 2009). Conversely, novel anti-angiogenic treatments have led to the radiological concept of pseudoresponse, whereby the anti-vascular endothelial growth factor treatment affects vascular permeability but may not significantly alter tumour progression, as evidenced by continued enlargement of hyperintensity signal on FLAIR and rapid relapse after interruption of treatment (Norden et al., 2008; Brandsma et al., 2009). In order to improve preoperative glioma grading and delineation, as well as to improve treatment response assessment, research in glioma imaging has focused on direct detection of biological tumoural changes by targeting local changes in metabolite composition, glucose metabolism, amino acid uptake and hypoxic markers.

2.3 Advanced MRI techniques

The use of advanced MRI techniques has the advantage of being available in most clinical settings and does not require additional, and often expensive and with limited half-lives, radioactive tracers. MRI can currently provide information on water mobility within tissue (diffusion imaging), chemical composition (proton MR spectroscopy) as well as cerebral blood volume (CBV) and permeability (perfusion MR) (Cao et al., 2006).

2.3.1 Diffusion imaging

Diffusion imaging exploits the variation of micromotion properties of water protons in different environments. Pathological changes such as increased cellularity, necrosis, cytotoxic and vasogenic edema, osmolarity and active transport mechanisms affect these properties. These changes have an impact on proton diffusivity and mobility, which can be measured by diffusion imaging (Bammer, 2003). Diffusion imaging consists of standard diffusion weighted imaging (DWI), apparent diffusion coefficient (ADC) map and diffusion tensor imaging (DTI). DTI is a measurement of diffusion along different axes and can be used to determine fractional anisotropy (the preferential movement of water protons in certain direction), from which white matter tractography can be extrapolated.

Although DWI has established its clinical use in the diagnosis of several cerebral pathologies, including acute stroke (Warach et al., 1992; Adams et al., 2007) and in differentiating necrotic tumours from cerebral abscesses (Kim et al., 1998; Desprechins et al., 1999), its role in glioma grading and delineation is uncertain. Kono et al. (2001) found an inverse relation between tumour cellularity and the ADC value in astrocytic tumours, but the DWI and ADC imaging values were unable to discriminate between non-enhancing tumour invasion and peritumoural edema.

Early cellular changes following treatment, such as cytotoxic edema and necrosis, can be measured using DWI and have been shown to predict clinical efficacy (Moffat et al., 2005).

Indeed, in twenty glioma patients undergoing radiotherapy, chemotherapy or combined treatment, the percentage of tumour volume having undergone a change in ADC signal after three weeks of treatment (compared to a pre-treatment MRI) was compared between the different radiographic outcome groups after completion of treatment. These values were found to be significantly different between the partial response (n = 6), stable disease (n = 6) and progressive disease (n = 8) groups. Although survival statistics were not provided, the early identification of response to treatment might allow the treatment team to offer therapeutic alternatives to non-responders at an earlier timepoint in the course of the disease.

Using measurements of mean diffusivity (MD) and fractional anisotropy (FA), DTI has a potential role in delineating tumour margins within white matter. A tumour infiltration index (TII), derived from MD and FA values, was presented as a potential tool to discriminate "pure" vasogenic edema from tumour infiltrated edema (Lu et al., 2004). They observed that peritumoural edema FA values were lower (relative to MD values) in glioma patients than in meningioma and metastasis patients. They hypothesized that this was due to concomitant white matter disruption by tumoural invasion. This suggestion was not confirmed pathologically in the study, and a more recent study failed to replicate this hypothesis (Kinoshita et al., 2010), although a positive correlation was found between the TII and the standard uptake value (SUV) on ^{11}C-methionine PET imaging (a marker of tumour infiltration) in peritumoural hyperintense T2 areas.

2.3.2 Perfusion MR

Dynamic MR imaging during intravenous injection of gadolinium can be used to calculate regional CBV and vascular permeability with a spatial resolution similar to DWI (Cao et al., 2006). Both CBV and vascular permeability have been shown to correlate with glioma histological grade, but with significant overlap between grades (Roberts et al., 2000; Law et al., 2004). The use of perfusion MR in delineating tumour margins or response to treatment has not been explored.

2.3.3 Proton MR Spectroscopy (MRS)

The resonance frequency of hydrogen atoms in a magnetic field varies in function of their chemical microenvironment (the molecule that contains them). MRS expresses these differences as a chemical shift. Various metabolites commonly detected in brain tissue have relevance in glioma imaging because they correlate with specific metabolic events. These include choline-containing compounds (cell membrane turnover), creatine (energy metabolism), lactate (hypoxia), lipids (necrosis), and n-acetyl-aspartate (neuronal cell integrity).

The MRS choline peak may provide information to delineate gliomas. The choline/NAA ratio has been shown to correlate with the degree of tumoural invasion (tumour cell density)(Croteau et al., 2001), and a cutoff choline/NAA index (CNI) of 2.5 has been suggested to differentiate tumour from non-tumour MRI changes in untreated patients (McKnight et al., 2002). However, the role of MRS in pre-operative tumour delineation is limited by the poor spatial resolution of the technique (0.8 to 1 cm^3 voxel size). This limitation might eventually be resolved with development of higher resolution MRIs.

MRS may also play a role in treatment outcome prediction. In 28 glioblastoma patients undergoing combined radiotherapy and chemotherapy, the volume of metabolic abnormality (determined as areas of CNI > 2.5) within the tumour correlated negatively with survival. Another retrospective study of 26 glioblastoma patients undergoing radiosurgery (following previous radiation) demonstrated increased survival when more than 50% of the MRS tumour volume (CNI > 2) was included in the radiosurgery target (Chan et al., 2004). The latter finding suggests that MRS may be of benefit in defining radiosurgical (and perhaps conventional radiation) target volumes.

MRS, more specifically the Cho/NAA and NAA/Cr ratios, has shown some diagnostic value in differentiating tumour recurrence from radiation necrosis (Rock et al., 2004; Weybright et al., 2005; Sundgren, 2009). However, MRS is unreliable in the common cases of mixed recurrent tumour and radiation change (Sundgre, 2009). In a recent report, Zhou et al. (2011) observed that viable glioma could be differentiated from normal tissue and radiation necrosis using a novel amide proton transfer (APT) MRI technique in an irradiated U87MG glioma rat model.

2.4 Positron emission tomography

2.4.1 The choice of radioactive label

The most common radioactive labels used in PET are ^{18}F and ^{11}C. Although comparative studies of ^{18}F and ^{11}C labels using the same tracer were not found, studies comparing SUVs of O-(2-[^{18}F]fluoroethyl)-L-tyrosine (FET) (Weber et al., 2000) or [^{18}F]fluorodopa(FDOPA) (Becherer et al., 2003) with L-[methyl-^{11}C]methionine (MET) in patients with intracerebral lesions found similar uptake values in normal brain and tumour between the two tracers. Therefore, the main advantage of ^{18}F labelled tracers seems to be the longer half-life (110 minutes) compared to ^{11}C (20 minutes), which allows centers without on-site cyclotrons to perform PET studies.

2.4.2 The choice of labelled tracer

The most commonly used PET radioactive tracer remains FDG. However, the physiologically high glucose metabolism of normal brain produces a high background FDG uptake which decreases the signal-to-noise ratio in FDG-PET imaging, decreasing the detectability of low-grade or recurrent gliomas (Chen & Silverman, 2008; Klasner et al., 2010). In the search for alternative tracers, amino acids were found to be ideal because most CNS tumours show high uptake of amino acids compared to normal brain tissue, which has much lower amino acid requirements due to its low proliferative potential. Many different amino acids, such as ^{11}C-methionine (MET), ^{11}C-leucine and ^{11}C-tyrosine, as well as amino acid analogs (^{18}F-FDOPA, ^{18}F-FET), have been synthesized (Klasner et al., 2010). As noted earlier, comparative studies showed similar uptake values between the ^{11}C-MET, ^{18}F-FET and ^{18}F-FDOPA tracers (Weber et al., 2000; Becherer et al., 2003). Other tracers, such as ^{18}F-fluoromisonidazole (FMISO), specifically target hypoxic cells (Bruehlmeier et al., 2004), while nucleotide analogs, such as [^{18}F]fluorothymidine (FLT), target cell proliferation.

2.4.3 PET in tumour diagnosis and grade

Various amino acid PET studies have demonstrated increased tracer uptake in tumours compared to non-tumoural lesions, but the differential diagnosis between tumour types could not be made (Herholz et al., 1998; Jacobs et al., 2005; Pauleit et al., 2005). An increased uptake of 1.5-1.6 compared to the contralateral hemisphere was suggested as a threshold for viable tumoural tissue (Jacobs et al., 2005). Some studies observed a significantly higher uptake in HGGs compared to LGGs using ^{11}C-MET PET[32,34], whereas other groups identified a non-significant trend of higher tracer uptake in higher glioma grades using ^{18}F-FET[2] and ^{18}F-FET PET[35]. Fueger et al. (2010) recently demonstrated that ^{18}F-FDOPA PET SUVs were significantly different between all grades in newly diagnosed gliomas, but not in previously treated gliomas. They calculated an SUV_{max} of 2.72 to discriminate between LGG and HGG. Furthermore, the ^{18}F-FDOPA values correlated with Ki-67 values in pathological samples. Identifying metabolic "hot spots" within non-enhancing lesions was shown to accurately target higher grade areas in suspected LGGs (Kunz et al., 2011). As well, combining PET findings with gadolinium-injected images increase the diagnostic yield of stereotactic biopsies in HGG (Pauleit et al., 2005).

2.4.4 PET and tumour delineation

Tumour margins determined by conventional MRI and PET tracer uptake often yield different but overlapping tumour volumes. In a report of 103 consecutive cases, Pirotte et al. (2006) used combined FDG-PET, MET-PET and MRI to define the planned surgical resection in 63 LGGs and 40 HGGs. They observed that the PET-defined tumour volume complemented the MRI-defined tumour volume in 96% of cases. PET imaging data altered the planned resection volume in 80% of cases. One of two trends was usually observed: either the planned resection volume was increased to achieve a complete removal of the tumour, or the resection volume was decreased in cases where the aim was to resect only the metabolically active (anaplastic) portion of the tumour. In LGG, PET imaging increased the planned resection volume in 57% of cases and decreased it in 27% of cases. In HGG, the resection volume was increased in 28% and decreased in 48% of cases. Unfortunately, pathological data regarding tissue in areas with discordant PET/MRI findings was not documented.

Importantly, in a subsequent study using the same combined PET/MRI to plan the resection, the same group reported an increased survival in HGG patients when a complete resection of the area of increased tracer uptake on PET had been achieved (mean = 32.5 vs 17.6 months, $p = 0.0001$) (Pirotte et al., 2009). Complete resection of the planned metabolically active volume was achieved in 70% of cases. Nariai et al. (2005) observed a similar survival advantage in their cohort of patients with HGGs when there was no residual area of elevated PET uptake.

2.4.5 PET and evaluation of response to treatment

An important aspect of imaging follow-up during the treatment of patients with glioma is the early identification of response to treatment. This allows the treating team to continue current treatment when it is appropriate, or to offer different treatment options as early as possible to non-responders. PET imaging using the nucleotide tracer ^{18}F-FLT has shown promise in this respect. In a group of twenty patients with recurrent glioma treated with bevacizumab and irinotecan, significant tracer uptake decreases in previous metabolically active areas at 2 weeks and 6 weeks following initiation of treatment were only observed in patients surviving > 12 months (Schiepers et al., 2010).

Another important aspect of glioma treatment follow-up is the ability to differentiate tumour recurrence from radiation-induced changes. In a series of 45 patients, Rachinger et al. (2005) report 93% specificity and 100% sensitivity for ^{18}F-FET PET in detecting tumour recurrence (compared to 93.5% specificity and 50% sensitivity for MRI). In this study, the ultimate diagnosis of radiation change was determined histopathologically in only 2 of 14 patients. Similarly, Nariai et al. (2005) found a significant difference in SUVs between recurrent glioma (n = 47) and radiation changes (n = 4, as defined histopathologically or by resolution of radiological findings) using ^{18}F-DOPA PET.

In summary, PET imaging provides complementary information to MRI in the diagnosis, tumour delineation and treatment follow-up of gliomas. Amino acid tracers are better suited to study brain cancers due to the greater signal to noise ratio compared to normal cerebral tissue. Nucleotide tracers such as FLT might be more sensitive to tumoural proliferation and may play an important role in the identification of treatment response and the discrimination of tumour recurrence from radiation-induced changes.

3. Intraoperative tools in glioma surgery

3.1 Extent of resection

The usefulness of aggressive resection of malignant gliomas has not been established. Many studies have shown no lengthening of progression free survival or overall survival with aggressive resection versus limited resection. The major limitation of these studies is that they relied on surgeon opinion to quantify the extent of resection; using qualitative terms such as gross total resection, subtotal resection, debulking, and biopsy. In fact, many of the studies predate MRI. Since malignant gliomas are highly invasive, the distinction between tumor and normal brain is typically not obvious. Thus, the intraoperative impression is often not concordant with the actual degree of resection.

More recent studies using early postoperative MRI, less than 48 hour postoperatively, to accurately quantify extent of resection have shown an advantage to aggressive resection. In fact, not only do patients with complete resection experience long survival, patients with incomplete but larger resection fair better than patients with incomplete but smaller resections (Stummer et al., 2006; McGirt et al., 2009).

Based on these findings and others there is a growing consensus that the extent of resection should be a primary concern, even where full resection is not possible, as the degree of tumor resection is associated with better patient outcomes when combined with chemotherapy and radiotherapy (Stummer et al., 2008). However, even for experienced surgeons, it can be difficult to define the tumor margins, as in many cases there is no demarcation between tumor and normal tissue.

3.2 Image guided surgery: Neuronavigation

Image guided surgery refers to a technique in which a point in a patient's space can be located on preoperative imaging. In neurosurgery, image guided surgery, or neuronavigation, refers to the ability to use a probe to locate a particular scalp, skull, or brain region on the preoperative MRI or computed tomography (CT) image. Advantages of neuronavigation include tailored craniotomy planning, and direct correlation of cortical anatomy with preoperative imaging. Neuronavigation is also useful in guiding the initial stages of resection, close to the cortical surface. Its usefulness in accurately identifying deeper tumor boundaries is dependent upon maintained accuracy with preoperative imaging. Since the preoperative imaging is static, and brain positioning is dynamic throughout an operation, there can be, and often is, a loss of accuracy over the course of the operation. Brain movement during surgery, or brain shift, can be caused by tumor removal, intracranial pressure reduction manoeuvres such as diuretic administration, cerebrospinal

fluid evacuation and gravity. Since malignant gliomas tend to be large and invade along deep white matter tracts, the utility of navigation to accurately locate deep tumor borders is limited by a loss of accuracy during the surgery.
Wirtz et al. (2000) studied the impact of navigation in 52 patients with grade four glioma. Early post-operative MRI was used to quantify the extent of resection. They found that a complete resection was achieved in 31% of cases in which navigation was used, whereas a complete resection was achieved in only 18% of cases without navigation. In contrast, Litofsky et al. (2006) reported that in 486 patients, the use of navigation resulted in fewer gross total resections. Willems et al. (2006) conducted a prospective randomized study in which 45 patients, each harbouring a solitary contrast-enhancing intracerebral tumor, were randomized for surgery with or without neuronavigation. Quantification of the extent of resection was determined using magnetic resonance imaging. They found that the mean amount of residual tumor tissue was 28.9% when navigation was not used and 13.8% when navigation was used. The corresponding mean amounts of residual gadolinium enhancing tumor tissue were 29.2 and 24.4%, respectively. These differences were not significant. They also found that gross total resection was achieved in five patients who underwent surgery without navigation and in three who underwent surgery with navigation. They concluded that there is no rationale for the routine use of neuronavigation to improve the extent of tumor resection.
Although a consensus has not been reached, most neurosurgeons agree that neuronavigation is valuable in surgical planning and the early stages of resection and that its accuracy is dependent on the dynamics of brain positioning throughout the operation. Developing techniques to update the navigation system during the operation, accounting for brain shift, will be increase the utility of navigation in glioma surgery.

3.3 Intraoperative MRI

Although not actually used as a guidance tool during the time of surgical resection, intraoperative MRI (iMRI) can be considered a tool to increase the extent of resection since it is performed within the same operative setting. Typically, the surgery is taken to the point at which the surgeon believes the resection has been completed. The dura and skin are then closed in a temporary fashion and the patient is then transferred into the adjacent iMRI or the iMRI is brought to the patient. Upon imaging, the decision is then made if residual resectable tumor remains, and if so, the skin and dura are reopened and the resection completed.
Advantages of this technique are that the image quality is excellent, neurosurgeons are familiar with this mode of imaging, and residual tumor is readily identifiable. Disadvantages of iMRI include the significant upfront infrastructure costs and additional surgical time required. Hirschberg et al. (2005) reported that the average operating time using iMRI was 5.1 hours and was significantly longer than in the conventional OR (3.4 hours). Importantly, iMRI is not an online technique, it does not guide the surgery or help to distinguish tumor from normal brain, it is used to evaluate the extent of resection at a surgeon defined time point.
Over the last 10 years, many centres have acquired, used, and are now reporting their experience with iMRI. Senft et al. (2010) reported their experience in using an iMRI system in glioma surgery. Between July 2004 and May 2009, a total of 103 patients harbouring gliomas underwent tumor resection with the use of a mobile low field iMRI. All patients underwent early postoperative high field MRI to determine the extent of resection. They

found that all tumors could be reliably visualized on intraoperative imaging. Intraoperative imaging revealed residual tumor tissue in 51 patients (49.5%), leading to further tumor resection in 31 patients (30.1%). Importantly, extended resection did not translate into a higher rate of neurological deficits. When analyzing survival of patients with glioblastoma, patients undergoing complete tumor resection did significantly better than patients with residual tumor (50% survival rate at 57.8 weeks vs. 33.8 weeks, log rank test p=0.003). Hatiboglu et al. (2009) studied the impact of iMRI on the decision to proceed with additional glioma resection during surgery and to maximize extent of resection. Patients who underwent craniotomy for glioma resection with high-field iMRI guidance were prospectively evaluated over a 1 year period. Volumetric analysis and extent of resection were assessed with iMRI, using gadolinium enhanced T1-weighted images for tumors showing contrast enhancement and T2-weighted images or nonenhancing tumors. Surgery was terminated after iMRI in 23 patients (52%) because gross total resection was achieved or because of residual tumor infiltration in an eloquent brain region. Twenty-one patients (47%) underwent additional resection of residual tumor after iMRI. For enhancing gliomas, the median extent of resection increased significantly from 84% (range, 59%-97%) to 99% (range, 85%-100%) with additional tumor removal after iMRI ($P < 0.001$). Gross total resection was achieved after additional tumor removal after iMRI in 15 of 21 patients (71%). Overall, 29 patients (65%) experienced gross total resection, and in 15 (52%), this was achieved with the contribution of iMRI.

To examine whether iMRI combined with neuronavigation contributes to a significantly improved extent of resection in glioma surgery Kuhnt et al. (2011) analysed 293 glioma patients who underwent craniotomy and tumor resection with the aid of 1.5 T iMRI and integrated multimodal navigation. In cases of remnant tumor, an update of navigation was performed with intraoperative images. Tumor volume was quantified pre- and intra-operatively by segmentation of T2-abnormality in low-grade and contrast enhancement in high-grade gliomas. They found that in 25.9% of all cases examined, additional tumor mass was removed as a result of the information provided by iMRI. This led to complete tumor resection in 20 cases, increasing the rate of gross-total removal from 31.7% to 38.6%. In 56 patients, additional but incomplete resection was performed due to close location to eloquent brain areas.

Leuthardt et al. (2011) recently reported their experience with the combination of awake craniotomy and iMRI for resection of gliomas in close proximity to eloquent cortex. They studied 12 patients undergoing this procedure. They found that the extent of resection was limited because of proximity to eloquent areas in 5 cases: language areas in 3 patients and motor areas in 2 patients. Additional tumor was identified and resected after iMRI in 6 cases. Average operating room time was 7.9 hours (range 5.9 - 9.7). They concluded that awake craniotomy and iMRI can be safely performed to maximize resection of tumours near eloquent language areas.

In summary, many centres have now reported significant improvements in extent of resection, without increased rates of neurologic deficit, using iMRI in glioma surgery. Most importantly, this surgical improvement has lead to longer survival.

3.4 Ultrasound co-registered with MRI

The first reports of the use of intraoperative brain ultrasonography (US) to image the brain were published well over 50 years ago (French et al., 1950; Ballantine et al., 1950; Balantine et al., 1950). Reports using real-time B-mode 2D US imaging, as we know it today, were published in the early 80s (Voorhies & Patterson, 1980; Rubin et al., 1980). 2D US can be used at the beginning of the operation, while on dura, to image the tumor and its relationship to brain structures including ventricles, blood vessels, gyri, sulci and rigid structures such as the falx and tentorium. Such imaging, prior to dural opening, is similar to the preoperative MRI since tumor resection has not yet taken place and brain shift is minimal. US can also be used on the surface of the brain or within the resection cavity provided an adequate probe-fluid interface can be maintained. US is useful as an intraoperative imaging tool since it can be used throughout the operation to update the surgeon with respect to residual tumor and help identify the surgical location. Imaging in real-time compensates for the problem of brain shift which compromises neuronavigation techniques since they are based on the static preoperative images. A major drawback of 2D US is that the real-time images are displayed in a plane corresponding to probe positioning and not the conventional axial, sagittal and coronal planes commonly used by neurosurgeons. Such arbitrary orientation can be confusing and unsettling for many neurosurgeons.

To address this issue, tracked US or 3D US was developed. In this technique, the US probe is registered to the neuronavigation system and the 2D images are acquired and reformatted into 3D. These images can then be displayed with the corresponding MR images to better orient the user, an attractive solution for most neurosurgeons. To assess the usefulness of 3D US in detected tumor, Unsgaard et al. (2005) compared 3D ultrasound with preoperative MR images in 28 tumor cases and found that ultrasound was at least as good as MRI in identifying tumor borders. Other studies have also validated the accuracy of US in brain tumor surgery. Gerganov et al. (2008) compared 3D US reconstructions with iMRI during brain tumor resection procedures and found that the image quality before the resection to be of similar quality with both modalities. Similarly, van Velthoven et al. [23] found that ultrasound is as reliable as MRI to delineate gliomas, metastases and meningiomas. In fact, it may even be superior to MRI in defining low-grade tumor boundaries (Unsgaard et al., 2005).

Three dimensional US may be useful in identifying tumor, but does its lead to an increased extent of resection? To answer this question, Unsgaard et al. (2002) reported on their series of cases in which the operation was taken to the point at which the impression was that no residual tumor remained. At this time 3D US imaging was used and revealed previously unidentified residual tumor was found in 53% of cases.

More recently, 3D US has been improved to take into account brain shift during the course of the operation. Using a non-linear algorithm, Mercier et al. (2011) have shown that they are able to fit the US taken during and at the end of the operation with the preoperative MRI taking into account brain shift so as to provide the surgeon with real-time imaging referenced to the preoperative MRI. They found that interpreting the post-resection ultrasound is easier when properly registered with the preoperative MRI and with the pre-resection ultrasound. Further studies are necessary to determine if this translates into increased extent of resection.

3.5 Fluorescence guided resection

The ability to visualize the tumor intraoperatively, and distinguish it from normal brain would present an ideal situation allowing for maximal resection of brain cancers. Such a technique would require high sensitivity and specificity.

5-aminolevulinic acid (5-ALA) is a natural biochemical precursor of hemoglobin that elicits synthesis and accumulation of fluorescent porphyrins in various epithelia and cancerous tissue (Mlkvy et al., 1998). The topical form of this agent is FDA approved for and has been employed for dermatologic surgery (Roberts & Cairnduff, 1995; Lang et al., 2001; Sadick, 2010). 5-ALA is produced at the cytosolic surface of the mitochondrial membrane and then transported to the cellular cytosol for hemebiosynthesis (Kennedy et al., 1990; Kennedy & Potter, 1992; Henderson et al., 1995; Kloek et al., 1996). The availability of 5-ALA in the cell cytoplasm is the rate limiting factor in heme biosynthesis in all but erythopoetic cells. Heme biosynthetic enzymes are more active in brain cancer than in normal brain tissue. As a result, addition of ALA (the rate-limiting agent and precursor) to malignant glial cells leads to an increase in the intracellular accumulation of protoporphorin IX, a fluorescent intermediary in heme biosynthesis (Kennedy et al., 1990; Kennedy & Potter, 1992; Henderson et al., 1995; Kloek et al., 1996). As a result, malignant glial cells fluoresce red relative to normal brain tissue when visualized under ultraviolet light.

Stummer et al. (1998) reported on the sensitivity and specificity of 5-ALA. Intraoperatively detected areas of weak or strong fluorescence are tumor-cell positive in the majority of cases [84.8% (90% CI: 70.7% - 93.8%)], and only a low number of fluorescent (all weakly) biopsies are tumor cell negative (3.8% of all biopsies taken). The minimum tumor cellularity of 4.5% is requried for 5-ALA detectable under fluorescence light. Approximately two thirds of non-fluorescent biopsies taken from normal adjacent tissue are tumor-cell positive, demonstrating the invasive growth pattern of malignant glioma. 5-ALA-induced fluorescence detection sometimes fails to identify areas that show contrast-enhancement in postoperative MR, especially in those areas that are not accessible by the blue light source.

Several European centers have investigated the role of 5-aminolevulinic acid in fluorescence guided resection of newly diagnosed Grade III/IV astrocytomas (Stummer et al., 1998; Stummer et al., 2000; Stummer et al., 2006). Stummer et al. (2006) demonstrated in their randomized multicenter phase III trial (n = 322 patients, dose of 20 mg/kg body weight) a gross total resection rate of 63.6% in the experimental arm (5-ALA guided resection) versus 37.6% in the control arm (standard white light resection). Clinically, this translated into a higher 6 month progression free survival than those allocated to white light resection (41.0% versus 21.1%). This trial is the first study that showed prospectively that fluorescence-guidance increases the completeness of resection of malignant gliomas.

In the clinical studies 5-ALA has proven to be safe. Events have been classified according to their relationship to the drug, and those related to the combination of drug and procedure. During the last 2 years in the post marketing studies in Europe under a stringent risk management program, no significant adverse effects have been reported to regulatory authorities in Europe.

In 2006 it was reported that the use of 5-ALA was associated with improved gross tumor resection when used as a fluorescent agent in high grade glioma (Stummer et al., 2006). This European registration trial for 5-ALA as a fluorescent guided probe for tumor visualization, revealed a marked improvement in percentage of patients achieving gross total resection compared to normal operating white light (64% vs 38%, $p < 0.001$). Randomized control trials in both Canada and United States of America are in the final stages of preparation.

4. Conclusion

Since the routine use of early post-operative MRI to accurately quantify extent of resection has become common, studies are now being reported revealing that increased extent of resection yields improvements in overall survival. However, even in cases of complete resection of the MRI based gadolinium-enhancing portion of the tumor, tumors always recur and the prognosis is poor.

While MRI based imaging is the current standard for tumor imaging, labelled tracer PET imaging is emerging as a complimentary technique to better visualize the entirety of the tumor. Just as it is difficult to visualize the entirety of the tumor on imaging, it is also difficult to visualize the tumor, and distinguish it from normal brain, intraoperatively. Imaging tools that can be used to increase the rate of resection include iMRI, 3D US, and fluorescence guided surgery.

5. References

Adams, H. Jr., del Zoppo, G. et al. Guidelines for the Early Management of Adults With Ischemic Stroke: A Guideline From the American Heart Association/American Stroke Association Stroke Council, Clinical Cardiology Council, Cardiovascular Radiology and Intervention Council, and the Atherosclerotic Peripheral Vascular Disease and Quality of Care Outcomes in Research Interdisciplinary Working Groups: The American Academy of Neurology affirms the value of this guideline as an educational tool for neurologists. Circulation 2007;115:e478-534.

Ballantine HTJr, Bolt RH, Hueter TF, Ludwig GD (1950) On the detection of intracranial pathology by ultrasound, vol 112. Science, New York, pp 525 - 528

Ballantine HT, Jr, Ludwig GD, Bolt RH, Hueter TF (1950) Ultrasonic Localization of the cerebral ventricles. Trans Am Neurol Assoc 51:38–41

Bammer R. Basic principles of diffusion-weighted imaging. Eur J Radiol 2003;45:169-84.

Becherer A, Karanikas G, Szabó M, et al. Brain tumour imaging with PET: a comparison between [^{18}F]fluorodopa and [^{11}C]methionine. Eur J Nucl Med Mol Imaging 2003;30:1561-7.

Brandsma D, van den Bent MJ. Pseudoprogression and pseudoresponse in the treatment of gliomas. Curr Opin Neurol 2009;22:633-8.

Brandsma D, Stalpers L, Taal W, Sminia P, van den Bent MJ. Clinical features, mechanisms, and management of pseudoprogression in malignant gliomas. Lancet Oncol 2008;9:453-61.

Bruehlmeier M, Roelcke U, Schubiger PA, Ametamey SM. Assessment of Hypoxia and Perfusion in Human Brain Tumors Using PET with 18F-Fluoromisonidazole and 15O-H2O. J Nucl Med 2004;45:1851-9.

Cao Y, Sundgren PC, Tsien CI, Chenevert TT, Junck L. Physiologic and Metabolic Magnetic Resonance Imaging in Gliomas. J Clin Oncol 2006;24:1228-35.

Chan AA, Lau A, Pirzkall A, et al. Proton magnetic resonance spectroscopy imaging in the evaluation of patients undergoing gamma knife surgery for Grade IV glioma. J Neurosurg 2004;101:467-75.

Chen W, Silverman DHS, Delaloye S, et al. 18F-FDOPA PET Imaging of Brain Tumors: Comparison Study with 18F-FDG PET and Evaluation of Diagnostic Accuracy. J Nucl Med 2006;47:904-11.

Chen W, Silverman DHS. Advances in Evaluation of Primary Brain Tumors. Semin Nucl Med 2008;38:240-50.

Croteau D, Scarpace L, Hearshen D, et al. Correlation between magnetic resonance spectroscopy imaging and image-guided biopsies: semiquantitative and qualitative histopathological analyses of patients with untreated glioma. Neurosurgery 2001;49:823-9.

Desprechins B, Stadnik T, Koerts G, Shabana W, Breucq C, Osteaux M. Use of Diffusion-Weighted MR Imaging in Differential Diagnosis Between Intracerebral Necrotic Tumors and Cerebral Abscesses. AJNR Am J Neuroradiol 1999;20:1252-7.

de Wit MC, de Bruin HG, Eijkenboom W, Sillevis Smitt PA, van den Bent MJ. Immediate post-radiotherapy changes in malignant glioma can mimic tumor progression. Neurology 2004;63:535-7.

French LA, Wild JJ, Neal D (1950) Detection of cerebral tumors by ultrasonic pulses; pilot studies on postmortem material. Cancer 3:705 - 708

Fueger BJ, Czernin J, Cloughesy T, et al. Correlation of 6-18F-Fluoro-L-Dopa PET Uptake with Proliferation and Tumor Grade in Newly Diagnosed and Recurrent Gliomas. J Nucl Med 2010;51:1532-8.

Gerganov VM,Akbarian A, SamiiA, Samii M, FahlbuschR (2008) Intraoperative visualization of tumor resection in patients with intracranial tumors—a comparison of two-dimensional ultrasound and high-field MRI. 59th annual meeting of the German society of neurosurgery (DGNC), Würzburg

Hatiboglu MA, Weinberg JS, Suki D, Rao G, Prabhu SS, Shah K, Jackson E, Sawaya R. Impact of intraoperative high-field magnetic resonance imaging guidance on glioma surgery: a prospective volumetric analysis. Neurosurgery. 2009 Jun;64(6):1073-81;

Henderson BW, Vaughan L, Bellnier DA, van Leengoed H, Johnson PG, Oseroff AR. Photosensitization of murine tumor, vasculature and skin by 5-aminolevulinic acid-induced porphyrin. PhotochemPhotobiol. Oct 1995;62(4):780-789.

Herholz K, Hölzer T, Bauer B, et al. 11C-methionine PET for differential diagnosis of low-grade gliomas. Neurology 1998;50:1316-22.

Minim Invasive Neurosurg. 2005 Apr;48(2):77-84. Impact of intraoperative MRI on the surgical results for high-grade gliomas. Hirschberg H, Samset E, Hol PK, Tillung T, Lote K.

Jacobs AH, Kracht LW, Gossmann A, et al. Imaging in Neurooncology. Neurorx 2005;2:333-47.

Kim Y, Chang K, Song I, et al. Brain abscess and necrotic or cystic brain tumor: discrimination with signal intensity on diffusion-weighted MR imaging. Am J Roentgenol 1998;171:1487-90.

Kinoshita M, Goto T, Okita Y, et al. Diffusion tensor-based tumor infiltration index cannot discriminate vasogenic edema from tumor-infiltrated edema. J Neurooncol 2010;96:409-15.

Kläsner BD, Krause BJ, Beer AJ, Drzezga A. PET imaging of gliomas using novel tracers: a sleeping beauty waiting to be kissed. Expert Rev Anticancer Ther 2010;10:609-13.

Kennedy JC, Pottier RH, Pross DC. Photodynamic therapy with endogenous protoporphyrin IX: basic principles and present clinical experience. J PhotochemPhotobiol B. Jun 1990;6(1-2):143-148.

Kennedy JC, Pottier RH. Endogenous protoporphyrin IX, a clinically useful photosensitizer for photodynamic therapy. J PhotochemPhotobiol B. Jul 30 1992;14(4):275-292.

Kloek J, Beijersbergen van H. Prodrugs of 5-aminolevulinic acid for photodynamic therapy. PhotochemPhotobiol. Dec 1996;64(6):994-1000.

Kono K, Inoue Y, Nakayama K, et al. The Role of Diffusion-weighted Imaging in Patients with Brain Tumors. AJNR Am J Neuroradiol 2001;22:1081-8.

Kuhnt D, Ganslandt O, Schlaffer SM, Buchfelder M, Nimsky C. Quantification of glioma removal by intraoperative high-field magnetic resonance imaging - an update.. Neurosurgery. 2011 May 26. [Epub ahead of print]

Kunz M, Thon N, Eigenbrod S, et al. Hot spots in dynamic18FET-PET delineate malignant tumor parts within suspected WHO grade II gliomas. Neuro-oncol 2011;13:307-16.

Law M, Yang S, Babb JS, et al. Comparison of Cerebral Blood Volume and Vascular Permeability from Dynamic Susceptibility Contrast-Enhanced Perfusion MR Imaging with Glioma Grade. AJNR Am J Neuroradiol 2004;25:746-55.

Lang K, Schulte KW, Ruzicka T, Fritsch C. Aminolevulinic acid (Levulan) in photodynamic therapy of actinic keratoses. Skin Therapy Lett. Sep 2001;6(10):1-2, 5.

Leuthardt EC, Lim CC, Shah MN, Evans JA, Rich KM, Dacey RG, Tempelhoff R, Chicoine MR.. [Epub ahead of print] Utilization of Movable High Field Strength Intraoperative Magnetic Resonance Imaging with Awake Craniotomies for Resection of Gliomas. A Preliminary Experience. Neurosurgery. 2011 Apr 14

Lu S, Ahn D, Johnson G, Law M, Zagzag D, Grossman RI. Diffusion-Tensor MR Imaging of Intracranial Neoplasia and Associated Peritumoral Edema: Introduction of the Tumor Infiltration Index1. Radiology 2004;232:221-8.

McGirt MJ, Chaichana KL, Gathinji M, et al. Independent association of extent of resection with survival in patients with malignant brain astrocytoma. J Neurosurg. Jan 2009;110(1):156-162.

McKnight TR, von dem Bussche MH, Vigneron DB, et al. Histopathological validation of a three-dimensional magnetic resonance spectroscopy index as a predictor of tumor presence. J Neurosurg 2002;97:794-802.

Mercier L, Del Maestro RF, Petrecca K, Kochanowska A, Drouin S, Yan CX, Janke AL, Chen SJ, Collins DL.

New prototype neuronavigation system based on preoperative imaging and intraoperative freehand ultrasound: system description and validation. Int J Comput Assist Radiol Surg. 2011 Jul;6(4):507-22.

Mlkvy P, Messmann H, Regula J, et al. Photodynamic therapy for gastrointestinal tumors using three photosensitizers--ALA induced PPIX, Photofrin and MTHPC. A pilot study.Neoplasma. 1998;45(3):157-161.

Moffat BA, Chenevert TL, Lawrence TS, et al. Functional diffusion map: A noninvasive MRI biomarker for early stratification of clinical brain tumor response. Proc Natl Acad Sci U S A 2005;102:5524-9.

Nariai T, Tanaka Y, Wakimoto H, et al. Usefulness of L-[methyl-11C] methionine-positron emission tomography as a biological monitoring tool in the treatment of glioma. J Neurosurg 2005;103:498-507.

Norden AD, Young GS, Setayesh K, et al. Bevacizumab for recurrent malignant gliomas: efficacy, toxicity, and patterns of recurrence. Neurology 2008;70:779-87.

Pauleit D, Floeth F, Hamacher K, et al. O-(2-[18F]fluoroethyl)-l-tyrosine PET combined with MRI improves the diagnostic assessment of cerebral gliomas. Brain 2005;128:678-87.

Pirotte B, Goldman S, Dewitte O, et al. Integrated positron emission tomography and magnetic resonance imaging-guided resection of brain tumors: a report of 103 consecutive procedures. J Neurosurg 2006;104:238-53.

Pirotte BJ, Levivier M, Goldman S, et al. Positron emission tomography-guided volumetric resection of supratentorial high-grade gliomas: a survival analysis in 66 consecutive patients. Neurosurgery 2009;64:471-81; discussion 81.

Rachinger W, Goetz C, Popperl G, et al. Positron emission tomography with O-(2-[18F]fluoroethyl)-l-tyrosine versus magnetic resonance imaging in the diagnosis of recurrent gliomas. Neurosurgery 2005;57:505-11; discussion -11.

Roberts DJ, Cairnduff F. Photodynamic therapy of primary skin cancer: a review. Br J Plast Surg. Sep 1995;48(6):360-370.

Roberts HC, Roberts TPL, Brasch RC, Dillon WP. Quantitative Measurement of Microvascular Permeability in Human Brain Tumors Achieved Using Dynamic Contrast-enhanced MR Imaging: Correlation with Histologic Grade. AJNR Am J Neuroradiol 2000;21:891-9.

Rock JP, Scarpace L, Hearshen D, et al. Associations among Magnetic Resonance Spectroscopy, Apparent Diffusion Coefficients, and Image-Guided Histopathology with Special Attention to Radiation Necrosis. Neurosurgery 2004;54:1111-9 10.227/01.NEU.0000119328.56431.A7.

Rubin JM, Mirfakhraee M, Duda EE, Dohrmann GJ, Brown F (1980) Intraoperative ultrasound examination of the brain. Radiology137:831 - 832

Sadick N. An open-label, split-face study comparing the safety and efficacy of levulankerastick (aminolevulonic acid) plus a 532 nm KTP laser to a 532 nm KTP laser alone for the treatment of moderate facial acne. J Drugs Dermatol. Mar;9(3):229-233.

Schiepers C, Dahlbom M, Chen W, et al. Kinetics of 3'-Deoxy-3'-18F-Fluorothymidine During Treatment Monitoring of Recurrent High-Grade Glioma. J Nucl Med 2010;51:720-7.

Clin Neurol Neurosurg. 2010 Apr;112(3):237-43. Epub 2009 Dec 24. Low field intraoperative MRI-guided surgery of gliomas: a single center experience. Senft C, Franz K, Ulrich CT, Bink A, Szelényi A, Gasser T, Seifert V.

Stummer W, Stocker S, Wagner S, et al. Intraoperative detection of malignant gliomas by 5-aminolevulinic acid-induced porphyrin fluorescence. Neurosurgery. Mar 1998;42(3):518-525; discussion 525-516.

Stummer W, Novotny A, Stepp H, Goetz C, Bise K, Reulen HJ. Fluorescence-guided resection of glioblastoma multiforme by using 5-aminolevulinic acid-induced porphyrins: a prospective study in 52 consecutive patients. J Neurosurg. Dec 2000;93(6):1003-1013.

Stummer W, Pichlmeier U, Meinel T, Wiestler OD, Zanella F, Reulen HJ. Fluorescence-guided surgery with 5-aminolevulinic acid for resection of malignant glioma: a randomised controlled multicentre phase III trial. Lancet Oncol. May 2006;7(5):392-401.

Stummer, W., Reulen, H., Meinel, T., Pichlmeier, U., Schumacher, W., &Tonn, J. (2008).Extent of resection and survival in GlioblastomaMultiforme; Identification of and adjustment of bias. Neurosurgery, 62, 564-576.

Stupp R, Mason WP, van den Bent MJ, et al. Radiotherapy plus concomitant and adjuvant temozolomide for glioblastoma. N Engl J Med. Mar 10 2005;352(10):987-996.

Sundgren PC. MR Spectroscopy in Radiation Injury. AJNR Am J Neuroradiol 2009;30:1469-76.

Taal W, Brandsma D, de Bruin HG, et al. Incidence of early pseudo-progression in a cohort of malignant glioma patients treated with chemoirradiation with temozolomide. Cancer 2008;113:405-10.

Unsgaard G, Ommedal S, Muller T, Gronningsaeter A, Nagelhus Hernes TA (2002) Neuronavigation by intraoperative three-dimensional ultrasound: initial experience during brain tumor resection. Neurosurgery 50:804 - 812; discussion 812

Acta Neurochir (Wien). 2005 Dec;147(12):1259-69; discussion 1269. Epub 2005 Sep 19. Ability of navigated 3D ultrasound to delineate gliomas and metastases--comparison of image interpretations with histopathology. Unsgaard G, Selbekk T, Brostrup Müller T, Ommedal S, Torp SH, Myhr G, Bang J, Nagelhus Hernes TA.

Voorhies RM, Patterson RH (1980) Preliminary experience with intra-operative ultrasonographic localization of brain tumors. Radiol Nucl Med 10:8 - 9

Warach S, Chien D, Li W, Ronthal M, Edelman RR. Fast magnetic resonance diffusion-weighted imaging of acute human stroke. Neurology 1992;42:1717.

Weber WA, Wester H-J, Grosu AL, et al. O-(2-[^{18}F]Fluoroethyl)-L-tyrosine and L-[methyl-^{11}C]methionine uptake in brain tumours: initial results of a comparative study. Eur J Nucl Med Mol Imaging 2000;27:542-9.

Weybright P, Sundgren PC, Maly P, et al. Differentiation Between Brain Tumor Recurrence and Radiation Injury Using MR Spectroscopy. Am J Roentgenol 2005;185:1471-6.

Neurosurg. 2006 Mar;104(3):360-8.Effectiveness of neuronavigation in resecting solitary intracerebral contrast-enhancing tumors: a randomized controlled trial.Willems PW, Taphoorn MJ, Burger H, Berkelbach van der Sprenkel JW, Tulleken CA.

Wirtz CR, Albert FK, Schwaderer M, Heuer C, Staubert A, Tronnier VM, Knauth M, Kunze S. The benefit of neuronavigation for neurosurgery analyzed by its impact on glioblastoma surgery. Neurol Res. 2000 Jun;22(4):354-60.

Zhou J, Tryggestad E, Wen Z, et al. Differentiation between glioma and radiation necrosis using molecular magnetic resonance imaging of endogenous proteins and peptides. Nat Med 2011;17:130-4.

8

Podocalyxin in the Diagnosis and Treatment of Cancer

Kelly M. McNagny[1], Michael R. Hughes[1], Marcia L. Graves[1], Erin J. DeBruin[1], Kimberly Snyder[1], Jane Cipollone[1], Michelle Turvey[2], Poh C. Tan[1], Shaun McColl[2] and Calvin D. Roskelley[1]

1. Introduction

Although their functions in tumour development and progression are not well understood, several secreted and membrane-associated mucins have proven to be valuable diagnostic and prognostic markers in human cancer and many of these are targets for cancer vaccines and therapies (Singh et al., 2008; Chauhan et al., 2009; Kufe, 2009). Podocalyxin-like protein 1 (**podocalyxin**, gene name ***PODXL***) is a member of the CD34 family of sialomucins. Podocalyxin (PC), also called PCLP1, gp135, MEP21, and thrombomucin, is a single-pass type I transmembrane protein primarily expressed by vascular endothelia, specialized kidney epithelial cells called podocytes, and a limited set of hematopoietic progenitor cells in adult mice and humans (Nielsen & McNagny, 2009b). Expression of PC has also been noted on the luminal face of kidney tubule cells, breast and ductal lumens, oviductal luminal cells, mesothelial cells and neurons in normal mammalian tissues. Polymorphisms and inappropriate or increased expression of PC is linked to several human cancers including germ-line cancers, several carcinomas, malignant astrocytoma and leukemia. In many of these cancers, detection of high levels of PC expression is associated with high-grade, aggressive tumours, increased risk of metastases and poor prognosis. In this review, we will examine the known and proposed functions of PC in normal (adult and embryonic) and cancerous cells, the molecular mechanisms regulating these functions, and potential applications of PC as a molecular marker in the diagnosis, prognosis and treatment of cancer.

2. Podocalyxin expression and normal function in mammals

2.1 Podocalyxin has an essential role in the development and function of the kidney glomerulus

PC is named for its expression on specialized kidney epithelial cells called podocytes. On these cells, PC is required for the development of the foot process that, together with fenestrated vascular endothelia, form the filtration apparatus of the glomerulus (reviewed in Nielsen & McNagny, 2009b). Unlike vascular and hematopoietic tissues where other members of the CD34 family are co-expressed, PC is the only CD34-family sialomucin

[1]*The University of British Columbia, Canada*
[2]*The University of Adelaide, Australia*

expressed on podocytes and therefore serves a non-redundant function in podocyte development. Germ-line deletion of *Podxl* in mice results in anuria and death within 24 hours of birth due to the failure of embryonic podocytes to undergo appropriate morphogenesis and form foot processes - one of the most potent mucin-dependent knockout phenotypes described (Doyonnas et al., 2001).

Although many tissue types and cell lineages express PC during mouse embryogenesis (and presumably human), PC's only essential function identified so far is the formation of the glomerular filtration apparatus of the kidney. However, we are beginning to discover more subtle roles for PC in the development, morphogenesis, polarization and motility of cells that form the lumen of tubules and ducts (or boundary elements in tissues) including kidney tubules, ovary ducts, mammary ducts and vascular lumens. For example, germ-line deletion of *Podxl* in mice causes a delay in the formation of lumens between adjacent endothelial cells of the developing aorta (Strilic et al., 2009) and reduces the adhesion of the mesothelia lining of the gut surface mesothelia to the umbilicus during embryogenesis (Doyonnas et al., 2001). From these and other embryonic analyses we have developed the concept that podocalyxin acts a general anti-adhesive that aids in the demarcation of tissue boundaries (McNagny et al., 1997; Doyonnas et al., 2001). PC expression is also required for efficient neurite outgrowth and branching in the developing brain (Vitureira et al., 2005, 2010). Despite these subtle developmental delays or abnormalities, in all tissues we have examined so far, save the kidney, *Podxl*$^{-/-}$ mouse neonates appear to be remarkably normal.

In adult mice and humans, PC is primarily restricted to vascular endothelia, kidney podocytes and a subset of hematopoietic stem cells. In addition, PC expression has also been reported on some mature blood types including mouse "stress" erythroid progenitors (and anemia-induced erythroblasts) (Doyonnas et al., 2005; Sathyanarayana et al., 2007; Maltby et al., 2009) and activated rat platelets (Miettinen et al., 1999). Although others and we have proposed a role for PC (and the CD34 antigen) in facilitating the trafficking of hematopoietic progenitors cells to the bone marrow (BM) as well as more mature blood cells from the BM or periphery to sites of inflammation (Nielsen & McNagny, 2008, 2009a, 2009b), the function of PC expression on normal hematopoietic cells remains enigmatic.

In summary, although PC has a critical role in kidney development, PC appears to be dispensable for the normal development of other tissues we have examined including vascular endothelia, breast duct epithelia and hematopoietic tissues. However, after increasingly more detailed analyses, we have also found that PC has subtle roles in these tissues under conditions of tissue remodeling and development that may have consequences in disease pathogenesis (unpublished observations).

2.2 Transcriptional regulation of *PODXL* expression

The regulation of *PODXL* expression is modulated by several transcription factors, epigenetic methylation of CpG islands in the *PODXL* promoter and by expression of micro RNA (miR-199a2). Depending on the cell lineage and disease state, *PODXL* expression can be induced by Sp1 (specificity protein 1) and Wilms' tumour suppressor protein 1 (WT1). The *PODXL* promoter contains multiple binding sites for Sp1 and there is evidence of direct binding of WT1 to the *PODXL* promoter (Palmer et al., 2001; Butta et al., 2006). While Sp1 is expressed in many cell types and has many targets in the human genome, Sp1 is upregulated in many cancers including epithelial carcinomas (reviewed in Li & Davie, 2010). WT1 is primarily expressed in developing kidney and in the podocytes of the glomerulus in normal kidney. However, WT1 is overexpressed in cancers of the kidney, lung and breast and in acute leukemia and myelodysplastic syndromes. Thus, both Sp1 and WT1 may influence the expression of *PODXL* in cancers.

Adult erythroid cells express PC in response to anemic stress via erythropoietin receptor (EpoR)-dependent activation of the signal transducer and activator of transcription 5 (STAT5) (Sathyanarayana et al., 2007). Although *PODXL* expression via STAT5 has not been demonstrated in other cell types, STAT5 activation can be induced in epithelial cells by a variety of mechanisms. For example, with respect to the pathogenesis of carcinomas (especially prostate and breast cancers) STAT5 activation downstream of the prolactin receptor activation is one possible route to enhanced PC expression (Jacobson et al., 2010).

Transcriptional repressors of *PODXL* include the ubiquitously expressed tumour suppressor transcription factor p53 (*TP53*) and the integrin-associated adaptor protein PINCH1 (*LIMS1*) (Stanhope-Baker et al., 2004; Wang et al., 2011). PINCH1 is normally associated with focal adhesion complexes in podocytes but becomes dissociated from these in response to transforming growth factor beta (TGFβ) stimulation (Wang et al., 2011). PINCH1 then enters the nucleus and antagonizes WT1 transcriptional activation of *PODXL* (Wang et al., 2011). Since TGFβ can induce *PODXL* expression in a human lung adenocarcinoma cell line (**see §3.5.1**) (Meng et al., 2011), the role of TGFβ and PINCH1 in the regulation of *PODXL* expression may be specific to podocytes (or normal, adherent epithelia). Finally, *PODXL* is a target for miR-199a2, a micro RNA that is normally expressed in epithelial cells of many tissues (Cheung et al., 2011). miR-199a2 targets (represses) a collection of transcripts and has a putative role as a tumour suppressor in several human cancers (**see §3.7.2**).

3. Podocalyxin is a diagnostic marker and prognostic indicator in cancer

Within the last 5-7 years, retrospective analysis of tumour tissue archives by histology, protein and transcript expression analyses have identified increased PC expression or *PODXL* gene polymorphisms in several human cancers. In this section, we will outline what is known of PC expression patterns in human cancers including epithelial carcinomas (kidney, breast, thyroid, lung, ovarian, prostate and gastrointestinal cancer), germ-cell tumours (testicular cancer), astrocytomas (brain cancer) and leukemia (**Table 1**). In general, in studies where PC expression has been correlated with tumour behaviour and patient outcome data, PC expression in primary tumour cells is associated with increased tumour aggressiveness, risk of distant metastases and poor prognosis. Mechanistic studies using human cancer cell lines suggest that PC expression in tumour cells is not just merely correlative with aggressiveness, but may have a direct contribution to tumour progression, survival and metastases. In addition to the potential this wealth of data offers for the development of PC-targeted adjuvant treatments for systemic cancer, these findings and accompanying mechanistic studies provide insights into the molecular mechanisms of tumour progression and metastases. While it is clear that there remain many technical challenges for the development of PC-targeted cancer treatments, implementation of clinically beneficial diagnostics is feasible and compatible with existing technology and methods, requiring only a concerted validation effort.

Review Section (§) Primary Tissue	Podocalyxin expression profile	Diagnostic & Prognostic Significance
§3.1.1 Kidney (Renal cell carcinoma)	• PC protein expression 4-fold higher in cancerous cells of rare subset of RCC tumours (~10%) • PC expression in primary RCC correlates with risk of metastasis and poor patient outcome. Hazard ratios (HR) (PC^+ *vs.* PC^- RCC primary tumors) HR = 3.6 (metastasis-free survival) HR = 7.5 (disease-specific survival) (Hsu et al., 2010)	• PC expression in tumor cells correlates with increased risk of aggressive tumor phenotype, and is an independent predictor of distant metastases and poor prognosis
§3.1.2 Kidney (Nephroblastoma)	• Higher PC transcript expression (↑ 1.5 fold) in more aggressive anaplastic (advanced grade) compared to low grade nephroblastoma (Stanhope-Baker et al., 2004)	• Diagnostic marker (transcript) of anaplastic grade nephroblastoma
§3.2 Breast carcinoma	• High PC protein expression in rare "node-negative" subset of breast carcinoma (~6%) • PC overexpression in primary breast tumours associated with increased relative risk of poor outcome (RR = 8.45) (Somasiri et al., 2004)	• PC expression in tumor cells correlates with increased risk of aggressive tumor phenotype, and is an independent predictor of distant metastases and poor prognosis
§3.3 Ovarian carcinoma	• High expression of PC on tumour cells in 67% of all ovarian epithelial tumours and 87% of high-grade serous epithelial ovarian carcinoma • PC cytoplasmic expression not associated with disease-outcome in high-grade serous ovarian tumours, but cell surface expression of PC is an independent predictor of poor patient outcome with HR ~ 1.6 (compared to PC-negative high-grade serous ovarian tumor) (Cipollone et al, submitted)	• Prognostic marker of poor outcome in high-grade serous ovarian cancer when PC overexpression is cell surface localized
§3.4 Thyroid carcinoma	• High expression of PC protein common (~52% cases) in undifferentiated thyroid carcinoma (UTC) subtype but not detected in normal thyroid epithelia or other thyroid cancer cells (Yasuoka et al., 2008)	• Diagnostic and staging marker of undifferentiated thyroid carcinoma
§3.5 Lung (small-cell lung carcinoma)	• PC protein expression detected in tumour cells in majority (~87.5%) in small-cell lung carcinoma (SCLC) (Koch et al., 2008)	• Diagnostic marker (tissue biopsy)
§3.6 Prostate carcinoma	• *PODXL* germ-line polymorphism and SNP are associated with increased risk of developing prostate cancer with an aggressive tumor. In-frame single or double deletion polymorphism in exon 1 associated with increased risk of prostate cancer Odds ratio (OR) = 2.14-2.58 (all prostate cancer) OR = 3.04-4.42 (aggressive disease) SNP (G340A) resulting in missense mutation associated with increased risk of prostate cancer OR = 1.48 (all prostate cancer) (Neville et al., 2002) • Possible increased PC expression in metastatic tumor but not primary prostate tumours (**Fig. 5**) (Yu et al., 2004; Chandran et al., 2007)	• Genetic marker of prostate cancer risk • High expression of PC a potential prognostic marker of tumour aggressiveness and metastases

Review Section (§) Primary Tissue	Podocalyxin expression profile	Diagnostic & Prognostic Significance
§3.7 Testicular (germ cell tumour)	• PC antigens (GCTM-2, TRA-1-60/81) detected in serum of testicular cancer patients (35-75% NSGCT cases) (Schopperle et al., 2003) • *PODXL*-targeting miR-199a downregulated in testicular cancer (Cheung et al., 2011)	• Potential serum marker for testicular cancer • PC potentially equally or more robust marker of testicular cancer compared to α-fetoprotein or chorionic gonadotrophin
§3.8.1 Liver (hepatocellular carcinoma (HCC))	• High expression of PC protein detected in sinusoidal endothelial associated with HCC but not normal adjacent tissue or cirrhotic lesions (Chen et al., 2004; Heukamp et al., 2006)	• Differential diagnosis of HCC *vs.* cirrhotic lesions (tissue biopsy)
§3.8.2 Pancreatic ductal adenocarcinoma	• PC protein expressed in primary tumours of 42% pancreatic ductal adenocarcinoma (PDAC) and 30% ampullary ductal carcinoma but rarely in other primary tumours of GI origin (e.g., liver, colon, esophagus) • High PC expression more often detected in high-grade PDAC (53% Grade 3, 48% Grade 2 and 18% Grade 1) (Ney et al., 2007)	• Possible identification of primary tissue of metastatic tumours from a suspected GI source
§3.8.3 Colon carcinoma	• PC protein and peptides detected in media and lysate of colon carcinoma cell lines. Expression not yet determined in colon cancer primary tumours. (Thomas et al., 2009)	• Potential serum marker for colon cancer
§3.9 Hematopoietic	• PC protein expression commonly detected (77-87% cases) in diffuse pattern (immunohistology) in formalin-fixed bone marrow biopsy in majority cases of AML, ALL and myeloid sarcoma (Kelley et al., 2005). • Cell surface expression in 20% AML from fresh blood or bone marrow samples (flow cytometry) • (Riccioni et al., 2006).	• Potential diagnostic marker (tissue biopsy), however significance to disease phenotype and outcome not known • Potential surface marker of AML blasts in peripheral blood
§3.10 Brain (astrocytoma)	• High PC protein and transcript expression in ~50% cases of high-grade malignant astrocytomas (anaplastic astrocytoma and glioblastoma) but not low-grade astrocytic tumours (Hayatsu et al., 2008).	• Diagnostic marker of high grade/anaplastic astrocytoma

Table 1. Summary of podocalyxin expression profiles in human cancers.

3.1 Kidney cancer

3.1.1 Renal cell carcinoma

Renal cell carcinoma (RCC), which accounts for 85% of renal cancers, originates from epithelial cells of the renal tubules (Cohen & McGovern, 2005). In a retrospective study, PC protein expression was examined in a collection of 303 formalin-fixed, paraffin-embedded RCC tumours (Hsu et al., 2010). Of these, 29 tumour specimens (9.6%) were found to express PC protein in cancerous cells (4-fold over non-expressors) (Hsu et al., 2010). In contrast, in normal kidney and the majority of RCC patient tumours, PC is only detected in the glomerulus and vascular endothelia (Hsu et al., 2010). Patient outcome data showed that PC-positive RCC tumours were much more likely to be high-grade, advanced-stage tumours (Hsu et al., 2010). Importantly, patients with PC-positive RCC also had decreased disease-specific and metastasis-free survival and PC-positive RCC tumours (stage I-III) were more likely to result in distant metastases (i.e., non-lymph node sites) (Hsu et al., 2010). These findings suggest that PC expression in primary RCC tumours is a strong and independent predictor of distant metastasis and poor prognosis (Hsu et al., 2010). Thus, by identifying a rare, high-risk RCC sub-type, evaluation of PC expression has clear potential diagnostic and prognostic value.

3.1.2 Wilms' tumor (Nephroblastoma)

Wilms' tumour, or nephroblastoma, the most common pediatric kidney cancer, has a unique histological presentation indicative of aberrant or incomplete kidney development during embryogenesis (Huff, 2011). Unlike most of the cancers discussed in this review, PC expression (transcript) is significantly *reduced* in 64 patient nephroblastoma samples (relative mean 0.29) compared to pooled normal fetal kidney (Stanhope-Baker et al., 2004). Although WT1 is a positive regulator of *PODXL* expression (Palmer et al., 2001), and loss of WT1 expression is associated with some Wilms' tumours, there was no evidence of a correlation between *PODXL* and *WT1* expression in this study (Stanhope-Baker et al., 2004). However, perhaps of diagnostic value, this same study showed that *PODXL* expression was increased in more aggressive, anaplastic tumours compared to 40 non-anaplastic tumors (Stanhope-Baker et al., 2004). Notably, functional loss of p53 is associated with the most aggressive, anaplastic nephroblastomas with poor prognosis. As p53 negatively regulates *PODXL* expression (Stanhope-Baker et al., 2004), enhanced *PODXL* expression in anaplastic nephroblastomas may be explained directly by this genetic pathway. Although more study is required to know if enhanced *PODXL* expression in anaplastic nephroblastoma has a direct role in promoting tumour aggressiveness, expression of PODXL in nephroblastoma may be useful as a marker of poorly differentiated, anaplastic tumours.

3.2 Breast carcinoma

3.2.1 Expression of podocalyxin is an independent predictor of poor outcome in invasive breast carcinoma

In normal human breast tissue, expression of PC protein is relatively low and restricted to the apical face of the luminal duct epithelia and, as in most tissues, PC also marks the lumen of vascular endothelia in the breast (Somasiri et al., 2004). However, in a survey of tissue microarray constructed from 272 primary tumour samples from patients with locally invasive breast cancer, high expression of PC protein was detected in a small subset (6%) of invasive breast carcinomas (Somasiri et al., 2004). Notably, PC-positive primary tumours were associated with significantly higher risk of poor outcome (decreased disease-specific survival) compared to patients with tumours expressing little or no PC (Somasiri et al., 2004). PC-positive tumours were not significantly different in histological classification, size or risk of lymph node metastasis. However, PC expressing tumours were more likely to present at an advanced tumour grade, express p53, and be negative for estrogen receptor (ER) (*ESR1*) and HER-2 (*ERBB2*) (Somasiri et al., 2004). These data reveal that high expression of PC in primary, locally invasive breast carcinoma is a strong and independent predictor of poor outcome (Somasiri et al., 2004). As with its detection of rare RCC subsets, evaluation of PC expression in primary breast carcinomas may have immediate diagnostic and prognostic value in guiding treatment or surveillance strategies in breast cancer. In addition, detailed profiling of PC-tumours may provide a deeper understanding of tumour progression mechanisms. Related to these efforts, in the next section we discuss some of the molecular mechanisms that underlay PC's role in promoting progression of invasive breast cancer to metastatic breast carcinoma.

3.2.2 Podocalyxin regulates breast cancer tumour cell invasiveness and migration *in vitro*

In order to gain insight into the biological role of PC in breast cancer, we, as well as other investigators, have surveyed the expression of *PODXL* and its intracellular ligands, NHERF-1 and -2, in human breast cancer cell lines and examined the effects of altering its expression on the behavior of these cells *in vitro* and *in vivo*. Recent microarray analysis of a collection of 50 human breast cancer cell lines revealed a wide range of expression of *PODXL*, NHERF-1 (*SLC9A3R1*) and NHERF-2 (*SLC9A3R2*) transcripts (Kao et al., 2009) **(Fig. 1)**. *PODXL* tends to be highly expressed in estrogen receptor- and progesterone receptor (PR)-negative (ER^-/PR^-) basal-like breast cancer lines. Conversely, high NHERF-1 and NHERF-2 expression correlates with luminal-type, ER^+ breast cancers. MCF7 cells are a line of luminal-like breast epithelial cells (Neve et al., 2006; Kao et al., 2009) obtained by pleural effusion (i.e., lung metastases) of a patient with metastatic invasive ductal adenocarcinoma (ER^+/PR^+)(Soule et al., 1973). Relative to other breast cancer cell lines, MCF7 expresses low-moderate levels of endogenous *PODXL* transcripts and high levels of NHERF-1 (and low to moderate expression of NHERF-2) (Kao et al., 2009) (**Fig. 1**). MDA.MB.231 cells, which express high levels of endogenous PODXL, are a basal B-subtype breast cancer cell line derived from pleural effusion of human metastatic breast adenocarcinoma (Kao et al., 2009) **(Fig. 1)**. In contrast to MCF7 cells, MDA.MB.231 are ER^-/PR^- and have a highly invasive phenotype in *in vitro* assays and *in vivo* xenograft models (Lacroix and Leclercq, 2004; Neve et al., 2006).
By overexpressing exogenous PC and structural mutants in MCF7 cells or by suppressing endogenous PC in MDA.MB.231 cells using RNA-interference (RNAi) methods, we (and others) have found that PC promotes a more aggressive, invasive phenotype *in vitro* and *in vivo* (Somasiri et al., 2004; Sizemore et al., 2007). In addition, our preliminary results corroborate a role for PC in breast cancer invasion since suppression of endogenous *PODXL* in MDA.MB.231 impairs serum-dependent migration *in vitro* (Turvey & McColl, unpublished observations). We are currently working to determine if silencing *PODXL* expression down regulates invasion-associated adhesion molecules and matrix proteinases and how loss of *PODXL* alters the morphology and cytoskeletal dynamics in MDA.MB.231.

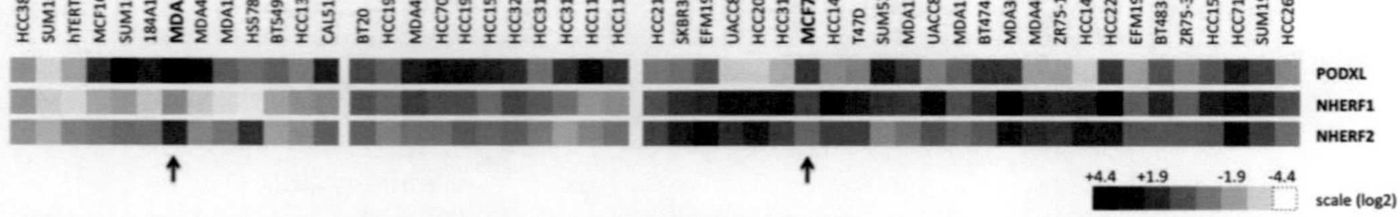

Fig. 1. Transcript expression levels of PODXL, NHERF1 and NHERF2 in a collection of human breast cancer cell lines. Arrows indicate the luminal-like MCF7 and basal (B)-like MDA.MB.231 breast cancer cell lines commonly used in the study of PC function. The transcript expression heat map was generated from meta-analysis of publically available microarray gene expression profiles of human breast cancer cell lines (Kao et al., 2009) using Gene Cluster 3.0 and Java TreeView.

3.2.3 Podocalyxin modulates EMT-independent breast cancer progression and metastatic potential

Epithelial-to-mesenchymal transition (EMT) is an important paradigm in the understanding of tumor progression to systemic, metastatic cancer (discussed in more detail in **§3.5.1**). However, EMT is not an obligate pathway to metastases (Wicki et al., 2006), and invasive ductal breast carcinomas, which form the great majority of locally invasive breast lesions, retain epithelial characteristics and epithelial differentiation markers (Cleton-Jansen, 2002; Sarrio et al., 2008). Thus, a better understanding of EMT-independent mechanisms of tumour invasion and metastasis is critical for developing therapeutic strategies in ductal breast carcinoma in particular, but also other cancers in general.

By expressing exogenous *PODXL* in MCF7 cells, we have found that PC promotes altered morphogenesis, loss of adhesion and impaired tumour cell aggregation in 3D spheroid cultures (Graves and Roskelley, manuscript in preparation). Importantly, altered adhesion is not associated with disruption of cell-cell junctions, impaired expression or re-localization of cell-cell junction regulators (e.g., E-cadherin, β-catenin, ZO-1) or, disruption of extra-cellular matrix (ECM) adhesion complexes (e.g., β1-integrin, activated focal adhesion kinase (FAK)). Rather, expression of PC in polarized cells enhances the exclusion of β1-integrins from the free, apical surface of MCF7 and recruits F-actin from the basolateral ECM-adhesion complexes to an expanded apical membrane domain. We hypothesize that PC-mediated redistribution of F-actin and other cortical actin components weakens adhesion of the basolateral membrane domain to ECM. Moreover, when single cells are shed from the epithelial sheets, PC is redistributed in a global pattern that blocks homotypic adhesion. Expression of PC on shed, single cells may also promote chemotaxis, enhance adhesion-free survival or participate in the homing to distant tissue sites (**Fig. 2**). Thus, while PC expression in some epithelial tissues may help to define the apical domain and reinforce polarization, dysregulated mistargetting or overexpression of PC disrupts normal tissue architecture of epithelial sheets and spheroids and may promote invasive and metastatic characteristics.

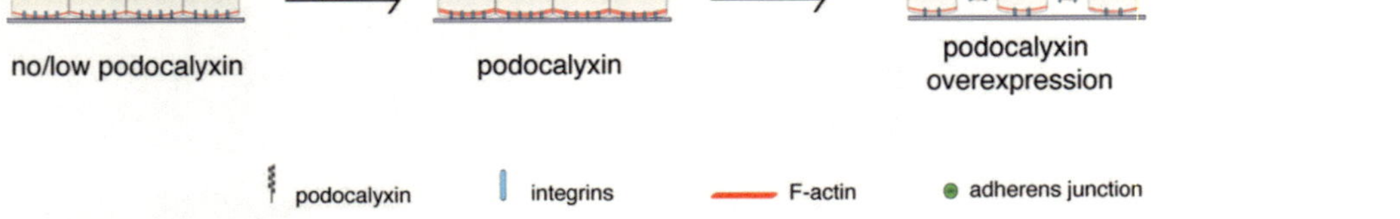

Fig. 2. Podocalyxin expression defines the apical domain of polarized epithelia but promotes non-EMT loss of adhesion and shedding when overexpressed.

Finally, to gain some insight into the *in vivo* function of PC in the growth, local invasion and metastatic potential of human breast cancers, we have used tumor xenograft models. In preliminary experiments, sub-cutaneous transplantation of MCF7 or PC-overexpressing MCF7 cells into immunodeficient mice (Rag2M) suggests that expression of high levels of

PC enhance tumour growth and density (Graves and Roskelley, manuscript in preparation). In addition, although the PC–positive MDA.MB.231 cell line forms lung tumors in NOD-SCID *Il2rγ* -/- (NSG) mice 6-8 weeks after intravenous injection, PC-deficient MDA.MB.231 cells fail to form lung tumours (Turvey and McColl, unpublished observations). Because equal numbers of PC-positive and PC-negative MDA.MB.231 tumor cells appear in the pulmonary parenchyma at early time points (3-14 days), we hypothesize that PC promotes survival in recipient lung tissue (Snyder, Hughes and McNagny, unpublished observations). We are continuing to use these models, and orthotopic mammary fat pad transplant breast tumour models, to fully characterize PC's role in breast tumour invasion and metastases. In summary, the data suggest PC plays a key role in enhancing breast carcinoma growth and invasiveness *in vivo*.

3.3 Ovarian carcinoma

Ovarian cancer remains the most lethal gynecological cancers and, like most epithelial carcinomas, systemic spread generally has a poor prognosis since there are currently no curative interventional therapies. PC is expressed in normal mesothelia-derived tissues that encase the ovaries and make up the free luminal surface of cells that line the oviducts and endometrium (Cipollone and Roskelley, manuscript submitted). In addition, PC protein is detectable in the tumor cells of approximately two-thirds of human ovarian carcinoma cases. Although the mere presence of PC protein in ovarian carcinomas does not correlate with disease outcome, expression of PC on the cell surface (as opposed to intracellular localization) is predictive of poor outcome for high-grade serous ovarian carcinoma, 87% of which express significant amounts of the mucin.

As with breast cancer cell lines, PC expression in ovarian cancer lines is variable (Cipollone and Roskelley, *ibid*). To evaluate PC's molecular functions in ovarian carcinoma, we ectopically expressed PC in the serous carcinoma-derived cell line (OVCAR-3) originally derived from malignant ascites (Hamilton et al., 1983). OVCAR-3 cells express epithelial differentiation markers, form well-structured adherent epithelial sheets in culture, and are generally non-invasive and have low motility *in vitro* (Comamala et al., 2011). Forced expression of PC in OVCAR-3 cells reduced *in vitro* adhesion to extracellular matrices including; mesothelial-cell layers, immobilized β1-integrin antibodies and fibronectin. As with other epithelial cells, exogenously expressed PC is preferentially localized to the apical free surface of OVCAR-3 cell layers in 2D culture and spheroids in 3D culture. As observed in MCF7 cells, PC excludes β1-integrin from free apical domains. Thus, when expressed at the cell surface, PC may act as an anti-adhesin in serous ovarian carcinoma by sterically masking integrin-extracellular matrix interactions, and, by promoting cortical cytoskeletal rearrangements that weaken adhesion to ECM. This PC-induced morphogenesis may be of critical importance to ovarian carcinoma progression, as these tumors very often metastasize after small nodules are shed, in an anti-adhesive (non-EMT dependent) fashion, into the abdominopelvic cavity. Thus, while PC-driven non-EMT shedding and migration may be rare in some epithelial cancers (breast and renal), PC expression may be a common, and critically important molecular mechanism driving tumour metastasis in high-grade serous ovarian carcinoma.

3.4 Thyroid carcinoma

Thyroid carcinomas (non-lymphoma, squamous cell or sarcoma) are classified according to histological characteristics and origin. The most common "differentiated" subtypes (papillary and follicular) are highly treatable and responsive to therapy. The medullary and undifferentiated (anaplastic) sub-types, although more rare, have a less favorable prognosis. Although PC is normally absent on thyroid epithelia and is not detected in well-differentiated thyroid carcinoma tumour subtypes or squamous cell carcinoma (thyroid), in immunohistological analyses of 238 thyroid tumours, PC was detected on tumours of over half the cases (n=69) of undifferentiated thyroid carcinoma (UTC). In addition, in cases where the thyroid tumours have a mixed histological type (UTC adjacent to differentiated tumour cells), PC was detected only on cells with UTC phenotype (Yasuoka et al., 2008). We note that the pattern of PC expression on thyroid carcinoma and small-cell lung carcinoma (**§3.5**) (correlates with a "de-differentiated" tumour phenotype consistent with an EMT transformation. Thus, although PC may not be sufficient to drive EMT, high expression on UTC and other mechanistic studies (**§3.5.1**) suggest that PC expression may be upregulated as part of an EMT program. If this is so, similar to its function in EMT-independent tumours, PC may help to promote a non-cohesive, invasive phenotype during EMT.

3.5 Small-cell lung carcinoma

Small-cell lung carcinomas (SCLC) (16% of lung cancers) are malignancies that typically arise from epithelial cells of the proximal airways (bronchus). SCLC tumours consist of multipotent epithelial ("stem-like") cells that form typically diffuse and non-cohesive clusters. Analysis of formalin-fixed, paraffin-embedded bronchial-tumour biopsies (and adjacent normal bronchial tissues) reveals that the majority of SCLC but not normal bronchial epithelia expresses PC and its expression in SCLC correlates with non-methlyated CpG islands in the *PODXL* gene (Koch et al., 2008).

Although PC is not detected in normal adult bronchial epithelium, clusters of PC-positive epithelial cells can be detected in deep pockets of developing proximal bronchi and trachea of fetal lung (Koch et al., 2008). The authors suggest the intriguing hypothesis that *PODXL* marks multipotent bronchial epithelial cells during lung development and that SCLC "cancer stem cells" may retain or acquire the characteristics of this stem-like population. There are currently no studies that correlate PC expression with patient outcome or response to chemotherapy in lung cancers. PC expression in non-small cell lung carcinomas (NSCLC) was not performed in this study so it is not yet known if PC also marks primary NSCLC tumours of the lung. For these reasons, the diagnostic value of PC expression in lung cancer is less certain than in other cancers. However, although many technical challenges remain, identification of tumour-specific glycoforms of PC (see following sections) may provide targets for adjuvant therapy in lung cancer. This is particularly important in SCLC where surgical resection of tumours is more difficult. Alternatively, if PC expression is consistently associated with type 3 EMT processes in lung cancer (see below), or other EMT-dependent cancer metastases, expression of PC (assessed by biopsy or *in vivo* imaging) may herald a switch from locally invasive to a more advanced disease stage.

3.5.1 Podocalyxin in TGFβ-mediated epithelial-to-mesenchymal transition (EMT)

Epithelial-mesenchymal transition (EMT) (type 3) is a paradigm of tumour invasion and metastasis whereby epithelial cells lose their apical and basal polarization and robust cell-cell contacts to become mesenchymal in morphology and adopt an invasive, migratory behaviour (Kalluri and Weinberg, 2009). Among many other alterations in gene expression patterns, EMT is associated with loss of the adherens-junction regulator E-cadherin (*CDH1*), stabilization and nuclear-localization of β-catenin (*CTNNB1*), and upregulation of the intermediate filament protein vimentin (*VIM*), a mesenchymal marker (Zeisberg and

Neilson, 2009). As we have noted above, PC does not appear to be capable of initiating EMT on its own. However, Wilkins et al. have recently demonstrated that it may contribute to the EMT that is initiated by transforming growth factor beta (TGFβ) (Meng et al., 2011).

Although TGFβ has tumour suppressing activity in some cancers, especially at the early stages of tumour progression, TGFβ, in the context of enhanced phosphatidylinositol-3-kinase (PI3K)/Akt and other survival signalling pathways can drive EMT processes (Ouyang et al., 2010). TGFβ-induced de-differentiation is not limited to malignant cells, as normal human and mouse podocytes undergo an EMT-like transition in response to TGFβ (Herman-Edelstein et al., 2011; Li et al., 2008; Wang et al., 2011). A549, a human lung adenocarcinoma cell line, undergoes EMT-like transformation in the presence of TGFβ, with prototypical EMT features including down regulation of E-cadherin, upregulation of vimentin, expression of MMP2 and fibronectin and, secretion of collagens (type I, III and IV) (Kasai et al., 2005). These alterations in gene expression pattern are accompanied with altered cell morphology, loss of cell-cell contact and enhanced migration (Kasai et al., 2005; Meng et al., 2011).

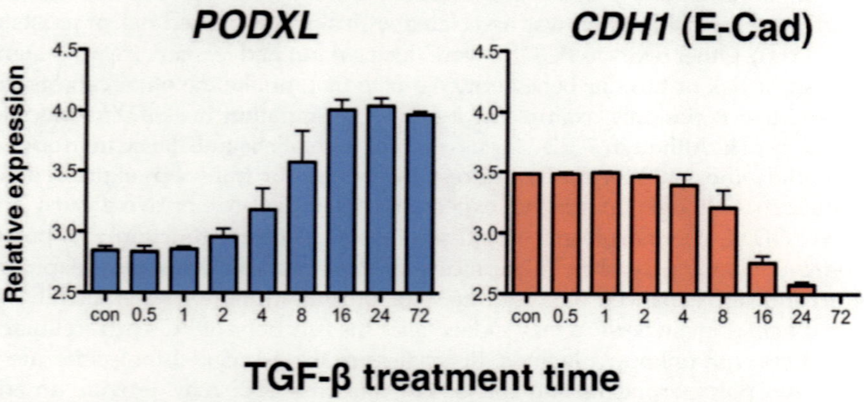

Fig. 3. *PODXL* expression is upregulated during TGFβ-induced EMT of a lung adeno-carcinoma cell line (A549). Expression profiles where generated by meta-analysis of publically available gene expression data using the Gene Expression Omnibus (GEO) dataset GDS3710 (Sartor et al., 2010).

Meng et al recently demonstrated that PC protein expression is upregulated in response to TGFβ1 (Meng et al., 2011) . A query of a publically available gene expression dataset of A549 cells undergoing TGFβ1-induced EMT corroborates their findings and shows that the kinetics of PODXL transcript expression are similar to EMT-associated down regulation of E-cadherin (*CDH1*) transcript (Sartor et al., 2010) **(Fig. 3)**. Intriguingly, using a gene-silencing approach (shRNA), Meng et al show that PC is required for at least some EMT-related processes including mesenchyme-like morphogenesis, cell migration and changes in expression of E-cadherin and vimentin (Meng et al., 2011). PC was also found to co-distribute with newly secreted collagen I at the leading edge of migrating TGFβ-treated A549 cells. In addition, collagen I could be co-precipitated with anti-PC antibodies in TGFβ-treated A549 cells. Notably, the collagen I-binding integrins (α1β1 and α2β1) were not identified in collagen I-PC complexes or detected in PC-collagen membrane domains. Thus, one possible role for PC in a collagen-complex could be the exclusion of collagen- or matrix-binding integrins from the leading edge of migrating cells and intercellular destabilization of strong adhesion to ECM - themes consistent with our findings using breast and ovarian cancer cell lines (**§3.2.3 & 3.3**).

We note that in this example, PC expression is down-stream (or parallel) to TGFβ1-induced EMT. Thus, while high expression of PC in some tumour cells (e.g, breast carcinoma) can promote EMT-independent tumour progression, PC may also support the invasive and migratory functions of tumour cells that have undergone EMT.

3.6 Prostate carcinoma

A 1.1 Mb region of human chromosome 7q32-33 flanked by microsatellite markers D7S2452 and D7S684 strongly linked to prostate tumour aggressiveness contains the *PODXL* locus (Neville et al., 2002). In a sibling-pair study, a variable in-frame, germ-line deletion of one or two Ser-Pro repeats in the PC mucin domain (deletion of residues 23-24 or 23-26) was found to be associated with enhanced risk of developing prostate cancer (increased overall risk (OR)=2-2.5 fold) and increased tumour aggressiveness (OR=3-4.4 fold) (Casey et al., 2006). In addition, a missense single-nucleotide polymorphism (SNP, *G340A*) resulting in a Ser substitution at Gly114 (also in the mucin domain) was associated with a 50% increased risk of prostate cancer (Casey et al., 2006). Other SNPs in *PODXL* were detected but had lesser correlative significance to prostate cancer risk or tumour behaviour. We note that, unlike the other cancers discussed in this review, this is the only example of a germ-line mutation in *PODXL* associated with increased cancer risk. Although 7q32-33 is a region of high allelic imbalance in prostate cancer, this patient study did not specifically address PC protein or transcript expression levels in prostate tumours. Although we may not expect that deletion of one or two glycosylation sites arising from *PODXL* polymorphisms would significantly alter PC function, it is possible that such in-frame deletions may alter PC surface stability, apical localization or expression and therefore account for enhanced aggressiveness of prostate tumours. Alternatively, in-frame deletions of mucin domain Ser-Pro may indeed alter the functions of PC's extracellular domain or its association with unknown ligands. Regardless of the associated molecular mechanism, *PODXL* deletion polymorphisms and the *G340A* missense SNP may provide an additional genetic screening method to evaluate prostate cancer risk.

3.6.1 Forced expression of podocalyxin enhances the motility of prostate cancer cells

PC3 cells are a human prostatic adenocarcinoma cell line derived from bone metastases (Kaighn et al., 1979). PC3 cells, which are considered to have a relatively high metastatic potential and invasive phenotype in comparison to other prostate cancer lines, do not express detectable levels of PC by western analysis (Sizemore et al., 2007). However, as for other epithelial tumour cell lines, forced expression of full-length PC in this prostate cell line enhanced cell motility *in vitro* (Sizemore et al., 2007). This enhanced motility may depend on the activation of Rac1 that, in turn, requires the association with two intracellular binding proteins, NHERF1 and ezrin. Thus, as for other carcinomas discussed in this review, expression of PC in prostate epithelial has the potential to impart a more aggressive phenotype with potential clinical importance. Further study of PC expression profiles in primary or secondary prostate tumors, coupled to tumour phenotype and outcome data, are required to evaluate whether expression of PC has diagnostic value in prostate cancer. Query of microarray gene expression data from normal prostate tissue and primary and secondary prostate cancer suggest that *PODXL* expression may not be altered in primary prostate tumors (**Fig. 4**). Conversely, metastatic tumours originating from the prostate may have increased *PODXL* expression (~1.4 fold) (**Fig. 4**). Therefore, it is unclear if the increased risk and tumour aggressiveness associated with this *PODXL* polymorphism is related to altered PC function, expression or simply another marker that is linked to allelic imbalance of 7q32-33.

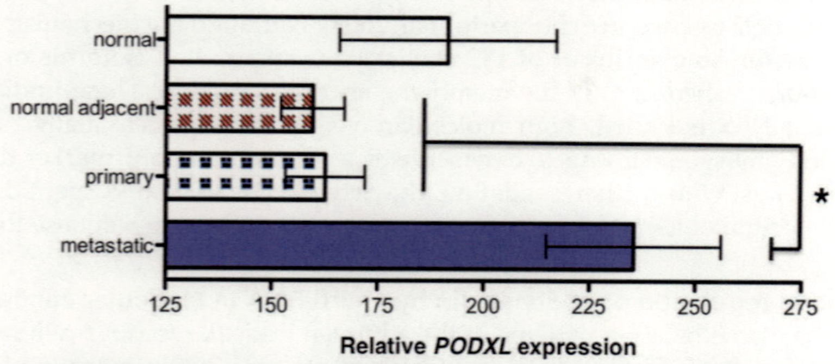

Fig 4. Expression of PODXL in normal human prostate tissue and prostate cancer (GEO dataset GSE6919) (Chandran et al., 2007; Yu et al., 2004). The metastatic tumour group is significantly different than the normal adjacent and primary tumour groups but not the normal donor group (*$p < 0.05$, Tukey one-way ANOVA analysis). All other group comparisons are not significantly different.

3.7 Testicular cancer and embryonal carcinoma

Testicular cancer, the most common cancer in young males, has a high cure rate even after systemic spread (reviewed in Winter & Albers, 2011). However, risk stratification and classification of the primary tumour by histological methods and determination of tumour marker levels is important for designing surveillance and systemic treatment strategy in the event of metastasis or re-lapses. The vast majority of testicular tumours (95%) can be broadly classified as either seminomatous- (SGCT) or non-seminomatous- (NSGCT) germ cell tumours. Seminomas are non-pluripotent, undifferentiated germ cell progenitors whereas non-seminomas tumours are comprised of several subtypes arising from embryonic or extraembryonic (e.g., yolk sac) lineages. Embryonal carcinomas and teratomas are examples of sub-types of NSGCT. Importantly, treatment strategies for SGCT and NSGCT cancers are different, with the major difference being that NSGCTs are generally resistant to radiotherapy.

PC is antigenically identical to tumour markers originally designated GCTM-2 (or gp200), TRA-1-60 and TRA-1-80 expressed on embryonal carcinoma (EC) cell lines and inner blastocyst-derived human embryonic stem cells (hESCs) (Schopperle et al., 2003; Schopperle & DeWolf, 2007). The TRA-1-60/81 epitopes are present only on a high molecular weight form of PC (200 kD) expressed by undifferentiated embryonal carcinoma or hESCs. Intriguingly, the antigenic sites detected by these antibodies disappear following retinoic acid (RA)-induced differentiation of ECs or following differentiation of ESCs into embryoid bodies (EBs) (Schopperle and DeWolf, 2007). However, EBs continue to express a lower molecular weight isoform (170 kD) of PC that can be detected using antibodies recognizing peptide epitopes, or by the terminal glycan, β-(D)-galactose (Galβ)-binding plant lectin, peanut agglutinin (PNA) (Schopperle and DeWolf, 2007). Thus, there is evidence to suggest that there are tumor and tissue type specific epitopes on PC. These epitopes are present on primitive or pluripotent germ-line tumours or hESCs.

GCTM-2 has been identified as a tumour marker of NSGCT and a soluble form of GCTM-2 has been detected in the sera in 7 of 20 patients diagnosed with NSGCT. In addition, TRA-1-

60 was present in the sera of over 75% of patients (n=42) with NSGCT and even in two-thirds of NSGCT patients negative for the "gold-standard" testicular cancer serum tumour markers, α-fetoprotein and chorionic gonadotrophin (Mason et al., 1991; Badcock et al., 1999; Gels et al., 1997 as cited in Schopperle et al, 2003). Although the mechanism has not yet been defined, serum-soluble forms of PC may arise from secreted isoforms or proteolytic cleavage (membrane shedding) of the membrane anchored protein. These findings suggest that PC; especially a modified, high molecular weight form preferentially expressed in undifferentiated embryonic lineages, may serve as a sensitive tumour marker detectable in patient serum. Thus, with further validation, the detection of soluble PC peptide fragments could aid in detection of testicular germ-line tumours and evaluating response to therapy.

3.7.1 Epigenetic regulation of podocalyxin by micro RNA in testicular cancer

In a screen of gene methylation patterns in the a human testicular tumour cell line (NT2) (an embryonic carcinoma), Cheung et al (Cheung et al., 2011) recently identified a hypermethylated region in intron 14 of the dynamin 3 locus (*DNM3*) located on chromosome 1(q24). This region codes for the expression of three micro RNAs (miR), including miR-199a2 (hsa-mir-199a-2) in an antisense orientation. miR-199a2, together with miR-199a-1 (located on hChr 19p13), encode the pre-microRNA species miR-199a. Reduced expression of miR-199a has previously been linked to poor prognosis in serous ovarian carcinoma (Nam et al., 2008) and pro-inflammatory and anti-apoptotic pathways in chemoresistant ovarian cancer stem cells (Yin et al., 2010). miR-199a, which is normally abundantly expressed in most human epithelial and non-epithelial tissues (with the notable exception of brain and peripheral blood mononuclear cells (Liang et al., 2007)), targets a cluster of genes that include transcripts encoding PC, HIF-1α, IKKβ and SIRT1α, mTOR, SMAD1 and c-MET and several others (Cheung et al., 2011). Note that regulation of these targets by miR-199a and expression of the miR-199a-1 and miR-199a-2 loci is tissue specific. For example, reduced expression of miR-199a (along with other miRs) has also been linked to bladder cancer (Ichimi et al., 2009). Conversely, miR-199a expression is upregulated with a cluster of other miRs in metastatic uveal melanoma and gastric cancer (Ueda et al., 2010; Worley et al., 2008).

The miR-199a2 pre-microRNA is processed to yield two mature miR species, miR-199a-5p and miR-199a-3p, and both are down regulated in malignant testicular tumours in comparison to normal or benign tumour tissue (Cheung et al., 2011). miR-199a-5p and -3p have distinct RNA targets, and only miR-199a-5p is a direct negative regulator of *PODXL*. Expression of miR-199a-5p negatively correlates with PC protein expression in malignant testicular tumors (both seminomatous and non-seminomatous) (Cheung et al., 2011). Ectopic expression of miR199-a in NT2 cells attenuates migration and invasion *in vitro* and tumour growth and metastatic potential in xenograft transplant models. Suppression of *PODXL* in NT2 cells by RNAi also attenuates matrix invasion in an *in vitro* assay. These data suggest that epigenetic regulation of the ha-miR-199a-2 locus by CpG methylation results in repression of miR-199a2 expression and upregulation of *PODXL* and that these events correlate with tumour malignancy in testicular cancer. Other targets of miR-199a-5p and -3p are also likely involved in the invasive phenotype of testicular tumours.

3.8 Gastrointestinal cancers

3.8.1 Hepatocellular carcinoma

Hepatocellular carcinoma (HCC) is a common adult liver malignancy associated with infection by hepatitis (HVB and HVC) and cirrhotic liver disease. Patients with cirrhosis from a variety of causes are at an increased risk of developing HCC. Unfortunately, the majority of HCC patients (>80%) present with systemic or locally advanced tumours that cannot be cured surgically. Although recently, the application of anti-angiogenic drugs (e.g., sorafenib) has shown promise in slowing tumour growth in HCC patients, chemotherapy and radiotherapy are ineffective, and HCC has a very low five-year survival rate (~5%). Prompt detection and diagnosis of HCC in cirrhotic liver by imaging methods or histological assessment of biopsy is critical for designing an effective treatment strategy.

Although one group showed that PC was only weakly present in 9% of HCC tumours (i.e., neoplastic liver epithelial cells) (Ney et al., 2007), PC and CD34 were commonly upregulated on sinusoidal endothelia associated with primary HCC tumour tissue (Chen et al., 2004; Heukamp et al., 2006). In contrast, in normal liver tissue, PC is restricted to hepatic arterioles (Heukamp et al., 2006). PC and CD34 are also present (in a more punctuate pattern) on the sinusoidal endothelia of hyperplastic focal nodules and liver adenomas (Heukamp et al., 2006). Thus, expression of PC (and CD34) may provide an additional diagnostic marker for the evaluation of liver biopsies in HCC. PC and CD34 are widely expressed in vascular endothelia in adult tissues but their function remains ill-defined. Although PC has been shown to play a role in the formation of vascular lumens in the developing embryo, it is not essential for the homeostatic maintenance of vascular endothelia in adults (at least in mice). Nevertheless, mounting evidence suggests that PC and CD34 have a role in the formation of new vessels during development and vascularization of solid tumours; and, the maintenance of vessel integrity in inflamed tissues (Blanchet et al., 2008; Maltby et al., 2011; Strilic et al., 2009). Thus, further study of the role of CD34 and PC in neovascularization and vessel homeostasis may provide new targets for anti-angiogenic treatments for solid tumours.

3.8.2 Pancreatic ductal adenocarcinoma

Pancreatic ductal adenocarcinoma (PDAC) is the most common pancreatic cancer, often detected at an advanced stage. Because there are no effective systemic therapies, PDAC diagnosis typically has a very poor prognosis (~3% 5-yr survival). Determining the primary source of adenocarcinoma is important in treatment strategies and prognosis. Neoplasms originating from the pancreatic duct, gall bladder, bile duct, ampulla of Vater and duodenum are difficult to distinguish by immunohistology alone since many express a similar profile of epithelial cytokeratin- and mucin-family proteins. Immunohistochemical analysis of primary adenocarcinoma and carcinoma tumours of gastrointestinal, pancreatic and extrapancreatic origin suggest expression of PC is associated with primary epithelial neoplasms of the pancreatic duct (44%) or ampullary origin (30%) (Ney et al., 2007). Although PC is expressed is less than half of these adenocarcinomas, it is not detected (or very weak) in normal or inflamed pancreas (chronic pancreatitis) or in most primary tumours from all other gastrointestinal sites including bile duct. Although these data suggest that expression of PC may be useful for the differential identification of primary adenocarcinoma, it is not known if PC expression at secondary tumour sites correlates with their primary origin. However, expression of PC does appear to correlate with more advanced histological tumour grade, as 53% of Grade 3, 48% of Grade 2 and 18% of Grade 1 tumours express PC (Ney et al., 2007). Thus, as with several other epithelial malignancies described in this review, expression of PC correlates with a more anaplastic, poorly differentiated phenotype and more aggressive (or advanced) cancers.

3.8.3 Colorectal cancer

Although the expression of PC has not been verified in primary or metastatic tumours in human colorectal cancer, two studies have identified PC expression in colon cancer cell lines, and PC protein as a shed, soluble component of colon cancer cell cultures (Ito et al., 2007; Thomas et al., 2009) In addition, Thomas et al (Thomas et al., 2009) demonstrated that PC, immunopurified from a colon cancer cell line (LS174T), can act as an E- and L-selectin ligand (but not P-selectin) using a PC-coated microbead flow adhesion assay. E/L-selectin binding was dependent on a sialofucosylated epitope of PC expressed in LS174T, similar to, but distinct from sulfated sLe^x epitopes present on sialomucins processed in HEV (see **§5.2**) (Thomas et al., 2009). Thus, tumor-specific modifications (glycosylation) of PC may allow for interaction with selectins.

Importantly, neither of these studies showed that PC protein is expressed on the surface of colon carcinoma cells (as opposed to intracellular), or that PC serves as an E/L-selectin adhesive ligand *in vitro* or *in vivo*. If PC were indeed shown to be a *bona fide* E/L-selectin ligand on these carcinomas, this would offer an attractive target for the development of adjuvant therapies. This is especially true if the unique modification of PC detected in human colon cancer cell lines is recapitulated in primary and metastatic colorectal adenomas and carcinomas. Retrospective analyses of tissue microarrays of primary colorectal carcinomas and adenocarcinomas (and perhaps metastatic, secondary tumour sites) similar to those performed for RCC and breast cancer are required to determine if expression of PC is associated with colorectal cancers and if expression correlates with patient outcome. At least one study (Ney et al., 2007) suggested that PC is not commonly expressed in gastrointestinal tumours, including colon-derived, with the exception of pancreatic cancers. Then again, this is also true for breast and renal cancer – the prognostic power of evaluating PC expression in human cancer appears to be in identifying rare, highly lethal sub-types.

3.9 AML, ALL and cutaneous myeloid sarcoma

PC expression has been reported on a human monocytic cell line (U937) after induced differentiation with vitamin D3 and transforming growth-factor beta (TGFβ) and on normal human monocytes treated with macrophage colony-stimulating factor (MCSF) for 3-6 days *in vitro* (Riccioni et al., 2006). In both cases, PC expression correlates with a more differentiated, monocytic cell-surface marker phenotype (e.g., CD14$^+$CD11b$^+$). However, PC expression has not been reported on human monocytes derived from normal bone morrow (BM) or peripheral blood (Kelley et al., 2005).

Kelley et al (Kelley et al., 2005) found that PC is often expressed on leukemic blasts including 77% (n = 39) of acute myeloid leukemia (AML), 81% (n = 27) acute lymphoid leukemia (ALL) and 87% (n=15) cases of cutaneous myeloid sarcoma (Kelley et al., 2005). Expression of PC was detected in all clinical sub-types of AML (M1-M7) and both T and B-cell lineage ALL. A second study reported a much lower frequency of PC-positive blasts in 73 cases of AML with approximately 20% of cases presenting with a moderate frequency of PC-positive cells (20-50% positive blasts (+)) and 18% displaying high frequency (>50% positive blasts (++)) (Riccioni et al., 2006). Importantly, while Kelley et al used immunohistochemical analysis of formalin-fixed BM biopsy tissue and PC was observed in a punctuate, cytoplasmic distribution; Ricconini et al used freshly isolated BM or peripheral blood-derived leukemic blasts and flow cytometery analysis (i.e., cell-surface expression of PC). Thus, while PC is commonly expressed in leukemic blasts in the BM, cell-surface exposure of PC is likely more rare (at least in AML).

There are no studies that address the clinical consequences of PC expression in leukemia. Expression of PC in hematopoietic malignancies may reflect transformation of an immature progenitor that normally expresses PC or a "de-differentiation" gene expression pattern of a leukemic stem cell. We have found that expression of PC in mouse hematopoietic stem or progenitor cells (HSC/Ps) enhances CXCR4-induced chemotaxis and BM-homing/retention (**see §6.2.3**) (Nielsen & McNagny, 2009a) (and our unpublished observations). Thus, one possible consequence of PC overexpression in leukemia may be that PC enhances close contact to CXCL12-secreting cells and, subsequently, an advantage (over normal hematopoietic progenitors or PC-negative leukemia) with to respect retention, proliferation, survival or chemo-resistance of leukemic cells.

3.10 Malignant astrocytic tumours

Astrocytomas, tumours originating from astrocytes of the brain and spinal cord, are the most common neoplasm of the central nervous system (Zhu & Parada, 2002). Often presenting at an advanced stage, astrocytic tumours are classified into four histological grades that broadly include benign (I), diffuse (low-grade) (II), anaplastic astrocytoma (III) and glioblastoma (IV). The most aggressive, glioblastoma (GBM), is also the most common malignant astrocytic tumour with a 5-year survival rate of less than 3%. Although systematic metastasis of astrocytomas is rare, aggressive local invasion into surrounding tissue, rapid growth and resistance to apoptosis accounts for the lethality of these brain cancers – tumour behaviours supported by aggressive angiogenesis (Anderson et al., 2008).

In a study of 51 astrocytomas using immunohistochemical staining of frozen sections, immunoblotting of tumour lysates and quantitative real-time PCR, PC expression was found to be present in approximately half of the cases of anaplastic astrocytoma and GBM, but none of the lower-grade astrocytomas (Hayatsu et al., 2008). The pattern of staining in the anaplastic astrocytomas is consistent with cell-surface expression of PC; however, PC localization in GBM was more diffuse and PC-positive tumour cells were associated with regions of microvascular proliferation. Using a lectin-binding microarray combined with a mass spectrometry approach, another group detected PNA-reactive PC abundantly expressed on the surface of a "stem cell like" human GBM cell line (GBM1), but not on an adherent GMB line (U373) (He et al., 2010).

Notably, the sialomucin podoplanin (*PDPN*), which shares some striking structural and functional properties with PC, is also highly expressed in glioblastoma (Mishima et al., 2006). Podoplanin is expressed on the outer/invasive edge of some tumours and is thought to have a role in the anti-adhesive phenotype of EMT-independent tumour invasion (Wicki and Christofori, 2007). Invoking a similar paradigm to breast and ovarian carcinoma (**§3.2.3 & 3.3**), we posit that high expression of PC may promote an EMT-independent morphogenesis that, combined with other transforming pathways, promotes an invasive phenotype in astrocytomas.

4. Podocalyxin marks embryonal carcinomas and embryonic stem cells

PODXL transcript and protein is down regulated in embryoid bodies (EB) and lineage-restricted EB cultures compared to undifferentiated human embryonic stem cells (hESCs) (Brandenberger et al., 2004; Cai et al., 2006). PC-binding antibodies TRA-1-60 and TRA-1-81, together with membrane surface, stage-specific embryonic antigens (SSEA)-3 and SSEA-4; and, intracellular markers alkaline phosphatase, telomerase, Oct4 and Nanog are routinely used to characterize undifferentiated hESC (De Miguel et al., 2010; Palecek, 2011). As mentioned previously, the TRA-1-60 and TRA-1-81 epitopes are present only on the high molecular weight form of PC detected in embryonal carcinoma (EC) cell lines and these markers are lost upon induced differentiation of EC or hESC. Thus, PC is a marker of undifferentiated human embryonal cells and PC is either alternately modified (e.g., glycosylation pattern) or its expression is reduced upon differentiation. In an effort to identify novel markers of undifferentiated hESC, Choo et al generated an anti-PC antibody (IgM isotype, mAb 84) cytotoxic to undifferentiated hESC (human embryonic stem (HES) cell lines HES-2, -3 and -4) and at least one embryonal carcinoma cell line (NCCIT) (Choo et al., 2008). Importantly, mAb 84 is not cytotoxic to mature human cell lines (HEK-293, HeLa) or hESC induced to differentiate by withdrawal of fibroblast growth factor 2 or following culture of hESC to form EB (day 22). Remarkably, mAb 84 rapidly (< 45 minutes) kills EC even at 4°C. The mechanism for mAb 84 cytotoxicity is not dependent on complement activation, hypercrosslinking of bound antibody or antibody internalization. Instead, mAb 84 mediates cell death by oncosis initiated by PC-mediated reassembly of cytoskeleton, degradation of cytoskeletal structural proteins (α-actinin, talin and paxillin), PC-aggregation and formation of large membrane pores (Tan et al., 2009). Since crosslinking other PC-specific antibodies bound to hESCs is not cytotoxic, the association of mAb 84 to a unique PC epitope (or potentially other additional unknown epitopes on hESCs) induces cytoskeletal reassembly in advance of PC aggregation and pore formation. Studies with antibody fragments revealed that cytotoxicity requires divalency with sufficient flexibility linking the antigen binding domains (Lim et al., 2011). Since pre-treatment of HES-3 hESC and NCCIT cultures with mAb 84 *in vitro* prevents teratoma formation in a severe combined immunodeficient (SCID) mouse xenograft model mAb 84 has potential applications in clearing tumour-forming undifferentiated hESCs from cultures of differentiated hESCs intended for cell-based, regenerative therapies (Choo et al., 2008; Tan et al., 2009). With respect to the treatment of cancer, a cytotoxic antibody like mAb 84 may also prove to be an effective oncolytic adjuvant therapy in germ-line tumours like testicular cancer (especially embryonal carcinoma subtype). This approach, of course, would require highly selective targeting of tumour-specific forms of PC to avoid renal toxicity. The encouraging example of mAb 84 suggests that highly selective targeting of PC expressing tumour cells *in vivo* may be possible.

5. Podocalyxin structure and function

In an effort to determine how expression of PC on cancer cells promotes tumour aggressiveness and metastasis, several groups, including our own, have performed structure-functional analyses in model cancer cell lines to delineate the specific roles of PC's protein domains in the regulation of cell morphology, motility and survival. The following sections summarize some of what is known of the molecular mechanisms regulated by PC. PC's highly charged and bulky extracellular domain imparts a biophysical anti-adhesive property that regulates cell morphology and cell-cell adhesion functions and, when appropriately modified, may also promote adhesion by binding to L- or E-selectin. The intracellular domain links apically-polarized PC to the cortical actin cytoskeleton. By recruiting ezrin and NHERF-1/2, PC's intracellular domain localizes signalling complexes at apical membrane domains. In general, expression of PC promotes cell motility and invasion functions in epithelial cells and promotes chemotaxis in hematopoietic cells.

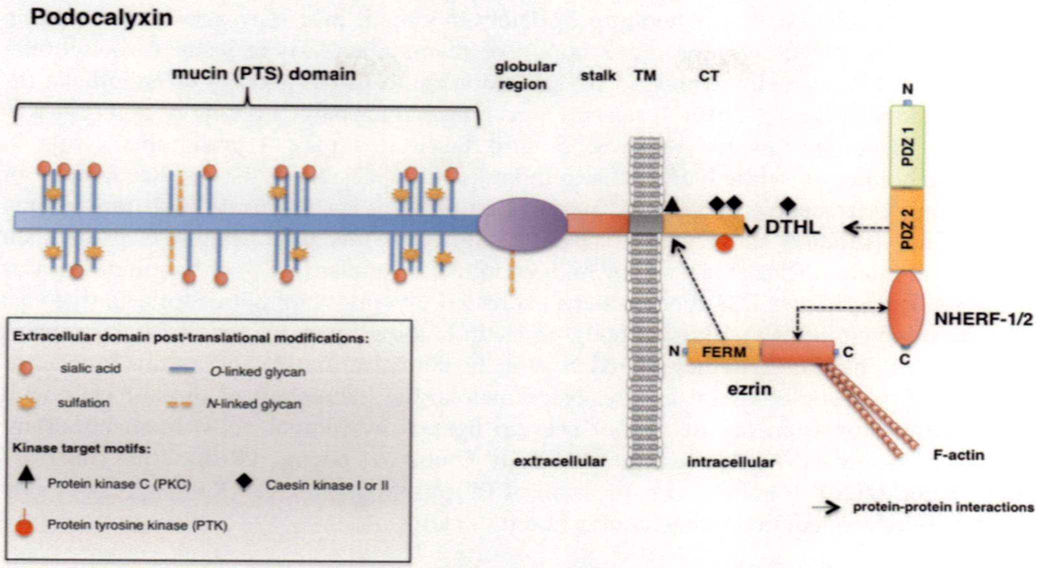

Fig. 5. Podocalyxin associates with NHERF-1/2 and ezrin to nucleate a variety of intracellular signalling complexes.

5.1 Podocalyxin is a CD34-family sialomucin

Podocalyxin is one of three members of the CD34-family of sialomucins that also includes CD34 and endoglycan (reviewed in Furness & McNagny, 2006). Mucins are members of a large class of secreted and type I transmembrane proteins that contain at least one extracellular domain rich in proline, serine and threonine residues (PTS domain). Mucin domains are extensively modified by post-translational addition of *O*-linked oligosaccharides (at S/T residues) and frequently modified by *N*-linked glycosylation and sulfation. Sialomucins, in particular, are also heavily modified by the addition of a terminal sialic acid to terminal *O*-linked glycans. PC is a sialomucin that, together with CD34 and endoglycan, makes up the CD34-family (reviewed in Furness and McNagny, 2006). The mature, cell surface expressed human PC protein is a 536 residue glycoprotein with a calculated peptide mass of 56 kilodaltons (kD); however, glycosylation and other post-translational modifications yield a product with an apparent molecular weight of 150-200 kD. The extracellular domain of PC consists of a heavily *O*-linked glycosylated, sialated and sulfated mucin domain, a globular domain containing a conserved four-cysteine (Cys) motif, and, a membrane-proximal stalk domain. Three or four sites of *N*-linked glycosylation also decorate the extracellular domain. Together, these modifications result in a highly negatively charged, sterically bulky glycoprotein (**Fig. 5**). Although the primary amino acid sequence of PC's extracellular domain is not well conserved by paralogs (or CD34-family homologs), the intracellular domain is highly conserved across species.

5.2 Extracellular ligands of podocalyxin

The only well-established extracellular ligand for CD34-family sialomucins is L-selectin (reviewed in (Furness & McNagny, 2006; Nielsen & McNagny, 2008)), however there are also reports to suggest that, when appropriately modified, they may also bind E-selectin (Thomas et al., 2009). Selectins are a family of mammalian C-type lectin carbohydrate-binding proteins normally expressed by hematopoietic cells (L- and P-) or endothelia (P- and E-) (Laubli & Borsig, 2010). L-selectin is responsible for naïve homing of leukocytes to secondary lymphoid organs; whereas, P- and E-selectins play a predominant role in mediating homing of white blood cells to inflamed (or specialized) tissues. Recognition of CD34-family sialomucins by selectins requires an unusual carbohydrate post-translational modification (sulfated sialyl Lewis-X (sLe^X)). Although this modification is present on CD34-family sialomucins expressed by high endothelial venules (HEV) of lymph nodes, it is not typically found on CD34-type proteins expressed by non-lymphoid endothelia (the vast majority of all endothelia). Thus, although selectin-binding functions for CD34 sialomucins (including PC) have been demonstrated *in vitro*, the biological significance of this function is unclear for most endothelium *in vivo*. Nevertheless, the interaction of tumour cells with selectins (or expression of selectins or selectin ligands by tumour cells) is an important paradigm in cancer metastases (reviewed in Laubli & Borsig, 2010). Thus, aberrant modification (sLe^X) or enhanced expression of PC in malignant cells (Kannagi, 2004) may facilitate selectin-mediated tissue homing and trafficking.

5.3 Intracellular binding partners of podocalyxin

The intracellular domain of PC contains a membrane proximal ERM (ezrin, radixin, moesin)-protein association domain, as well as putative target sites for serine and threonine (S/T) kinases (e.g., casein kinases I/II (CKI/II) and protein kinase C (PKC)) and protein tyrosine kinases (PTK) (**Fig. 5**). In addition, the four C-terminal amino acids of the intracellular domain, aspartate-threonine-histidine-leucine (DTHL) is an interaction motif for proteins containing a PSD-95/Dlg/ZO-1 (PDZ)-domain.

The best-characterized intracellular binding partners for PC are ezrin and NHERF isoforms 1 and 2 (solute carrier family 9 (Na^+/H^+ exchanger), member 3 regulator -1 and -2) (**Fig. 5**). Notably, dysregulated expression, localization and mutants of ezrin and NHERF-1 (also called EBP50) and -2 have been implicated in human cancers (Dai et al., 2004; Brambilla & Fais, 2009; Mangia et al., 2009; Hayashi et al., 2010). As adaptor proteins with diverse binding partners, ezrin and NHERF-1/2 have the potential to link PC to several signalling pathways (see **Table 2**). Likewise, by targeting ezrin and NHERF-1/2 to select apical membrane domains, PC may regulate the localization, function and availability of these complexes.

5.3.1 NHERF-1 and NHERF-2

NHERF-1 and -2 both have two tandem PDZ domains - the centrally located PDZ class II domain associates with PC's C-terminal DTHL motif, leaving NHERF's N-terminal PDZ class I domain free to interact with other binding partners. **Table 2** provides a partial list of known NHERF-1/2 binding partners. Ezrin can either directly binds to PC via the membrane proximal ERM protein-binding motif or indirectly via the C-terminal ERM motif of NHERF-1/2. NHERF-1/2 have a wide range of binding partners that include ion channels, G protein coupled receptors, receptor tyrosine kinases (RTKs), intracellular signalling intermediates and β-catenin, a transcription factor (**Table 2**). NHERF-1/2 may also homodimerize or polymerize via PDZ-domain interactions, or bind other PDZ domain containing proteins like PDZ K1 (Garbett et al., 2010).

NHERF-1/2 binding partners	Ezrin binding partners
Sialomucins Podocalyxin, endoglycan (but not CD34) *Receptor tyrosine kinases* Epidermal growth factor receptor (EGFR), Platelet derived growth factor receptor (PDGFR) *G protein coupled receptors* β2-adrenergic receptor, κ-opiod receptor, Frizzled isoforms (Wheeler et al., 2011), Parathyroid hormone receptor, P2Y1 purinergic receptor *Ion channels* Cystic fibrosis transmembrane conductance regulator (CTFR), Na^+/H^+ exchanger member 3 (NHE3) TRPC4 (transient receptor potential cation channel 4) (Lee-Kwon et al., 2005) Mrp2 (multidrug resistance-associated protein 2) (Li et al., 2010) *Transcription factors* β-catenin *PDZ domain proteins* PDZ K1 (Garbett et al., 2010), NHERF-1/2 (homodimer or polymer) *ERM proteins* Ezrin, radixin, moesin, merlin *PI3K pathway regulators* PTEN (Takahashi et al., 2006), Akt (Wang et al., 2008) *Rho-family regulators or downstream effectors* ARHGEF7 (Hsu et al., 2010), RACK1 (Liedtke et al., 2004)	*Sialomucins* Podocalyxin, CD44, CD43, PSGL-1 *Non-receptor tyrosine kinases* Focal adhesion kinase (FAK), Src-family kinase (SFKs) *Integrin-binding adhesion molecules* Intercellular-adhesion molecules (ICAMs) -1, -2 & -4 *Serine/threonine kinase* Protein kinase A (PKA) *Phosphatidylinositol 3-kinases* p85 of class I PI3Ks *Cytoskeleton/adaptors* F-actin, NHERF-1/2 *Membrane phospholipids* PI (4,5) P_2 *Ca^{2+} signaling effectors* S100P (Austermann et al., 2008) *Rho-family regulators or downstream effectors* RhoGDI (Schmieder et al., 2004)

Table 2. A partial list of reported binding partners of NHERF-1/2 and ezrin. Specific binding references are shown in the table. For reviews of NHERF-1/2 binding interactions see references Weinman et al., 2006; Georgescu et al., 2008; Nielsen and McNagny, 2009 & Hayashi et al., 2010. Ezrin binding interactions were recently reviewed in Bambilla & Fais, 2009.

5.3.2 Ezrin

Ezrin acts as an intracellular adaptor to provide linkage of integral membrane proteins with the cytoskeleton. Ezrin contains an N-terminal FERM protein-interaction domain capable of binding the intracellular domain of several type I transmembrane proteins, NHERF-1/2, RhoGDI and the membrane lipid, phosphatidylinositol-4,5-bisphosphate ($PI(4,5)P_2$), and a C-terminal domain that bind polymerized actin (F-actin) (**Table 2**). The C-terminal domain of ERM folds over to associate with its N-terminus in an inactive conformation and phosphorylation of a conserved Thr residue in the C-terminus, downstream of Rho kinase, protein kinase C isoforms (and other S/T kinases), induces an open conformation that permits ERM proteins to link complexes to polymerized actin (F-actin) (Fehon et al., 2010). Phosphorylation of Tyr residues (perhaps by RTKs or Src-family kinases) further enhances ezrin activation or activation of ezrin-dependent signalling events. By using NHERFs as an adaptor, ezrin can link several other transmembrane proteins to the cytoskeleton including ion channels and GPCRs. We note that PC is one of few transmembrane proteins that can bind ezrin both directly and indirectly through NHERF-1/2.

6. The molecular basis for podocalyxin function in tumour metastasis

At least some of PC's molecular functions in normal and neoplastic tissues can be explained by viewing PC as a key electrostatic anti-adhesive force between extracellular membrane surfaces (Gelberg et al., 1996; Takeda et al., 2000; Galeano et al., 2007; Strilic et al., 2009). However, since the intracellular domain of PC is phosphorylated on Ser/Thr and Tyr residues and PC assembles signalling complexes in response to cell activation, PC undoubtedly influences the behaviour of tumour cells by regulating intracellular signalling pathways. Some of these intracellular signalling complexes likely reinforce the localization of PC to the apical membrane of polarized cells. However, they may also enhance (or otherwise regulate) downstream signalling events important in the rearrangement of cytoskeleton and adhesion-independent survival. We propose the extracellular domain of PC is necessary and sufficient for PC's homotypic anti-adhesive functions and morphogenesis of apical membranes. However, stable apical localization of PC, and its effects on the migration and, potentially, survival-promoting functions depends on the intracellular domain and assembled signalling complexes. In the next section we will review the proposed molecular signalling mechanisms regulated by PC and relate these signalling functions to PC's role as a promoter of tumour progression and metastases.

6.1 Podocalyxin regulates adhesion and membrane morphogenesis in epithelial cells

Many of the molecular functions of PC, including signalling mechanisms mediated via ezrin and NHERF-1/2, have been elucidated using the human breast cancer cell line MCF7, the human prostate cancer line PC3 and the canine renal tubule cell line, Madin-Darby canine kidney (MDCK). Since human RCC arise from renal tubule cells, the MDCK model cell line may offer valuable insights into the molecular mechanisms of tumour progression and metastasis in RCC. Although renal tubules in human and rabbit do not express detectable levels of PC protein, MDCK cells and adult canine kidney tubular cells have detectable PC (Cheng et al., 2005; Meder et al., 2005). As mentioned in previous sections, MCF7 and PC3 cells are derived from metastatic breast and prostate tumours, respectively. Both of these cell lines express low to moderate levels of PC and are therefore useful for *in vitro* and *in vivo* assays using methods to force expression of PC or structural mutants of PC. Conversely, RNAi methods can be used to study the functions of endogenous PC in tumour cells or cell lines. Although there are discrepancies in the assignment of functional roles to PC's structural domains (see details below), taken together, these studies show that high expression of PC results in enhanced motility, invasiveness and destabilization of epithelial cell morphology in 2D- and 3D-cultures. These phenotypes are characteristics of aggressive epithelial tumours with propensity to metastasize.

6.1.1 Podocalyxin's function in epithelial architecture and morphogenesis

Although MCF7 cells express moderate levels of *PODXL* transcript (Kao et al., 2009) **(Fig. 1)**; by western blotting and immunofluorescence confocal microscopy, expression of PC is low or not detected, respectively (Nielsen et al., 2007; Sizemore et al., 2007; Somasiri et al., 2004). In order to study the molecular function of PC in breast epithelial cells, others and we have ectopically expressed full-length PC and a series of structural mutants in MCF7 (**Fig. 6**). Overexpression of full-length PC (FL) in MCF7 results in apical bulging of monolayers, reduced transepithelial resistance (i.e., disrupted cell junctions), delamination and shedding of cells from monolayers *in vitro* (Nielsen et al., 2007; Somasiri et al., 2004). Strikingly, expression of PC in MCF7 (and MDCK) potently induces formation of apical microvilli. Epithelial microvilli are common features in specialized epithelial layers involved in the secretion or absorption of nutrients, vesicles and proteins from the extracellular space (Lange, 2011).

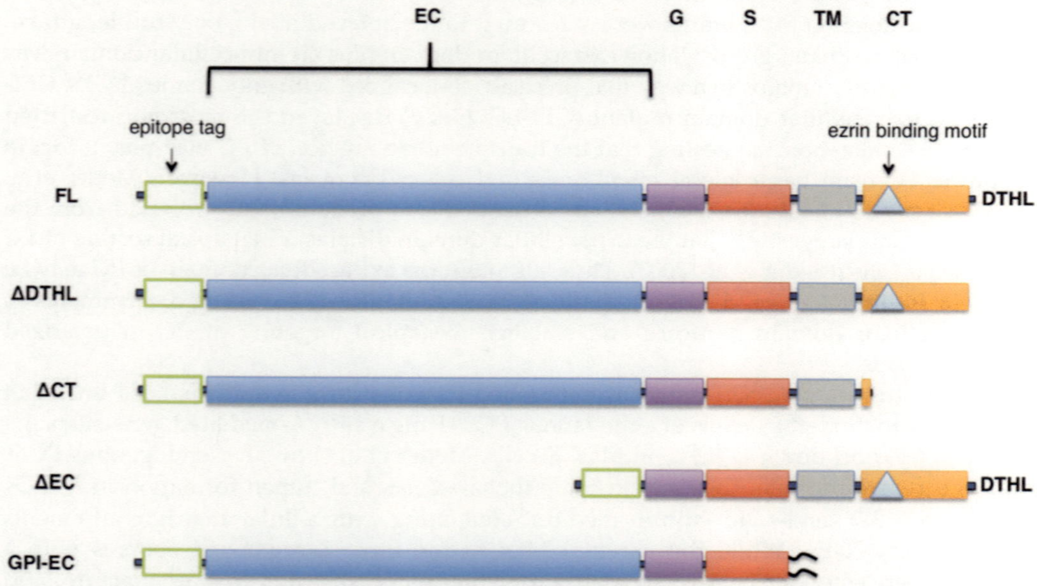

Fig. 6. Schematic of podocalyxin protein structural mutants used to delineate biological functions of specific protein domains. EC- extracellular (*O*-glycosylated mucin) domain, G - globular domain, S- stalk domain, TM- transmembrane domain, CT –cytoplasmic domain. Triangle in membrane proximal CT domain denotes ezrin-binding motif. Adapted from Meder et al, 2005 & Nielsen et al, 2007.

As we anticipated, full-length, exogenously expressed PC recruits NHERF-1, ezrin and F-actin to apical membrane domains and forms microvilli in MCF7 cells. However, surprisingly, the intracellular domain of PC is dispensable for the formation of microvilli since the transmembrane-anchored extracellular domain alone (ΔCT) is sufficient to drive morphogenesis and the recruitment of ezrin and F-actin to apical membranes and microvilli in MCF7 (Nielsen et al., 2007). Notably, NHERF-1 is not recruited to apical domains or microvilli in the absence of PC's C-terminal DTHL domain (ΔDTHL or ΔCT). This result suggests that the extracellular domain, likely by a biophysical charge- and steric-based intermolecular repulsion mechanism, can drive membrane morphogenesis and rearrangement of the cytoskeleton (including nucleation of ezrin and F-actin in microvilli) to support stable microvilli. We note that this biophysical mechanism requires high expression of PC since endogenous levels of PC in MDCK and MCF7 are not sufficient to drive microvillus formation. However, such high expression of PC may have relevance in some human epithelial cancers, including the rare sub-sets of high PC-positive metastatic breast cancer and renal cell carcinomas mentioned previously.

Although many investigators agree that PC, NHERF-1/2 and ezrin form a complex that marks apical membrane domains, the mechanism of PC's apical targeting is not yet certain. We have found that expression of full-length PC (FL), and PC mutants ΔCT, ΔDTHL and ΔEC (**Fig. 6**) in MCF7 result in sorting of these exogenously expressed proteins to the apical membrane domain. Conversely, using a similar series of PC mutants expressed in MDCK cells, two other laboratories show that precise apical targeting of PC requires its intracellular domain (Cheng et al., 2005; Meder et al., 2005). In these studies, although the majority of intracellular-deletion PC mutants were still sorted to the apical domain, only full-length PC with an intact *O*-linked glycosylation extracellular domain plus an intracellular domain was targeted to apical domains in a way that precisely co-localized with endogenous PC. A GPI-linked PC extracellular domain mutant (GPI-EC, **Fig. 6**) displayed the most non-restricted membrane localization, suggesting that the transmembrane region of PC may play a role in excluding PC from basal lateral membranes and cell-cell contacts. However, Meder et al show that a non-membrane anchored construct of PC is predominantly secreted from the apical face, thus suggesting that the extracellular domain dictates initial apical sorting of PC in epithelial cells (Meder et al., 2005). Thus, although the extracellular domain of PC may be sufficient for initial apical distribution, the ezrin and NHERF-1/2 binding determinants in the intracellular domain reinforce and stabilize the apical targeting of PC in polarized epithelial sheets.

The above studies were performed by expressing PC constructs in epithelial cell lines that express low to moderate levels of endogenous PC. Using a siRNA-mediated gene-silencing approach to knockdown *PODXL* in MDCK cells, Meder et al show that endogenous PC is required for appropriate polarization of epithelial sheets and lumen formation in MDCK clusters in a 3D semi-solid culture medium containing extracellular matrix components (Meder et al., 2005). While the parental MDCK line formed organized spheres with a central lumen when suspended in matrix, deletion of PC disrupts this architecture, and MDCK fail to form an organized lumen (Meder et al., 2005). Correspondingly, using siRNA-mediated knockdown of endogenous PC in MDCK, Cheng et al show that endogenous PC is required for hepatocyte growth factor (HGF)-induced tubulogenesis (Chen et al., 2005). Transfection with siRNA-resistant PC (FL) and mutant constructs reveals that tubule formation of MDCK requires the intracellular domain. However, PC's extracellular *O*-linked glycosylated mucin domain has a role in refining the architecture of tubule lumens. Finally, enforced expression of PC in MDCK cells inhibits cell-cell adhesion and disrupts junctional complexes. This effect is dependent on sialylation of PC, suggesting a charge-repulsion mechanism.

6.1.2 NHERF-herding function of podocalyxin's intracellular domain

Although the mechanisms responsible for the apical localization of PC require further investigation, it is clear that one of PC's functional roles is the recruitment of adaptor proteins to apical domains. By binding ezrin and NHERF-1/2, PC has the potential to impact the activity or compartmentalization of a variety of signalling pathways. While some of PC's functions can be explained purely by invoking a biophysical charge/steric-repulsion paradigm, several biological functions of PC undoubtedly require recruitment of ezrin and NHERF into apical-domain signalling complexes. Since PC can recruit and restrict NHERF and ezrin (and potentially their numerous binding partners (**Table 2**)) to apical membrane domains, we posit that many of PC's functions stem from the concentration of signalling complexes – either down regulating signals in other membrane domains (e.g., adherens junctions or focal adhesions) or enhancing signals in the apical domains.

Cortactin (*CTTN*) is an F-actin- and Arp2/3-binding adaptor involved in the branching and nucleation of the cortical actin cytoskeleton and formation of membrane protrusions (reviewed in Weaver, 2008). Cortactin's localization and functional activation is regulated by a large number of binding partners. Importantly, cortactin is enriched in cell protrusions called "invadopodia" and has a role in the invasion of tumour cells through extracellular matrix (Weaver, 2008). PC was found to co-localize with cortactin (and perhaps directly or indirectly bind) at the apical domain of rat podocytes (Kobayashi et al., 2009). Effacement of podocytes caused phosphorylation of cortactin, dissociation of cortactin from PC/apical domains and translocation of cortactin to the basolateral face (Kobayashi et al., 2009). Although the interaction of cortactin and PC in invasive tumours has not yet been examined, PC localizes to "invadopodia"-like protrusions in *in vitro* assays. Furthermore, cortactin is known to regulate the secretion of MMPs at invadopodia. In this way, and by recruitment of NHERFs and ezrin, PC may regulate changes in cortical actin assembly associated with tumour invasion and metastasis. This idea is supported by an experiment showing that forced expression of PC in MCF7 enhances expression and secretion of matrix metalloproteinases (MMP)-1 and MMP-9 (Sizemore et al., 2007).

6.2 Podocalyxin's role in the regulation of tumour growth, adherence-independent survival and cell motility

6.2.1 Regulation of Rho-family GTPases

In MDCK cells, formation of a PC-NHERF-1-ezrin ternary complex regulates RhoA activation (Schmieder et al., 2004). As part of a regulatory cycle controlling activation state of RhoA, RhoGDI maintains RhoA in an inactive GDP-bound state. Redistribution of RhoGDI to the apical membrane domain complex PC-NHERF-1-ezrin frees RhoA for activation by guanine exchange factors. Although sequestration of RhoGDI is not dependent on the interaction of PC and NHERF-1 (but does depend on ezrin), activation of RhoA requires NHERF-1 association with PC's C-terminal DTHL motif (**Fig. 7**).

A recent study corroborates and extends this finding by showing that the PC-NHERF-ezrin ternary complex also regulates activation of Rac1 (a Rho-family member) by a mechanism whereby the N-terminal PDZ1 domain of NHERF-1 recruits the Rho guanine nucleotide exchange factor 7 (*ARHGEF7*) to this complex via ARHGEF7's C-terminal ENTL (a PDZ-binding motif) (**Fig. 7**) (Hsu et al., 2010). Cell motility requires a coordinated reorganization of the cytoskeleton, a process regulated in part by Rho-family GTPases. By regulating the activity and apical localization of RhoGDI, and ARHGEF7, PC may promote motility in some circumstances. Thus, in addition to dramatic morphogenic changes in the apical domain of epithelial cells resulting in reduced cell-cell and cell-matrix adhesion, inappropriate or unregulated expression of PC may promote cell motility by regulating the activity of small GTPases. Although the above studies were conducted in MDCK cells, others have shown that Rac1 mediates PC-enhanced invasion and motility of PC3 and MCF7 cells (Sizemore et al., 2007).

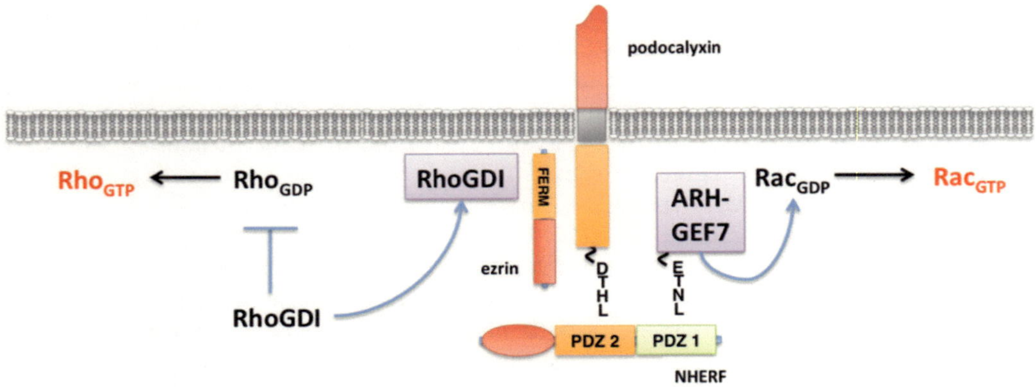

Fig. 7. Podocalyxin enhances activation of Rho-family GTPases by sequestration of RhoGDI and recruitment of a guanine exchange factor (ARHGEF7) to a PC-ezrin-NHERF complex assembled at membrane domains.

6.2.2 ERK and PI3K pathways

Forced expression of PC in MCF7 and PC3 cells induces ezrin-dependent activation of the Akt and Erk1/2 pathways (Sizemore et al., 2007). Moreover, activation of PI3K/Akt and Erk1/2 is required for PC-enhanced invasiveness of MCF7 and PC3. Invasiveness of PC-expressing cells was mediated in part by expression and secretion of matrix metalloproteinase -9 (MMP-9) and MMP-1, which in turn, required expression of ezrin and activation of PI3K and Erk1/2 (Sizemore et al., 2007).

Tyrosine phosphorylation of ezrin at central residue (Y353) has been shown to bind the regulatory subunit (p85) of class I PI3Ks and this association, in turn, induces activation of the PI3K pathway (Fievet et al., 2004; Gautreau et al., 1999). In addition, tyrosine phosphorylation of a residue (Y567) in ezrin's C-terminal domain disrupts the active conformation of ezrin and promotes intermolecular interactions with F-actin and other binding partners (Brambilla & Fais, 2009). Expression of PC in MCF7 and PC3 enhances phosphorylation of both the PI3K-activating Y353 and Y567 residues of ezrin (perhaps by Src-family kinases) (Sizemore et al., 2007). Activation of Erk1/2 via ezrin may be more indirect, proceeding through activation of Rho-family GTPases (Sahai and Marshall, 2002).

6.3 Podocalyxin enhances CXCL12-mediated migration of hematopoietic cells

CXCL12 (formerly known as stromal derived factor 1 (SDF1)) is a critical chemotatic factor for the maintenance of hematopoietic cells in the BM niche and also for the maintenance of secondary lymphoid organ architecture. CXCL12 is a ligand for two GPCR chemokine receptors, CXCR4 and CXCR7 (reviewed in Teicher and Fricker, 2010). CXCR4 has a well-established role in mediating CXCL12 chemotatic cues in cells, whereas CXCR7 does not appear to be a competent signalling receptor on its own, but may regulate CXCR4 activity. Importantly, CXCR4 and CXCR7 expression or function is dysregulated in many human cancers, including (but not limited to) myleloid and lymphoid leukemias and many of the carcinomas discussed in this review. Expression or dysregulated signalling of CXCR4 and CXCR7 promote the metastasis and survival of cancers to (or within) tissues rich in CXCL12 (Sun et al., 2010).

In our efforts to understand the function of PC expression on hematopoietic stem and progenitor cells (HSC/Ps), we have used an RNAi approach to knockdown *Podxl* expression in a mouse myeloid-progenitor, factor dependent cell line, FDCP-1. We have previously shown that PC is highly expressed in FDCP-1 and, upon stimulation with interleukin-3 (IL3), PC is redistributed from a global membrane expression pattern to a polarized membrane domain that also recruits NHERF-1 (Tan et al., 2006). Recently, we have found that silencing *Podxl* in FDCP-1 inhibits CXCL12-mediated migration (manuscript submitted). In corroboration of this finding, primary hematopoietic cells derived from *Podxl-/-* fetal liver (day 15.5 embryos) also display impaired migration to CXCL12 in an *in vitro* assay. Although we have not yet uncovered the molecular mechanisms underlying PC-enhanced migration to CXCL12, we have found that stimulation of FDCP-1 (or mouse fetal liver) with stem cell factor induces enhanced surface exposure CXCR4 that then becomes distributed with PC to a common polarized membrane domain. This distribution suggests that PC and CXCR4 can physically associate at the cell surface. Indeed, CXCR4 can be co-precipitated with PC antibodies under some conditions (unpublished observations). We hypothesize that PC, as exemplified by the related sialomucins CD34, PSGL-1 and CD164 (endolyn) (Forde et al., 2007; Veerman et al., 2007; Blanchet et al, 2011), has an active role in hematopoietic cell migration and tissue homing by stabilizing or enhancing chemokine receptor signalling. Although we currently favour a mechanism by which PC associates with, and physically stabilizes, CXCR4 at a polarized membrane domain, PC may also enhance intracellular CXCR4 signalling pathways including activation of Rho GTPase, PI3K and Erk1/2 (**see §6.2.1 & 6.2.2**).

6.4 Stabilization of the glucose-3-transporter (GLUT3)

GLUT3 (*SLC2A3*), one of 14 glucose transporter family members (GLUT1-14), was originally identified as a neuronal-specific glucose transporter but is also expressed in other tissues with high-energy demands, including cancer cells (Macheda et al., 2005; Thorens & Mueckler, 2010; Cairns et al., 2011). PC was recently found to form a stable complex with GLUT3 in human embryonal carcinoma cells (Tera-1 and NCITT) since GLUT3 can be co-precipitated from cell lysates using PNA or anti-PC antibody (and, inversely, podocalyxin is co-precipitated with anti-GLUT3 antibody) (Schopperle et al., 2010). Suppression of *PODXL* expression via siRNA also reduced GLUT3 protein concentrations in NCITT (Schopperle et al., 2010) – suggesting that PC may stabilize GLUT3 protein or regulate expression of GLUT3.

7. Conclusion

7.1 Podocalyxin drives tissue morphogenesis and promotes tumour invasion, metastasis and survival

By expressing full-length and mutant forms of PC in cancer cell lines and assessing cell morphology, apical targeting of proteins, motility and invasion, we and others begun to assign specific functions to PC structural domains. An emerging theme is that the highly charged and glycosylated extracellular domain of PC helps to define the apical domain of epithelial sheets – perhaps purely by a biophysical charge- and steric-repulsion mechanism. However, when overexpressed at high concentration, PC can drive epithelial cell morphogenesis and trigger intracellular cytoskeletal rearrangements that support formation of microvilli (possibly as a mechanism for coping with apical domain expansion), reduce adhesion to extracellular matrix and adjacent cells; and, facilitate cell shedding from monolayers. In this way, overexpression of PC promotes EMT-independent tumour invasion and metastasis. **Table 3** summarizes these and other tumour-promoting mechanisms regulated by PC.

Mechanism of invasion & metastasis	Podocalyxin functions in tumour cells
Morphogenesis & detachment from basement membranes	• Inter- and intra-cellular biophysical charge-repulsion • Recruitment/sequestration of cortical actin complexes to apical membrane and weakening of ECM adhesion • Exclusion of integrins from the apical domain
Invasion of surrounding tissue	• PC association with collagen at leading edge • Recruitment and apical localization of cortactin and induced expression and secretion of MMPs at the leading edge
High motility	• Enhanced CXCL12/CXCR4 axis signalling and chemotaxis • Activation and localization of Rho-family GTPases • Enhanced activation of PI3K and ERK1/2
Homing and to distant tissue sites	• Potential E/L-selectin ligand in some tumours • CXCL12/CXCR4 mediated engraftment and survival in secondary tissue
Adherence-independent survival	• Enhanced activation of PI3K/Akt and Erk 1/2 pathways • Promote expression/stabilization of GLUT3

Table 3. Mechanisms of podocalyxin-enhanced tumour progression.

Although the initial apical domain-sorting of PC may be, in part, a property of extracellular or transmembrane determinants, the prevailing evidence suggests that association of PC's intracellular domain with ezrin and NHERF-1/2 (and consequently to F-actin and the cytoskeleton), is responsible for fine-tuning or stabilizing the apical localization of PC in epithelial cells. In other words, NHERF-1/2 and ezrin enhance the efficient and functionally appropriate apical targeting of PC. Subsequently, PC engagement of NHERF-1/2 and ezrin can serve to nucleate signalling complexes at these apical domains and regulate the spatial signaling by these complexes. For example, NHERF-1/2 and ezrin promote activation of Rho-family GTPases, and cooperate to promote the activation of the Erk1/2 and PI3K/Akt pathways. In addition, since NHERF-1/2 and ezrin themselves have multiple protein-protein interaction domains, regulatory motifs and associate with numerous signalling intermediates (**Table 2**), the potential function of PC in regulating apical signalling events is likely much more extensive. By recruiting NHERF-1/2 and ezrin, PC has a role in the temporal and spatial localization of signalling intermediates that contribute to enhanced invasion, motility and adhesion-independent survival of tumor cells.

PC recruits cortactin, to apical membrane domains by an as-yet undetermined mechanism that may be independent of NHERF-1/2 and ezrin. Cortactin is commonly localized to leading edge tumour cell protrusions, called invadopodia, where it promotes invasive functions, including the secretion of matrix metalloproteinase and regulates cortical actin rearrangements that promote cell morphogenesis and motility. In addition, by stabilizing GLUT3, PC may not only support a metabolic switch to oxygen-poor glycolysis, but also alter downstream glycosylation machinery. Both of these events have the potential to promote adhesion-independent survival and metastasis of tumour cells.

Since some sialomucins, including endolyn (CD164) and PSGL-1, have been implicated in enhanced chemokine-mediated migration of hematopoietic cells (Forde et al., 2007; Veerman et al., 2007), we have also examined PC's role in mediating the migration of hematopoietic precursor cells to specific chemokines. Our preliminary work suggests that PC promotes the

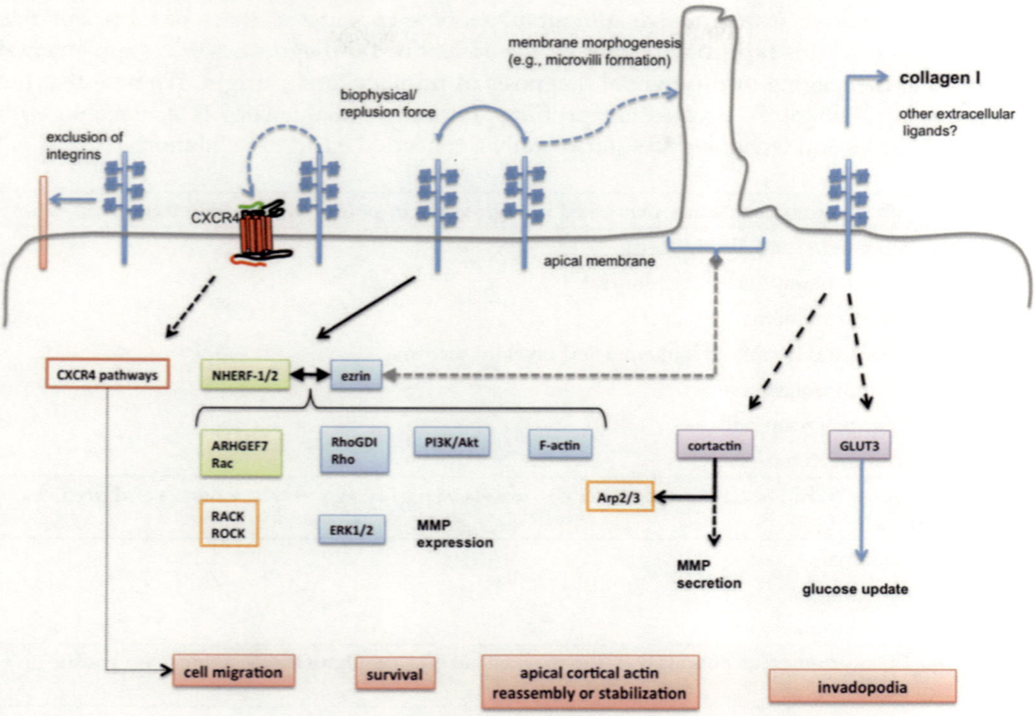

Fig. 8. Summary of podocalyxin-mediated molecular mechanisms promoting tumour growth, invasion, migration and adhesion-independent survival.

migration of hematopoietic cells and possibly tumor cells to CXCL12, perhaps by stabilizing the surface expression (and localization) of CXCR4. Thus, upregulation of PC on tumors may herald the acquisition of a great capacity for migration to CXCL12 rich tissues including bone, lung and brain.

7.2 Podocalyxin poorly differentiated tumours and promotes EMT and EMT-independent invasion and metastasis in human cancers

Evaluation of PC expression in human cancers, coupled with tumour characteristics and patient outcome data, reveals four cancer-indication "profiles" where high PC expression in primary tumours provides important diagnostic and prognostic information (**Table 4 (I-III)**) or polymorphisms in *PODXL* exons predicts cancer risk and tumour aggressiveness (**Table 4, IV**). These tumour-expression profiles, combined with *in vitro* and *in vivo* mechanistic studies, support the contention that PC promotes tumour invasion and metastases. In some human cancers, high PC expression is commonly detected in poorly differentiated, anaplastic tumour subtypes but not in lower grade tumours that retain differentiation markers and characteristics (Profile I). PC expression is also commonly detected in testicular cancer, a germ-line tumour. In these cases, PC may serve as a marker of immature or "de-differentiated" cells that have undergone EMT or retained a more primitive gene expression profile (perhaps derived from tissue stem cells). However, a causal link between PC expression and tumour progression and invasion is not proven in these profile I cancers. Nevertheless, drawing on *in vitro* studies, we hypothesize that PC may contribute to (but not initiate) the invasive or aggressive tumour phenotype in some of these cancers. For this reason, cancers of this type may benefit by the advent of PC diagnostics as a supplemental approach to the staging or differential diagnosis of primary tumor origin. We note that the clinical application of PC expression profiling for cancer diagnostics is achievable with existing reagents and technology, requiring only a concerted effort of validation.

Profile I. Podocalyxin is commonly expressed in high-grade or poorly differentiated tumours
• Thyroid carcinoma (undifferentiated)
• Pancreatic ductal/ampullary carcinoma
• Small-cell lung carcinoma
• Acute myeloid and lymphoid leukemia and myeloid sarcoma
• Anaplastic nephroblastoma
• Testicular cancer (germ cell)
• Malignant astrocytoma
Profile II. Podocalyxin is overexpressed in rare subsets of highly aggressive tumours and predicts poor prognosis
• Breast carcinoma
• Ovarian carcinoma
• Renal cell carcinoma
Profile III. PC expression as potential serum marker but clinical significance expression profile is undetermined
• Testicular cancer
• Colon cancer (cell line)
Profile IV. *PODXL* polymorphisms and SNPs associated with cancer risk and tumor aggressiveness
• Prostate carcinoma

Table 4. Podocalyxin expression profiles in human cancer.

In some cancers, PC overexpression in rare, highly aggressive tumour subtypes clearly correlates with enhanced tumour invasion, risk of metastasis and poor patient outcome (Profile II). In these cases, we propose that PC expression directly promotes EMT-independent invasion and metastases. We anticipate that further detailed analyses of aggressive tumor sub-types, especially for epithelial carcinomas, will expand the examples of rare, PC expressing, aggressive tumours in profile II. For instance: Because forced expression of PC in a prostate tumour cell line enhances invasive and migration potential, and PC is expressed in malignant prostate tumours (but not primary or normal adjacent tumours) (**Fig. 4**), we predict that a subset of high PC-expressing primary prostate tumours will display high risk of metastases. Evaluation of PC expression in primary tumours of profile II has the most value for prognostic assessment and the design of treatment and surveillance strategy. Furthermore, we hope that it will be possible to exploit PC expression in these indications for the development of targeted adjuvant therapies (**see §7.3**).

The detection of PC (or fragments) in serum may also provide a noninvasive biomarker of tumour progression or treatment progress in some cancers (profile III). The case is strongest for testicular cancer where serum PC (aka GCTM-2 or TRA-1-60) may be a more robust marker than current "gold-standard" biomarkers used in testicular cancer diagnostics. We suspect that cancers that commonly express high levels of PC (profile I) may also shed PC fragments into serum and continued research will likely confirm PC's utility as diagnostic serum marker. If so, PC detection in serum may be a generally useful for detecting disease or monitoring tumour progression and treatment efficacy.

Finally, genetic profiling of the *PODXL* locus reveals a fourth profile where polymorphisms in *PODXL* exons are associated with increase prostate cancer risk and tumor aggressiveness (**Table 4 (IV)**). Although it will be important to evaluate whether these genetic markers correlate with PC expression in prostate cancer or have any role in PC's functions in these tumours, screening for *PODXL* polymorphisms has potential theranostic applications in designing treatment strategies for prostate cancer patients.

7.3 Podocalyxin-targeted therapies for the treatment of metastatic cancer

There are several challenges to overcome in the development of PC-targeted adjuvant therapies for the treatment of high-risk primary tumours or oncolytic treatment of systemic cancers. First, we do not yet know if the high PC expression detected on primary tumours in the case of aggressive breast, renal cell and ovarian carcinoma is maintained on metastatic tumour cells or following engraftment at a secondary tissue site. However, evaluation of PC expression in breast and ovarian carcinoma cell lines, many of which were derived from metastatic tumours, suggests that PC expression might be a common feature of metastatic breast and ovarian cancer - especially, basal-type breast carcinomas (**Fig. 1**). Second, any PC-targeted therapies must carefully consider potential renal and vascular toxicity since PC is highly expressed on glomerular podocytes and on most vasculature. Fortunately, there are several examples of uniquely modified, tumour-specific forms of PC. These provide feasible targets for antibody-based drugs that are either directly oncolytic or block PC-mediated functions without affecting the function of normal cells.

8. Acknowledgement

The authors would foremost like to thank the patients that have donated tissues, genetic material and sacrificed some of their privacy to support the studies described in this review. KMM is a Senior Scholar of the Michael Smith Foundation of Health Research. KMM and CDR receive operating research funds for the study of podocalyxin's role in cancer biology from the Canadian Institutes of Health Research.

9. References

Anderson, J.C., McFarland, B.C. & Gladson, C.L. (2008). New molecular targets in angiogenic vessels of glioblastoma tumours. *Expert Reviews in Molecular Medicine.* Vol. 10, (Aug 7), pp. e23, ISSN 1462-3994

Austermann, J., Nazmi, A.R., Muller-Tidow, C., and Gerke, V. (2008). Characterization of the Ca2+ -regulated ezrin-S100P interaction and its role in tumor cell migration. *The Journal of Biological Chemistry.* Vol. 283, No. 43, (Oct 24), pp. 29331-29340, ISSN 0021-9258

Blanchet, M-R., Bennett J.L., Gold M., Levantini, E., Tenen, D.G., Girard M., Cormier Y. & McNagny, K.M. (2011). CD34 is required for dendritic cell trafficking and pathology in murine hypersensitivity pneumonitis. *American Journal of Respiratory and Critical Care Medicine.* In press, ISSN 1073-449X

Brambilla, D. & Fais, S. (2009). The Janus-faced role of ezrin in "linking" cells to either normal or metastatic phenotype. *International Journal of Cancer.* Vol. 125, No. 10, (Nov 15), pp. 2239-2245, ISSN 1097-0215

Brandenberger, R., Wei, H., Zhang, S., Lei, S., Murage, J., Fisk, G.J., Li, Y., Xu, C., Fang, R., Guegler, K., Rao, M.S., Mandalam, R., Lebkowski, J., and Stanton, L.W. (2004). Transcriptome characterization elucidates signaling networks that control human ES cell growth and differentiation. *Nature Biotechnology.* Vol. 22, No. 6, (Jun), pp. 707-716, ISSN 1087-0156

Butta, N., Larrucea, S., Alonso, S., Rodriguez, R., Arias-Salgado, E., Ayuso, M., Gonzalez-Manchon, C. & Parrilla, R. (2006). Role of transcription factor Sp1 and CpG methylation on the regulation of the human podocalyxin gene promoter. *BMC Molecular Biology.* Vol. 7, (Jan), pp. 17-29, ISSN 1471-2199

Cai, J., Chen, J., Liu, Y., Miura, T., Luo, Y., Loring, J.F., Freed, W.J., Rao, M.S., and Zeng, X. (2006). Assessing self-renewal and differentiation in human embryonic stem cell lines. *Stem Cells.* Vol. 24, No. 3, (Mar), pp. 516-530, ISSN 1066-5099

Cairns, R.A., Harris, I.S. & Mak, T.W. (2011). Regulation of cancer cell metabolism. *Nature Reviews.Cancer.* Vol. 11, No. 2, (Feb), pp. 85-95, ISSN 1474-1768

Casey, G., Neville, P.J., Liu, X., Plummer, S.J., Cicek, M.S., Krumroy, L.M., Curran, A.P., McGreevy, M.R., Catalona, W.J., Klein, E.A. & Witte, J.S. (2006). Podocalyxin variants and risk of prostate cancer and tumor aggressiveness. *Human Molecular Genetics.* Vol. 15, No. 5, (Mar 1), pp. 735-741, ISSN 0964-6906

Chandran, U.R., Ma, C., Dhir, R., Bisceglia, M., Lyons-Weiler, M., Liang, W., Michalopoulos, G., Becich, M. & Monzon, F.A. (2007). Gene expression profiles of prostate cancer reveal involvement of multiple molecular pathways in the metastatic process. *BMC Cancer.* Vol. 7, (Apr 12), pp. 64, ISSN 1471-2407

Chauhan, S.C., Kumar, D. & Jaggi, M. (2009). Mucins in ovarian cancer diagnosis and therapy. *Journal of Ovarian Research.* Vol. 2, (Dec 24), pp. 21-30, ISSN 1757-2215

Chen, X., Higgins, J., Cheung, S.T., Li, R., Mason, V., Montgomery, K., Fan, S.T., van de Rijn, M. & So, S. (2004). Novel endothelial cell markers in hepatocellular carcinoma. *Modern Pathology.* Vol. 17, No. 10, (Oct), pp. 1198-1210, ISSN 0893-3952

Cheng, H.Y., Lin, Y.Y., Yu, C.Y., Chen, J.Y., Shen, K.F., Lin, W.L., Liao, H.K., Chen, Y.J., Liu, C.H., Pang, V.F. & Jou, T.S. (2005). Molecular identification of canine podocalyxin-like protein 1 as a renal tubulogenic regulator. *Journal of the American Society of Nephrology.* Vol. 16, No. 6, (Jun), pp. 1612-1622, ISSN 1046-6673

Cheung, H.H., Davis, A.J., Lee, T.L., Pang, A.L., Nagrani, S., Rennert, O.M. & Chan, W.Y. (2011). Methylation of an intronic region regulates miR-199a in testicular tumor malignancy. *Oncogene.* (Mar 7), pp. 1-12, ISSN 1476-5594

Choo, A., Tan, H., Ang, S., Fong, W., Chin, A., Lo, J., Zheng, L., Hentze, H., Philp, R., Oh, S. & Yap, M. (2008). Selection against undifferentiated human embryonic stem cells by a cytotoxic antibody recognizing podocalyxin-like protein-1. *Stem Cells.* Vol. 26, No. 6, (Jun), pp. 1454-1463, ISSN 1066-509

Cleton-Jansen, A.M. (2002). E-cadherin and loss of heterozygosity at chromosome 16 in breast carcinogenesis: different genetic pathways in ductal and lobular breast cancer? *Breast Cancer Research.* Vol. 4, No. 1, pp. 5-8, ISSN 1465-5411

Cohen, H.T. & McGovern, F.J. (2005). Renal-cell carcinoma. *The New England Journal of Medicine.* Vol. 353, No. 23, (Dec 8), pp. 2477-2490, ISSN 1533-4406

Comamala, M., Pinard, M., Theriault, C., Matte, I., Albert, A., Boivin, M., Beaudin, J., Piche, A. & Rancourt, C. (2011). Downregulation of cell surface CA125/MUC16 induces epithelial-to-mesenchymal transition and restores EGFR signalling in NIH:OVCAR3 ovarian carcinoma cells. *British Journal of Cancer*. Vol. 104, No. 6, (Mar 15), pp. 989-999, ISSN 1532-1827

Dai, J.L., Wang, L., Sahin, A.A., Broemeling, L.D., Schutte, M. & Pan, Y. (2004). NHERF (Na+/H+ exchanger regulatory factor) gene mutations in human breast cancer. *Oncogene*. Vol. 23, No. 53, (Nov 11), pp. 8681-8687, ISSN 0950-9232

De Miguel, M.P., Fuentes-Julian, S. & Alcaina, Y. (2010). Pluripotent stem cells: origin, maintenance and induction. *Stem Cell Reviews*. Vol. 6, No. 4, (Dec), pp. 633-649, ISSN 1558-6804

Doyonnas, R., Kershaw, D., Duhme, C., Merkens, H., Chelliah, S., Graf, T. & McNagny, K. (2001). Anuria, omphalocele& perinatal lethality in mice lacking the CD34-related protein podocalyxin. *The Journal of Experimental Medicine*. Vol. 194, No. 1, (Jul), pp. 13-27, ISSN 0022-1007

Doyonnas, R., Nielsen, J., Chelliah, S., Drew, E., Hara, T., Miyajima, A. & McNagny, K. (2005). Podocalyxin is a CD34-related marker of murine hematopoietic stem cells and embryonic erythroid cells. *Blood*. Vol. 105, No. 11, (Jun), pp. 4170-4178, *ISSN* 0006-4971

Fehon, R.G., McClatchey, A.I. & Bretscher, A. (2010). Organizing the cell cortex: the role of ERM proteins. *Nature Reviews. Molecular Cell Biology*. Vol. 11, No. 4, (Apr), pp. 276-287, ISSN 1471-0080

Fievet, B., Gautreau, A., Roy, C., Del Maestro L, Mangeat, P., Louvard, D., and Arpin, M. (2004). Phosphoinositide binding and phosphorylation act sequentially in the activation mechanism of ezrin. *The Journal of Cell Biology*. Vol. 164, No. 5, (Mar), pp. 653-659, ISSN 0021-9258

Forde, S., Tye, B., Newey, S., Roubelakis, M., Smythe, J., McGuckin, C., Pettengell, R. & Watt, S. (2007). Endolyn (CD164) modulates the CXCL12-mediated migration of umbilical cord blood CD133+ cells. *Blood*. Vol. 109, No. 5, (Mar), pp. 1825-1833.

Furness, S.G. & McNagny, K. (2006). Beyond mere markers: functions for CD34 family of sialomucins in hematopoiesis. *Immunologic Research*. Vol. 34, No. 1, pp. 13-32, ISSN 0257-277X

Galeano, B., Klootwijk, R., Manoli, I., Sun, M., Ciccone, C., Darvish, D., Starost, M.F., Zerfas, P.M., Hoffmann, V.J., Hoogstraten-Miller, S., Krasnewich, D.M., Gahl, W.A. & Huizing, M. (2007). Mutation in the key enzyme of sialic acid biosynthesis causes severe glomerular proteinuria and is rescued by N-acetylmannosamine. *The Journal of Clinical Investigation*. Vol. 117, No. 6, (Jun), pp. 1585-1594, ISSN 0021-9738

Garbett, D., LaLonde, D.P. & Bretscher, A. (2010). The scaffolding protein EBP50 regulates microvillar assembly in a phosphorylation-dependent manner. *The Journal of Cell Biology*. Vol. 191, No. 2, (Oct 18), pp. 397-413, ISSN 1540-8140

Gautreau, A., Poullet, P., Louvard, D., and Arpin, M. (1999). Ezrin, a plasma membrane-microfilament linker, signals cell survival through the phosphatidylinositol 3-kinase/Akt pathway. *Proceedings of the National Academy of Sciences of the United States of America*. Vol. 96, No. 13, (Jun 22), pp. 7300-7305, ISSN 0027-8424

Gelberg, H., Healy, L., Whiteley, H., Miller, L.A. & Vimr, E. (1996). In vivo enzymatic removal of alpha 2-->6-linked sialic acid from the glomerular filtration barrier results in podocyte charge alteration and glomerular injury. *Laboratory Investigation.* Vol. 74, No. 5, (May), pp. 907-920, ISSN 0023-6837

Georgescu, M.M., Morales, F.C., Molina, J.R. & Hayashi, Y. (2008). Roles of NHERF1/EBP50 in cancer. *Current Molecular Medicine.* Vol. 8, No. 6, (Sep), pp. 459-468, ISSN 1566-5240

Hamilton, T.C., Young, R.C., McKoy, W.M., Grotzinger, K.R., Green, J.A., Chu, E.W., Whang-Peng, J., Rogan, A.M., Green, W.R. & Ozols, R.F. (1983). Characterization of a human ovarian carcinoma cell line (NIH:OVCAR-3) with androgen and estrogen receptors. *Cancer Research.* Vol. 43, No. 11, (Nov), pp. 5379-5389, ISSN 0008-5472

Hayashi, Y., Molina, J.R., Hamilton, S.R. & Georgescu, M.M. (2010). NHERF1/EBP50 is a new marker in colorectal cancer. *Neoplasia.* Vol. 12, No. 12, (Dec), pp. 1013-1022, ISSN 1476-5586

Hayatsu, N., Kaneko, M., Mishima, K., Nishikawa, R., Matsutani, M., Price, J. & Kato, Y. (2008). Podocalyxin expression in malignant astrocytic tumors. *Biochemical and Biophysical Research Communications.* Vol. 374, No. 2, (Sep), pp. 394-398, ISSN 0006-291X

He, J., Liu, Y., Xie, X., Zhu, T., Soules, M., DiMeco, F., Vescovi, A.L., Fan, X. & Lubman, D.M. (2010). Identification of cell surface glycoprotein markers for glioblastoma-derived stem-like cells using a lectin microarray and LC-MS/MS approach. *Journal of Proteome Research.* Vol. 9, No. 5, (May 7), pp. 2565-2572, ISSN 1535-3907

Herman-Edelstein, M., Thomas, M.C., Thallas-Bonke, V., Saleem, M., Cooper, M.E. & Kantharidis, P. (2011). Dedifferentiation of Immortalized Human Podocytes in Response to Transforming Growth Factor-{beta}: A Model for Diabetic Podocytopathy. *Diabetes.* (Apr 26), pp. 1-10, ISSN 1939-327X

Heukamp, L.C., Fischer, H.P., Schirmacher, P., Chen, X., Breuhahn, K., Nicolay, C., Buttner, R. & Gutgemann, I. (2006). Podocalyxin-like protein 1 expression in primary hepatic tumours and tumour-like lesions. *Histopathology.* Vol. 49, No. 3, (Sep), pp. 242-247, ISSN 1365-2559

Hsu, Y., Lin, W., Hou, Y., Pu, Y., Shun, C., Chen, C., Wu, Y., Chen, J., Chen, T. & Jou, T. (2010). Podocalyxin EBP50 ezrin molecular complex enhances the metastatic potential of renal cell carcinoma through recruiting Rac1 guanine nucleotide exchange factor ARHGEF7. *The American Journal of Pathology.* Vol. 176, No. 6, (Jun), pp. 3050-3061, ISSN 0002-9440

Huff, V. (2011). Wilms' tumours: about tumour suppressor genes, an oncogene and a chameleon gene. *Nature Reviews. Cancer.* Vol. 11, No. 2, (Feb), pp. 111-121, ISSN 1474-1768

Ichimi, T., Enokida, H., Okuno, Y., Kunimoto, R., Chiyomaru, T., Kawamoto, K., Kawahara, K., Toki, K., Kawakami, K., Nishiyama, K., Tsujimoto, G., Nakagawa, M. & Seki, N. (2009). Identification of novel microRNA targets based on microRNA signatures in bladder cancer. *International Journal of Cancer.* Vol. 125, No. 2, (Jul 15), pp. 345-352, ISSN 1097-0215

Ito, T., Maki, N., Hazeki, O., Sasaki, K. & Nekooki, M. (2007). Extracellular and transmembrane region of a podocalyxin-like protein 1 fragment identified from colon cancer cell lines. *Cell Biology International.* Vol. 31, No. 12, (Dec), pp. 1518-1524, ISSN 1065-6995

Jacobson, E.M., Hugo, E.R., Tuttle, T.R., Papoian, R. & Ben-Jonathan, N. (2010). Unexploited therapies in breast and prostate cancer: blockade of the prolactin receptor. *Trends in Endocrinology and Metabolism*. Vol. 21, No. 11, (Nov), pp. 691-698, ISSN 1879-3061

Kaighn, M.E., Narayan, K.S., Ohnuki, Y., Lechner, J.F. & Jones, L.W. (1979). Establishment and characterization of a human prostatic carcinoma cell line (PC-3). *Investigative Urology*. Vol. 17, No. 1, (Jul), pp. 16-23, ISSN 0021-0005

Kalluri, R. & Weinberg, R.A. (2009). The basics of epithelial-mesenchymal transition. *The Journal of Clinical Investigation*. Vol. 119, No. 6, (Jun), pp. 1420-1428, ISSN 1558-8238

Kannagi, R. (2004). Molecular mechanism for cancer-associated induction of sialyl Lewis X and sialyl Lewis A expression-The Warburg effect revisited. *Glycoconjugate Journal*. Vol. 20, No. 5, pp. 353-364, ISSN 0282-0080

Kao, J., Salari, K., Bocanegra, M., Choi, Y.L., Girard, L., Gandhi, J., Kwei, K.A., Hernandez-Boussard, T., Wang, P., Gazdar, A.F., Minna, J.D. & Pollack, J.R. (2009). Molecular profiling of breast cancer cell lines defines relevant tumor models and provides a resource for cancer gene discovery. *PloS One*. Vol. 4, No. 7, (Jul 3), pp. e6146, ISSN 1932-6203

Kasai, H., Allen, J.T., Mason, R.M., Kamimura, T. & Zhang, Z. (2005). TGF-beta1 induces human alveolar epithelial to mesenchymal cell transition (EMT). *Respiratory Research*. Vol. 6, (Jun 9), pp. 56, ISSN 1465-993X

Kelley, T.W., Huntsman, D., McNagny, K.M., Roskelley, C.D. & Hsi, E.D. (2005). Podocalyxin: a marker of blasts in acute leukemia. *American Journal of Clinical Pathology*. Vol. 124, No. 1, (Jul), pp. 134-142, ISSN 0002-9173

Kobayashi, T., Notoya, M., Shinosaki, T. & Kurihara, H. (2009). Cortactin interacts with podocalyxin and mediates morphological change of podocytes through its phosphorylation. *Nephron. Experimental Nephrology*. Vol. 113, No. 3, pp. e89-96, ISSN 1660-2129

Koch, L., Zhou, H., Ellinger, J., Biermann, K., Holler, T., von Rucker A, , Buttner, R. & Gutgemann, I. (2008). Stem cell marker expression in small cell lung carcinoma and developing lung tissue. *Human Pathology*. (Jul), pp. 1597-1605, ISSN 0046-8177

Kufe, D.W. (2009). Mucins in cancer: function, prognosis and therapy. *Nature Reviews. Cancer*. Vol. 9, No. 12, (Dec), pp. 874-885, ISSN 1474-1768

Lacroix, M. & Leclercq, G. (2004). Relevance of breast cancer cell lines as models for breast tumours: an update. *Breast Cancer Research and Treatment*. Vol. 83, No. 3, (Feb), pp. 249-289, ISSN 0167-6806

Lange, K. (2011). Fundamental role of microvilli in the main functions of differentiated cells: Outline of an universal regulating and signaling system at the cell periphery. *Journal of Cellular Physiology*. Vol. 226, No. 4, (Apr), pp. 896-927, ISSN 1097-4652

Laubli, H. & Borsig, L. (2010). Selectins promote tumor metastasis. *Seminars in Cancer Biology*. Vol. 20, No. 3, (Jun), pp. 169-177, ISSN 1096-3650

Lee-Kwon, W., Wade, J.B., Zhang, Z., Pallone, T.L., and Weinman, E.J. (2005). Expression of TRPC4 channel protein that interacts with NHERF-2 in rat descending vasa recta. *American Journal of Physiology. Cell Physiology*, Vol. 288, No. 4, (Apr 1), pp. C942-C949, ISSN 0363-6143

Li, L. & Davie, J.R. (2010). The role of Sp1 and Sp3 in normal and cancer cell biology. *Annals of Anatomy*. Vol. 192, No. 5, (Sep 20), pp. 275-283, ISSN 1618-0402

Li, M., Wang, W., Soroka, C.J., Mennone, A., Harry, K., Weinman, E.J., and Boyer, J.L. (2010). NHERF-1 binds to Mrp2 and regulates hepatic Mrp2 expression and function. *The Journal of Biological Chemistry*. Vol. 285, No. 25, (Jun 18), pp. 19299-19307, ISSN 1083-351X

Li, Y., Kang, Y.S., Dai, C., Kiss, L.P., Wen, X. & Liu, Y. (2008). Epithelial-to-mesenchymal transition is a potential pathway leading to podocyte dysfunction and proteinuria. *The American Journal of Pathology*. Vol. 172, No. 2, (Feb), pp. 299-308, ISSN 0002-9440

Liang, Y., Ridzon, D., Wong, L. & Chen, C. (2007). Characterization of microRNA expression profiles in normal human tissues. *BMC Genomics*. Vol. 8, (Jun 12), pp. 166, ISSN 1471-2164

Liedtke, C.M., Raghuram, V., Yun, C.C., and Wang, X. (2004). Role of a PDZ1 domain of NHERF1 in the binding of airway epithelial RACK1 to NHERF1. *American Journal of Physiolology. Cell Physiology*. Vol. 286, No. 5, (May), pp. C1037-44, ISSN 0363-6143

Lim, D.Y., Ng, Y.H., Lee, J., Mueller, M., Choo, A.B. & Wong, V.V. (2011). Cytotoxic antibody fragments for eliminating undifferentiated human embryonic stem cells. *Journal of Biotechnology*. Vol. 153, No. 3-4, (May 20), pp. 77-85, ISSN 1873-4863

Macheda, M.L., Rogers, S. & Best, J.D. (2005). Molecular and cellular regulation of glucose transporter (GLUT) proteins in cancer. *Journal of Cellular Physiology*. Vol. 202, No. 3, (Mar), pp. 654-662, ISSN 0021-9541

Maltby, S., Freeman, S., Gold, M.J., Baker, J.H., Minchinton, A.I., Gold, M.R., Roskelley, C.D. & McNagny, K.M. (2011). Opposing Roles for CD34 in B16 Melanoma Tumor Growth Alter Early Stage Vasculature and Late Stage Immune Cell Infiltration. *PloS One*. Vol. 6, No. 4, (Apr 11), pp. e18160, ISSN 1932-6203

Maltby, S., Hughes, M., Zbytnuik, L., Paulson, R. & McNagny, K. (2009). Podocalyxin selectively marks erythroid-committed progenitors during anemic stress but is dispensable for efficient recovery. *Experimental Hematology*. Vol. 37, No. 1, (Jan), pp. 10-18, ISSN 0301-472X

Mangia, A., Chiriatti, A., Bellizzi, A., Malfettone, A., Stea, B., Zito, F.A., Reshkin, S.J., Simone, G. & Paradiso, A. (2009). Biological role of NHERF1 protein expression in breast cancer. *Histopathology*. Vol. 55, No. 5, (Nov), pp. 600-608, ISSN 1365-2559

McNagny, K.M., Pettersson, I., Rossi, F., Flamme, I., Shevchenko, A., Mann, M. & Graf, T. (1997). Thrombomucin, a novel cell surface protein that defines thrombocytes and multipotent hematopoietic progenitors. *The Journal of Cell Biology*. Vol. 138, No. 6, (Sep 22), pp. 1395-1407, ISSN 0021-9525

Meder, D., Shevchenko, A., Simons, K. & Fullekrug, J. (2005). Gp135/podocalyxin and NHERF-2 participate in the formation of a preapical domain during polarization of MDCK cells. *The Journal of Cell Biology*. Vol. 168, No. 2, (Jan 17), pp. 303-313, ISSN 0021-9525

Meng, X., Ezzati, P. & Wilkins, J.A. (2011). Requirement of podocalyxin in TGF-beta induced epithelial mesenchymal transition. *PloS One*. Vol. 6, No. 4, (Apr 12), pp. e18715, ISSN 1932-6203

Miettinen, A., Solin, M.L., Reivinen, J., Juvonen, E., Vaisanen, R. & Holthofer, H. (1999). Podocalyxin in rat platelets and megakaryocytes. *The American Journal of Pathology*. Vol. 154, No. 3, (Mar), pp. 813-822, ISSN 0002-9440

Mishima, K., Kato, Y., Kaneko, M.K., Nishikawa, R., Hirose, T. & Matsutani, M. (2006). Increased expression of podoplanin in malignant astrocytic tumors as a novel molecular marker of malignant progression. *Acta Neuropathologica*. Vol. 111, No. 5, (May), pp. 483-488, ISSN 0001-6322

Nam, E.J., Yoon, H., Kim, S.W., Kim, H., Kim, Y.T., Kim, J.H., Kim, J.W. & Kim, S. (2008). MicroRNA expression profiles in serous ovarian carcinoma. *Clinical Cancer Research*. Vol. 14, No. 9, (May 1), pp. 2690-2695, ISSN 1078-0432

Neve, R.M., Chin, K., Fridlyand, J., Yeh, J., Baehner, F.L., Fevr, T., Clark, L., Bayani, N., Coppe, J.P., Tong, F., Speed, T., Spellman, P.T., DeVries, S., Lapuk, A., Wang, N.J., Kuo, W.L., Stilwell, J.L., Pinkel, D., Albertson, D.G., Waldman, F.M., McCormick, F., Dickson, R.B., Johnson, M.D., Lippman, M., Ethier, S., Gazdar, A. & Gray, J.W. (2006). A collection of breast cancer cell lines for the study of functionally distinct cancer subtypes. *Cancer Cell*. Vol. 10, No. 6, (Dec), pp. 515-527, ISSN 1535-6108

Neville, P.J., Conti, D.V., Paris, P.L., Levin, H., Catalona, W.J., Suarez, B.K., Witte, J.S. & Casey, G. (2002). Prostate cancer aggressiveness locus on chromosome 7q32-q33 identified by linkage and allelic imbalance studies. *Neoplasia*. Vol. 4, No. 5, (Sep-Oct), pp. 424-431, ISSN 1522-8002

Ney, J.T., Zhou, H., Sipos, B., Buttner, R., Chen, X., Kloppel, G. & Gutgemann, I. (2007). Podocalyxin-like protein 1 expression is useful to differentiate pancreatic ductal adenocarcinomas from adenocarcinomas of the biliary and gastrointestinal tracts. *Human Pathology*. Vol. 38, No. 2, (Feb), pp. 359-364, ISSN 0046-8177

Nielsen, J.S. & McNagny, K.M. (2009a). CD34 is a Key Regulator of Hematopoietic Stem Cell Trafficking to Bone Marrow and Mast Cell Progenitor Trafficking in the Periphery. *Microcirculation*. (May 27), pp. 1-10, ISSN 1549-8719

Nielsen, J.S. & McNagny, K.M. (2009b). The role of podocalyxin in health and disease. *Journal of the American Society of Nephrology*. Vol. 20, No. 8, (Aug), pp. 1669-1676, ISSN 1533-3450

Nielsen, J.S. & McNagny, K.M. (2008). Novel functions of the CD34 family. *Journal of Cell Science*. Vol. 121, No. Pt 22, (Nov 15), pp. 3683-3692, ISSN 0021-9533

Nielsen, J., Graves, M., Chelliah, S., Vogl, A., Roskelley, C. & McNagny, K. (2007). The CD34-related molecule podocalyxin is a potent inducer of microvillus formation. *PLoS One*. Vol. 2, No. 2, (Jan), pp. e227, ISSN 1932-6203

Ouyang, G., Wang, Z., Fang, X., Liu, J. & Yang, C.J. (2010). Molecular signaling of the epithelial to mesenchymal transition in generating and maintaining cancer stem cells. *Cellular and Molecular Life Sciences*. Vol. 67, No. 15, (Aug), pp. 2605-2618, ISSN 1420-9071

Palecek, S.P. (2011). Pluripotent Stem Cells: Sources and Characterization, In: *Tissue Engineering: From Lab to Clinic*, Pallua N. & Suschek, C.V. (eds.), pp. (69-82), Springer-Verlag, ISBN 978-3-642-02824-3, Berlin-Heidelberg.

Palmer, R.E., Kotsianti, A., Cadman, B., Boyd, T., Gerald, W. & Haber, D.A. (2001). WT1 regulates the expression of the major glomerular podocyte membrane protein Podocalyxin. *Current Biology*. Vol. 11, No. 22, (Nov 13), pp. 1805-1809, ISSN 0960-9822

Riccioni, R., Calzolari, A., Biffoni, M., Senese, M., Riti, V., Petrucci, E., Pasquini, L., Cedrone, M., Lo-Coco, F., Diverio, D., Foa, R., Peschle, C. & Testa, U. (2006). Podocalyxin is expressed in normal and leukemic monocytes. *Blood Cells, Molecules & Diseases*. Vol. 37, No. 3, (Nov-Dec), pp. 218-225, ISSN 1079-9796

Sahai, E., and Marshall, C.J. (2002). RHO-GTPases and cancer. *Nature Reviews. Cancer*. Vol. 2, No. 2, (Feb), pp. 133-142, ISSN 1474-175X

Sarrio, D., Rodriguez-Pinilla, S.M., Hardisson, D., Cano, A., Moreno-Bueno, G., and Palacios, J. (2008). Epithelial-mesenchymal transition in breast cancer relates to the basal-like phenotype. *Cancer Research.* Vol. 68, No. 4, (Feb 15), pp. 989-997, ISSN 1538-7445

Sartor, M.A., Mahavisno, V., Keshamouni, V.G., Cavalcoli, J., Wright, Z., Karnovsky, A., Kuick, R., Jagadish, H.V., Mirel, B., Weymouth, T., Athey, B. & Omenn, G.S. (2010). ConceptGen: a gene set enrichment and gene set relation mapping tool. *Bioinformatics.* Vol. 26, No. 4, (Feb 15), pp. 456-463, ISSN 1367-4811

Sathyanarayana, P., Menon, M., Bogacheva, O., Bogachev, O., Niss, K., Kapelle, W., Houde, E., Fang, J. & Wojchowski, D. (2007). Erythropoietin modulation of podocalyxin and a proposed erythroblast niche. *Blood.* Vol. 110, No. 2, (Jul), pp. 509-518, ISSN 0006-4971

Schmieder, S., Nagai, M., Orlando, R.A., Takeda, T. & Farquhar, M.G. (2004). Podocalyxin activates RhoA and induces actin reorganization through NHERF1 and Ezrin in MDCK cells. *Journal of the American Society of Nephrology.* Vol. 15, No. 9, (Sep), pp. 2289-2298, ISSN 1046-6673

Schopperle, W.M. & DeWolf, W.C. (2007). The TRA-1-60 and TRA-1-81 human pluripotent stem cell markers are expressed on podocalyxin in embryonal carcinoma. *Stem Cells.* Vol. 25, No. 3, (Mar), pp. 723-730, ISSN 1066-5099

Schopperle, W.M., Kershaw, D.B. & DeWolf, W.C. (2003). Human embryonal carcinoma tumor antigen, Gp200/GCTM-2, is podocalyxin. *Biochemical and Biophysical Research Communications.* Vol. 300, No. 2, (Jan 10), pp. 285-290, ISSN 0006-291X

Schopperle, W.M., Lee, J.M. & Dewolf, W.C. (2010). The human cancer and stem cell marker podocalyxin interacts with the glucose-3-transporter in malignant pluripotent stem cells. *Biochemical and Biophysical Research Communications.* Vol. 398, No. 3, (Jul 30), pp. 372-376, ISSN 1090-2104

Singh, A.P., Senapati, S., Ponnusamy, M.P., Jain, M., Lele, S.M., Davis, J.S., Remmenga, S. & Batra, S.K. (2008). Clinical potential of mucins in diagnosis, prognosis& therapy of ovarian cancer. *The Lancet Oncology.* Vol. 9, No. 11, (Nov), pp. 1076-1085, ISSN 1474-5488

Sizemore, S., Cicek, M., Sizemore, N., Ng, K.P. & Casey, G. (2007). Podocalyxin increases the aggressive phenotype of breast and prostate cancer cells in vitro through its interaction with ezrin. *Cancer Research.* Vol. 67, No. 13, (Jul 1), pp. 6183-6191, ISSN 0008-5472

Somasiri, A., Nielsen, J.S., Makretsov, N., McCoy, M.L., Prentice, L., Gilks, C.B., Chia, S.K., Gelmon, K.A., Kershaw, D.B., Huntsman, D.G., McNagny, K.M. & Roskelley, C.D. (2004). Overexpression of the anti-adhesin podocalyxin is an independent predictor of breast cancer progression. *Cancer Research.* Vol. 64, No. 15, (Aug 1), pp. 5068-5073, ISSN 1538-7445

Soule, H.D., Vazguez, J., Long, A., Albert, S. & Brennan, M. (1973). A human cell line from a pleural effusion derived from a breast carcinoma. *Journal of the National Cancer Institute.* Vol. 51, No. 5, (Nov), pp. 1409-1416, ISSN 0027-8874

Stanhope-Baker, P., Kessler, P.M., Li, W., Agarwal, M.L. & Williams, B.R. (2004). The Wilms tumor suppressor-1 target gene podocalyxin is transcriptionally repressed by p53. *The Journal of Biological Chemistry.* Vol. 279, No. 32, (Aug 6), pp. 33575-33585, ISSN 0021-9258

Strilic, B., Kucera, T., Eglinger, J., Hughes, M.R., McNagny, K.M., Tsukita, S., Dejana, E., Ferrara, N. & Lammert, E. (2009). The molecular basis of vascular lumen formation in the developing mouse aorta. *Developmental Cell.* Vol. 17, No. 4, (Oct), pp. 505-515. ISSN 1878-1551

Sun, X., Cheng, G., Hao, M., Zheng, J., Zhou, X., Zhang, J., Taichman, R.S., Pienta, K.J. & Wang, J. (2010). CXCL12 / CXCR4 / CXCR7 chemokine axis and cancer progression. *Cancer Metastasis Reviews.* Vol. 29, No. 4, (Dec), pp. 709-722, ISSN 1573-7233

Takahashi, Y., Morales, F.C., Kreimann, E.L., and Georgescu, M.M. (2006). PTEN tumor suppressor associates with NHERF proteins to attenuate PDGF receptor signaling. *The EMBO Journal.* Vol. 25, No. 4, (Feb 22), pp. 910-920, ISSN 0261-4189

Takeda, T., Go, W.Y., Orlando, R.A. & Farquhar, M.G. (2000). Expression of podocalyxin inhibits cell-cell adhesion and modifies junctional properties in Madin-Darby canine kidney cells. *Molecular Biology of the Cell.* Vol. 11, No. 9, (Sep), pp. 3219-3232, ISSN 1059-1524

Tan, H.L., Fong, W.J., Lee, E.H., Yap, M. & Choo, A. (2009). mAb 84, a cytotoxic antibody that kills undifferentiated human embryonic stem cells via oncosis. *Stem Cells.* Vol. 27, No. 8, (Aug), pp. 1792-1801, ISSN 1549-4918

Tan, P., Furness, S., Merkens, H., Lin, S., McCoy, M., Roskelley, C., Kast, J. & McNagny, K. (2006). Na+/H+ exchanger regulatory factor-1 is a hematopoietic ligand for a subset of the CD34 family of stem cell surface proteins. *Stem Cells.* Vol. 24, No. 5, (May), pp. 1150-1161, ISSN 1066-5099

Teicher, B.A. & Fricker, S.P. (2010). CXCL12 (SDF-1)/CXCR4 pathway in cancer. *Clinical Cancer Research.* Vol. 16, No. 11, (Jun 1), pp. 2927-2931, ISSN 1078-0432

Thomas, S., Schnaar, R. & Konstantopoulos, K. (2009). Podocalyxin-like protein is an E-/L-selectin ligand on colon carcinoma cells: comparative biochemical properties of selectin ligands in host and tumor cells. *American Journal of Physiology. Cell Physiology.* Vol. 296, No. 3, (Mar), pp. 505-513, ISSN 0363-6143

Thorens, B. & Mueckler, M. (2010). Glucose transporters in the 21st Century. *American Journal of Physiology. Endocrinology and Metabolism.* Vol. 298, No. 2, (Feb), pp. E141-5, ISSN 1522-1555

Ueda, T., Volinia, S., Okumura, H., Shimizu, M., Taccioli, C., Rossi, S., Alder, H., Liu, C.G., Oue, N., Yasui, W., Yoshida, K., Sasaki, H., Nomura, S., Seto, Y., Kaminishi, M., Calin, G.A. & Croce, C.M. (2010). Relation between microRNA expression and progression and prognosis of gastric cancer: a microRNA expression analysis. *The Lancet Oncology.* Vol. 11, No. 2, (Feb), pp. 136-146, ISSN 1474-5488

Veerman, K., Williams, M., Uchimura, K., Singer, M., Merzaban, J., Naus, S., Carlow, D., Owen, P., Rivera-Nieves, J., Rosen, S. & Ziltener, H. (2007). Interaction of the selectin ligand PSGL-1 with chemokines CCL21 and CCL19 facilitates efficient homing of T cells to secondary lymphoid organs. *Nature Immunology.* Vol. 8, No. 5, (May), pp. 532-539, ISSN 1529-2908

Vitureira, N., Andres, R., Perez-Martinez, E., Martinez, A., Bribian, A., Blasi, J., Chelliah, S., Lopez-Domenech, G., De Castro, F., Burgaya, F., McNagny, K. & Soriano, E. (2010). Podocalyxin is a novel polysialylated neural adhesion protein with multiple roles in neural development and synapse formation. *PloS One.* Vol. 5, No. 8, (Aug 10), pp. e12003, ISSN 1932-6203

Vitureira, N., McNagny, K., Soriano, E. & Burgaya, F. (2005). Pattern of expression of the podocalyxin gene in the mouse brain during development. *Gene Expression Patterns.* Vol. 5, No. 3, (Feb), pp. 349-354, ISSN 1567-133X

Wang, B., Yang, Y., and Friedman, P.A. (2008). Na/H exchange regulatory factor 1, a novel AKT-associating protein, regulates extracellular signal-regulated kinase signaling through a B-Raf-mediated pathway. *Molecular Biology of the Cell.* Vol. 19, No. 4, (Apr), pp. 1637-1645, ISSN 1939-4586

Wang, D., Li, Y., Wu, C. & Liu, Y. (2011a). PINCH1 is transcriptional regulator in podocytes that interacts with WT1 and represses podocalyxin expression. *PloS One.* Vol. 6, No. 2, (Feb 24), pp. e17048, ISSN 1932-6203

Weaver, A.M. (2008). Cortactin in tumor invasiveness. *Cancer Letters.* Vol. 265, No. 2, (Jul 8), pp. 157-166, ISSN 0304-383

Weinman, E.J., Hall, R.A., Friedman, P.A., Liu-Chen, L.Y., and Shenolikar, S. (2006). The association of NHERF adaptor proteins with g protein-coupled receptors and receptor tyrosine kinases. *Annual Review of Physiology.* Vol. 68, pp. 491-505, ISSN 0066-4278

Wheeler, D.S., Barrick, S.R., Grubisha, M.J., Brufsky, A.M., Friedman, P.A., and Romero, G. (2011). Direct interaction between NHERF1 and Frizzled regulates beta-catenin signaling. *Oncogene.* Vol. 30, No. 1, (Jan 6), pp. 32-42, ISSN 1476-5594

Wicki, A. & Christofori, G. (2007). The potential role of podoplanin in tumour invasion. *British Journal of Cancer.* Vol. 96, No. 1, (Jan 15), pp. 1-5, ISSN 0007-0920

Wicki, A., Lehembre, F., Wick, N., Hantusch, B., Kerjaschki, D., and Christofori, G. (2006). Tumor invasion in the absence of epithelial-mesenchymal transition: podoplanin-mediated remodeling of the actin cytoskeleton. *Cancer Cell.* Vol. 9, No. 4, (Apr), pp. 261-272, ISSN 1535-6108

Winter, C. & Albers, P. (2011). Testicular germ cell tumors: pathogenesis, diagnosis and treatment. *Nature Reviews. Endocrinology.* Vol. 7, No. 1, (Jan), pp. 43-53, ISSN 1759-5037

Worley, L.A., Long, M.D., Onken, M.D. & Harbour, J.W. (2008). Micro-RNAs associated with metastasis in uveal melanoma identified by multiplexed microarray profiling. *Melanoma Research.* Vol. 18, No. 3, (Jun), pp. 184-190, ISSN 0960-8931

Yasuoka, H., Tsujimoto, M., Hirokawa, M., Tori, M., Nakahara, M., Miyauchi, A., Kodama, R., Sanke, T. & Nakamura, Y. (2008). Podocalyxin expression in undifferentiated thyroid carcinomas. *Journal of Clinical Pathology.* Vol. 61, No. 11, (Nov), pp. 1228-1229, ISSN 1472-4146

Yin, G., Chen, R., Alvero, A.B., Fu, H.H., Holmberg, J., Glackin, C., Rutherford, T. & Mor, G. (2010). TWISTing stemness, inflammation and proliferation of epithelial ovarian cancer cells through MIR199A2/214. *Oncogene.* Vol. 29, No. 24, (Jun 17), pp. 3545-3553, ISSN 1476-5594

Yu, Y.P., Landsittel, D., Jing, L., Nelson, J., Ren, B., Liu, L., McDonald, C., Thomas, R., Dhir, R., Finkelstein, S., Michalopoulos, G., Becich, M. & Luo, J.H. (2004). Gene expression alterations in prostate cancer predicting tumor aggression and preceding development of malignancy. *Journal of Clinical Oncology.* Vol. 22, No. 14, (Jul 15), pp. 2790-2799, ISSN 0732-183X

Zeisberg, M. & Neilson, E.G. (2009). Biomarkers for epithelial-mesenchymal transitions. *The Journal of Clinical Investigation.* Vol. 119, No. 6, (Jun), pp. 1429-1437, ISSN 1558-8238

Zhu, Y. & Parada, L.F. (2002). The molecular and genetic basis of neurological tumours. *Nature Reviews. Cancer.* Vol. 2, No. 8, (Aug), pp. 616-626, ISSN 1474-175X

9

Using Clinical Proteomics to Discover Novel Anti-Cancer Targets for MAb Therapeutics

Erin G. Worrall and Ted R. Hupp
University of Edinburgh, Edinburgh Cancer Research Centre, Cell Signalling Unit, P53 Signal Transduction Laboratories, Edinburgh, Scotland

1. Introduction

1.1 A brief history of basic cancer research driven target discovery

The incidence of cancer has risen dramatically over the last century due to the improved treatments of chronic diseases and as a consequence of an ever aging population that results in elevated cancer development(Hanahan and Weinberg 2000). As a result of the dramatic rise in cancer incidence significant efforts have been placed on developing new strategies for the improved diagnosis and the treatment of cancer. Traditionally, ionizing radiation and/or cytotoxic chemotherapies like platinum derivatives and anti-metabolites have been most widely used as anti-cancer treatments and although these agents can still have significant effects on improving longevity in patients, the toxicity of these agents along with high frequency of acquired resistance requires the development of more specific anti-cancer agents.

International research efforts over the past thirty years have revolutionized our understanding of cancer developments. Pioneering distillation of this knowledge has led to the development of "the hallmarks of cancer" that specifies specific pathway perturbations in the development of the disease(Hanahan and Weinberg 2000). These rate-limiting stages are comprised of numerous biological systems that need to be perturbed during the multi-step evolution of the full cancer cell. The key systems maintaining tissue integrity and which are perturbed in cancer development include pathways that mediate genome instability, inflammation, sustained cell proliferation, evasion of tumour suppressor signals, death resistance, immortality, angiogenesis, metastasis, immune system silencing, and energy metabolism (Table 1).

This research knowledge summarized above has been acquired using a range of approaches including the study of cancer causing animal viruses like SV40 or human oncogenic viruses like HPV, the use of "model" organisms like bacteria, yeast, worms, and flies that recapitulate apoptosis and cell cycle concepts, and the development of human cancer cell lines that mimic certain aspects of cancers. Despite this enormous knowledge of cancer mechanisms, there have been relatively few anti-cancer drugs developed for routine clinical use from such information. In fact, the most "targetted" and common anti-cancer agents are those that either exploit knowledge of the physiology of cancer (like the anti-estrogen Tamoxifen) (Easton, Pooley et al. 2007) or those that exploit the use of natural products like

Cancer Hallmarks

I. Sustained Proliferation	growth factor ligands activate kinase growth signalling cascades growth factor independence via kinase activation or gene mutation genes include MAPK, B-RAF, AKT Therapeutic Mabs target tyrosine kinases
II. Evasion of Tumour Suppressors	mutation or inactivation of tumour suppressor proteins genes include p53, RB, NF2 Therapeutic Mabs target receptors elevated in p53^{-} cells like CD44
III. Inhibition of Cell Death Signalling	induction of anti-apoptotic programmes suppression of pro-apoptotic programmes genes includes bcl-2, bax, beclin
IV. Immortality	suppression of normal senescence programmes gene include Telomerase
V. Angiogenesis	reprogramming of tissue vascularization genes include vEGF, FGF, Thrombospondin Complex cell models required for further understanding Therapeutic Mabs target FGF receptor family
VI. Metastasis	reprogamming of cellular mechanisms of adhesion and migration genes incude E-Cadherin, EMT pathway (SNAIL, SLUG, TWIST) Complex cell models required for further understanding Therapeutic Mabs target integrins
VII. Immune System Evasion	Cellular resistance to cytotoxic T-cells and NK-cells genes include IRF-1, chemokine ligands, interluekins Complex animal models required for further understanding Therapeutic Mabs target T-cell receptors and CXC-receptors
VIII. Energy Metabolism	Reprogramming of cells to aerobic glycolysis Adaption of cells to hypoxia genes include GLUT1/3, HIF-1, TCA cycle gene mutation, CA-IX Therapeutic MAbs target Glucose transporters and CA-IX

Table 1.

Taxol (that targets microtubules and effects cell division)(Cowden and Paterson 1997). This is not to say that there are no novel agents being developed from our vast knowledge of cancer mechanisms; a large panel of small molecules have indeed been developed that target specific protein kinases, acetyltransferases, proteases, protein-folding enzymes, and other pro-oncogenic enzymes. Some of these small molecules form at the least proof-of-concepts in cancer models for the drug-ability of classes of enzyme: (i) cell cycle enzymes such as CDK1/2 are targeted by a small molecule named Roscovitine(Meijer, Borgne et al. 1997; Kim, Alarcon et al. 2009; Rule 2011); (ii) the protein folding enzyme HSP90 is targeted by the anti-tumour anti-biotic Geldanamycin (Kim, Alarcon et al. 2009); (iii) the protease component of the proteasome is targetted by a small peptide-mimetic Velcade (Rule 2011); (iv) a pro-apoptotic protein-protein interaction is mimicked by the tetra-peptide mimetic SMAC(Wang, Lu et al. 2011); (v) the E3 ubiquitin ligase MDM2 is targetted by a peptide mimetic named Nutlin(Vassilev, Vu et al. 2004); and (vi) histone de-acetylases are targeted by small molecules named Sirtuins(Medda, Russell et al. 2009). Although the majority of such drug-leads are not in the clinic, many of these pro-oncogenic enzymes will likely form important targeted therapies in the future. However, there is also some thought that the small molecule "landscape" that can be exploited to develop specific anti-cancer drugs has been relatively exhausted and that the new frontier involving "biologics" will provide a more revolutionary approach for treating large populations in the long-term.

2. The future of cancer therapeutics using clinical cancer models and biologics

In addition to the classic drug discovery process using small molecules that target enzyme pockets, the development of biologics, including the use of peptides, monoclonal antibodies, and aptamers, which has lagged the development of small anti-cancer molecules based on classic chemistry, will likely form a growing niche in the future. In part, this is due to the fact that the pharmaceutical industry has had one hundred years to develop the expertise of organic chemistry and has in a sense saturated the small molecule landscape. The exploitation of monoclonal antibodies that target extracellular receptors and/or peptide-aptamers that target the more difficult protein-protein interaction is only approximately 20 years old. However, the use of biologics like monoclonal antibodies and to a lesser extent protein-protein interaction inhibitors is emerging as a major market leader in all cancer based therapeutics. There are currently 10 FDA approved monoclonal antibodies for the treatment of cancer (Table 2).

Antibody	Brand name	Approval	Type	Target	Indication
Rituximab	Rituxan	1997	Chimeric	CD20	NHL
Trasuzumab	Herceptin	1998	Humanized	ErbB2	Breast Cancer
Gemtuzumab	Mylotarg	2000	Humanized	CD33	AML
Alemtuzumab	Campath	2001	Humanized	CD52	CLL
Ibritumomab tiuxetan	Zevalin	2002	Murine	CD20	NHL
Tositumomab	Bexxar	2003	Murine	CD20	NHL
Bevacizumab	Avastin	2004	Humanized	VEGF	Colorectal cancer
Cetuximab	Erbitux	2004	Chimeric	EGFR	Colorectal cancer, Head and Neck cancer
Panitumumab	Vectibix	2006	Human	EGFR	Colorectal cancer
Ofatumumab	Arzerra	2009	Human	CD20	CLL, NHL, DLBCL

Table 2. FDA approved mAbs for cancer treatment.

One of the largest sectors in the current pharmaceutical market is Oncology, which is largely due to the lack of targeted drugs for improved treatment of the vast number of different cancer types. Traditionally anti-cancer drugs fall into two loose categories either those which are cytotoxic (platinum based drugs) or those, which go after specific targets/proteins affecting a particular pathway. While traditionally the cytotoxic based chemotherapies have been most widely used there is now a need for the more targeted approach. Of these targeted therapies monoclonal antibodies (mAbs) are emerging as the market leaders in all cancer based therapeutics holding an 80% share of the US targeted cancer market (Aggarwal 2010) . Monoclonal based therapeutics have been around for the last 20 years with 30 immunoglobulins (IgGs) approved for a variety of conditions. One of the major limitations of monoclonal antibody therapeutics is target selection. While many companies first selected the clinically validated targets in the literature this area has become over crowded. Companies are now developing 2nd and 3rd generation antibodies towards these same targets either towards different epitopes, longer half-lives or with different scaffolds. (Beck, Wurch et al. 2010). However, the academic research and medical community has a key role to play in the target discovery process. This will greatly increase the pool of targets with which the pharmaceutical industry can exploit to begin to improve the costly process of developing novel anti-cancer treatments.

2.1 Targeting oncogenic kinase receptors using mAbs

Despite the fact that there are currently a paucity of well-defined, clinically accepted targets in oncology, a good example of a monoclonal antibody arising from physiologically relevant cancer model comes from the history of the development of the monoclonal that targets Her2, tratsuzumab (herceptin). Her2 was discovered as an ocogene activated by point mutations in chemically induced rat neroblastomas (Schechter, Stern et al. 1984). HER2 is a type 1 transmembrane glycoprotein divided into three domains: an N-terminal extracellular domain (ECD), a single α-helix transmembrane domain (TM), and an intracellular tyrosine kinase domain. The extracellular domain forms a large structure capable of binding a ligand although no known ligand has yet been found for Her2. Although no ligand is known for Her2 it is known that its dimerization with the other Her family members is required for its activation by inducing auto-phosphorylation of its intracellular tyrosine kinase domain. From its inception in the early 80's in rat neuroblastomas Her2 later went on to be shown to be overexpressed in a subset of breast cancers, with over-expression leading to poor prognosis (King, Kraus et al. 1985; Slamon, Clark et al. 1987). It was this association with overexpression and poor prognosis that led to the development of antibodies towards the extra-cellualar regions of these receptor tyrosine kinases. The resulting antibody named tratsuzumab was a humanized mouse monoclonal antibody and was later approved by the FDA in 1998 for treatment of metastatic breast cancer (Slamon, Leyland-Jones et al. 2001).

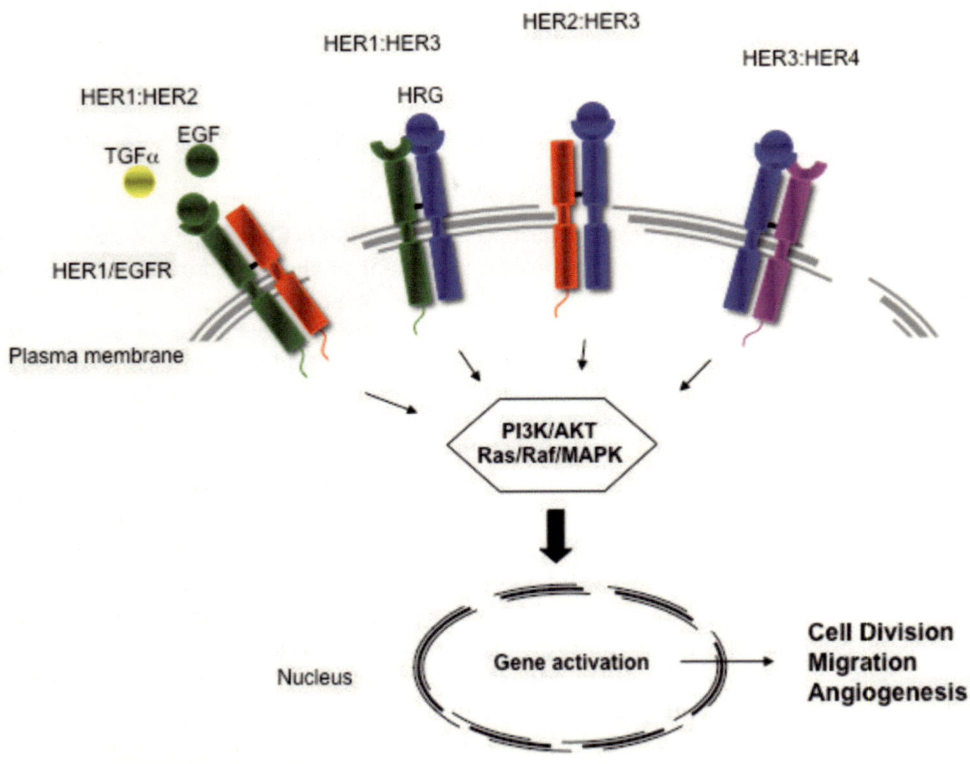

Fig. 1. **The Her2 Signalling pathway**. HER signaling pathway in breast cancer. There are four membrane receptor tyrosine kinases involved in Her signaling (HER1[EGFR],HER2, HER3 and HER4) and a number of known ligands (epidermal growth factor [EGF],transforming growth factor a [TGFa] and heregulins [HRG]). Ligand binding induces conformational changes in the receptor allowing homo and hetero-dimerization transmitting signals via phosphorylation on intra-cellular domain activating PI3K/AKT, RAS/MEK/MAPK cascades. The monoclonal antibody trastuzumab targets the HER2 receptor preventing it from dimerizing and activating its singaling pathways.

Tratsuzumab binds to a site close to the transmembrane region which is out with the potential ligand docking site effecting dimerization with other Her family members (Tai, Mahato et al. 2010). It was an instant success when used along side conventional chemotherapeutic agents with recurrence rates halved and mortality dropping by 30% which was seen to far out weigh the small risk of cardiotoxicity sometimes seen (Chang 2007). Such data highlight the utility of identifying receptors as anti-cancer targets and mAbs in particular as tools with which to develop specific and effective anti-cancer agents. However, this history highlights the time scale involved in the process from target discovery to clinically approved use of an agent.

2.2 Targeting hypoxic cells using mAbs

Another example of a physiologically relevant cancer target that is proving to be important in oncology is Carbonic anhydrase-IX (Thiry, Dogne et al. 2006). One of the key hallmarks of cancers is the change in metabolism linked in part to lowered oxygen supply (Hanahan and Weinberg 2011). In human cancers, hypoxia develops from an inadequate supply of oxygen, which is primarily a physiological change in the tissue due to structurally disturbed microcirculation and reduction in O_2 diffusion. Solid tumor growth is limited by vascularization and indeed promoted by angiogenesis, which is necessary for oxygen and nutrient supply. Hypoxia can induce the expression of many genes, including the key transcription factor HIF-1 that can in turn facilitate the induction of genes implicated in altered metabolism such as GLUT1/3 glucose importers and Carbonic Anhydrase IX (Figure 2).

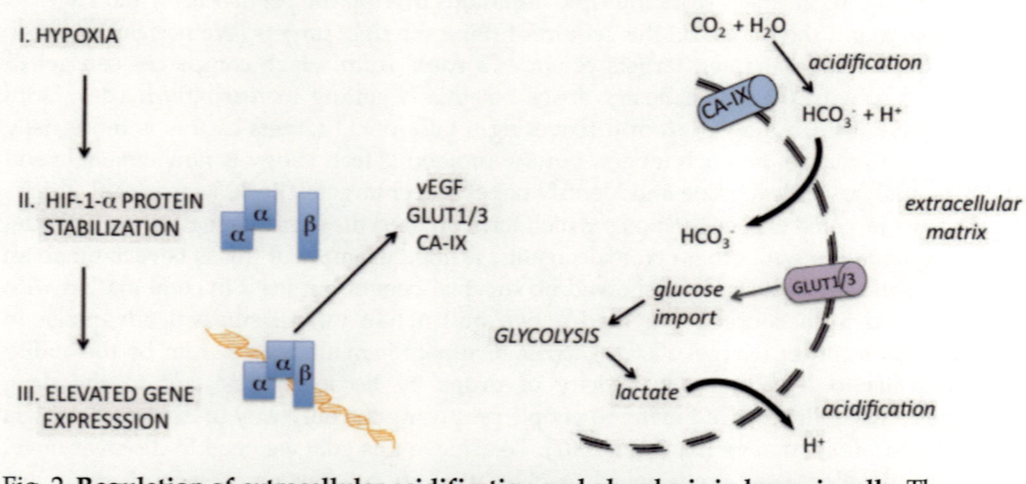

Fig. 2. **Regulation of extracellular acidification and glycolysis in hypoxic cells**. The transcription factor HIF-1a is degraded in normoxic cells through the VHL tumour suppressor protein. In response to lowered oxygen concentrations, HIF-1a is stabilized and forms a complex with HIF-lb to induce adaptive gene products. Some of these gene products include CA-IX and GLUT1/3 that coordinately mediate glycolysis and acidification that together drive survival in cancer cells. GLUT1/3 drives glucose transport where cellular energy is derived from glycolysis. CA-IX catalyzes extracellularly condensation of carbon dioxide and water to hydrogen ions and carbonate. Carbonate ions are transported intracellularly where CA-II neutralizes hydrogen ions and carbonate to carbon dioxide, which is transported from the cell.

The latter enzyme surprisingly functions as an intrinsic marker of cancer hypoxia and numerous mAbs and small molecule leads have been developed that target and exploit the hypoxia-specific nature of this isozyme. Many potent CA inhibitors derived from acetazolamide, ethoxzolamide and benzenesulfonamides have been shown to inhibit the growth of several tumor cell lines in vitro and in vivo(Vullo, Innocenti et al. 2005), although the specificity for isoforms and other enzymes like Aquaporin might add to the therapeutic responses. mAbs have also been developed independently to CA-IX and numerous studies have been developed showing that such mAbs can be used to target in vivo hypoxic regions of cancers (Zatovicova, Jelenska et al. 2010). Such mAbs might be used therapeutically as inhibitors of the enzyme or more possibly as carriers of cargo in a focussed attempt to increase local concentration of cyto-toxics.

2.3 Exploiting the immune system using mAbs

Immunological disorders have successfully been treated by targeting cytokines and associated receptors with a number of mAbs currently approved and many in clinical trials. A major imitation of most animal cancer models such as xenografts in immune compromised nude mice, not to mention the use of invertebrate model organisms or human cancer cell lines, is that the immune system is not taken into account as a variable factor. With so much known about the pathways involved in immunological conditions and so many mAbs in development and their success rate relatively high there is little need to identify new targets in this area. Cancer on the other hand is a different story due to its ever-evolving state. Cancer arises from multiple mutations driving the proliferation and survival of the cell so to put the brakes on this requires hitting the right targets (Weiner, Surana et al. 2010). Going for the validated targets provides a route from which companies can get to market quickly with their blockbuster drugs but this is getting increasingly harder. Until now many have steered away from discovering totally novel targets as this is more risky and the road to market is much longer, but the proteomic technology is now available and reliable to analyze clinical tissue and identify novel cancer targets. (Beck, Wurch et al. 2010)

To date most targeted cancer therapies which have entered the clinic have done so by being used in combination with other cytotoxic agents. A good example of this is bevacizumab an anti-VEGF antibody, which alone showed no survival benefit but used in combination with oxaliplatin and 5-fluorouracil provided a two and a half month survival advantage in metastatic colon cancer (Kerbel 2006) . Cancer treatment is made even harder by the ability of cancer cells to overcome the toxicity of drugs by becoming resistant to the drug themselves. This ability has led many to people proposing the only way to treat cancer is via a drug combination strategy (Sawyers 2007). To achieve this goal we need to discover novel targets and develop new drugs which can be used in synergy or as second, third line treatments to combat the ever evolving mechanisms of cancer to evade treatment.

2.4 BiTE therapy

Bi-specific antibodies are also being explored in the treatment of some malignancies with the aim to engage the patients' immune system to attack the tumor. The emerging leader in this field is blinataumomab, an anti CD19 and CD3 bi-specific single chain BiTE antibody (Bargou, Leo et al. 2008). With the knowledge that T cells are involved in the immune surveillance of cancer and their presence within tumors can effect the patients outcome, it is not surprising that exploiting T cells to control tumor growth is being explored (Swann and

Smyth 2007). Over the last 20 years many attempts have been made to achieve this such as vaccines, ex-vivo expanded T cells and T cell-activating antibodies, either alone or in combination with treatments such as IL2, IFN2a and GM-CSF to stimulate T cells (Nagorsen and Baeuerle 2011). These attempts thus far have yielded relatively low response rates presumably due to the nature of cancer to escape the pressure put on them by these treatments by losing molecules involved in T cell recognition for example.

Bi-specific antibodies can overcome the ability of cancer to evade such treatments by passing the need for a cancer cell to posses the ability to recognize T cells themselves. One arm of the the bi-specific antibody is targeted towards a surface antigen on cancer cells such as EGFR, Her2, or cell differentiation antigens such as CD20, CD22 or CD19. The second arm of the antibody is then targeted towards an activating component of the T cell such as CD3. The binding of both of these antigens brings together the cancer cells and T cells resulting in the activation of any cytotoxic T cells causing lysis of the tumor cells. The BiTE antibody blinatumomab is currently in clinical trials for use in NHL and ALL with promising results so far (Nagorsen and Baeuerle 2011).

3. Novel cancer target discovery using proteomic approaches

It is important to point out that many of the targets of monoclonal antibodies like those reviewed above were not discovered from basic cancer research using model organisms like yeast, worms, and flies, but were discovered from understanding using human cancer material the extracellular proteins driving cancer growth or resistance and exploiting knowledge of the immune system as a co-factor in cancer control. The development of "OMICS" platforms like transcriptomics and proteomics over the past ten years and the application of these OMICS approaches to human cancer tissue has revolutionized target discovery in the cancer field and has identified a large panel of novel anti-cancer targets that had not been previously realized. This highlights the need to develop approaches that can be used to interrogate clinical samples and place less emphasis on the use of model organisms like yeast, bacteria, and flies as doors to discover novel cancer targets. In fact, not only do such model organisms fail to model the "hallmarks" of cancer like immunity and metastasis, they do not express many of the oncogenic targets that are proving to be important in human cancer. This in part is due to the gene explosion in the animal lineage that accompanies complex vertebrate life; such advanced life is linked to complex problems faced by vertebrates that include multi-functional organs as well as much longer life spans and an immune system to combat pathogens that could easily colonize the rich tissue niches. It is also due to the surprising loss of some cancer genes on the evolutionary path of flies and worms. For example, the p53 tumour suppressor and its co-factor MDM2 appeared together very early in animal evolution and it was surprising to learn that the model organisms like flies and worms have lost these 2 key genes(Lane, Cheok et al. 2010). Thus, although an advantage of using invertebrate model organisms is that genetic screens coupled to rapid life span can be used to identify growth regulatory targets, such organisms do not have many of the oncogenic targets that are important for human cancer. An example of vertebrate-specific cancer gene discovered since the OMICS revolution was a gene named Anterior-Gradient-2. This gene and its orthologue AGR3 evolved from a founding gene that is in invertebrates named ERP18. The AGR2/AGR3/ERP18 family has since been under strict evolutionary control with no subsequent gene amplification and diversification, suggesting that the function of this family of vertebrate-specific genes is highly integrated and fixed. AGR2 specifically (i.e. not AGR3 not ERP18) plays a fundamental role in limb regeneration in amphibia, acts like a classic transforming oncogene, can mediate metastasis in animal models, and its expression can predict poor prognosis in various cancer types(Hrstka, Nenutil et al. 2010). Another important cancer gene that functions not only as a tumour suppressor but plays a key role in extending life span in mice, is a gene named ARF (p14 or p19 in human and mouse, respectively)(Maclaine and Hupp 2009). This gene interestingly is only in mammalian lineage and is one of the fastest adaptively evolving genes in mammals suggesting a key role in host-pathogen arms race that typifies genes under positive evolutionary pressure. There are other such cancer genes that are not present in classic invertebrate model organisms and highlights further the need for better clinical models to accurately understand the physiology of human cancer.

The limitation on the use of clinical tissue to identify novel and/or potential anti-cancer protein targets stems form the paucity of well-characterized and well collected clinical samples. That is to say, the methods for protein identification in clinical tissue are adequate, but the development of useful clinical models lag the technological developments. Traditionally or originally, examinations of differentially expressed proteins have utilized "tumour" vs "normal" tissue and exploited differential protein expression methods to identify proteins "over-expressed" in tumour vs normal tissue. Such protein differential display techniques (now called proteomics) including 2-d gel electrophoresis linked to mass-spectrometric fingerprinting has been available for almost twenty years. However, only with the full sequencing of human genome, software to annotate all potential open reading frames, and the use of MS/MS to sequence directly peptides and match peptides to the human proteome was relatively large scale proteomics screening useful. There are now many examples where differential protein expression can be quantitated in clinical tissue using mass spectrometric methods including iTRAQ(Collins, Lau et al. 2010) or label-free and data-independent methods like PAcIFIC (Panchaud, Scherl et al. 2009). Historically, most MS/MS protein sequencing has been performed using reversed-phase liquid chromatography (HPLC) tandem mass spectrometry (MS/MS) approaches with data-dependent ion selection. This so-called shotgun proteomics is combined with liquid or gas phase fractionation to increase coverage of the proteome, which is relatively speaking, still limiting. The recently described PAcIFIC has two advantages over these powerful, but traditional data-dependent shotgun proteomics approaches. First, because every *m/z* channel is evaluated systematically to collision induced dissociation (CID) there is an increase in the dynamic range of proteins identified. This permits detection of a larger number of low abundant proteins, such as kinases and transcription factors, that may have relatively weak precursor ions available for detection. Second, because of the thorough nature of PAcIFIC, protein sequence coverage is dramatically improved which increases confidence in protein identification, that is another contentious topic in the proteomics fields. Another generic limitation of full proteome coverage is in part due to biological issues like the fact that buffers used for lysis cannot extract all cellular proteins. Thus cutting edge proteomics approaches using mass spectrometry aim to elevate the coverage of proteins sequenced in a biological sample.

In addition to the strength and limitations of protein sequencing methods from biological tissue, it is also becoming apparent that examination of proteins differentially expressed in cancer versus normal tissue is not specifying adequate target-discovery. Many studies have compared cancer vs normal tissue in discovering differentially expressed proteins, but these data sets do not identify specific drivers of the disease because the tissues are very different from each other. More thoughtful approaches and study designs are required to identify higher-confidence anti-cancer drug targets that involve progression models where disease zones have evolved from precursor tissue regions. Some examples of such clinical proteomics approaches will be described below.

3.1 Discovering novel p53 regulators using clinical proteomics

Cancer development is a multi-step process which involves clonal evolution of cells under natural selection resulting in the survival of cells with an enhanced capacity to evade normal growth control (Rajagopalan, Bardelli et al. 2002). The core genetic blueprint of the cancer cell is being developed and involves universal perturbation in sets of signal transduction pathways regulated by well-studied proteins such as RAS, p16, and p53 (Hanahan and Weinberg 2000). Of these many pathways, one of the most frequently mutated and silenced genes in human cancers is p53 (Vousden and Lane 2007). The tumour suppressor protein p53 is a stress-activated transcription factor that mediates cellular response to a diverse range of environmental signals including DNA damage, virus infection, and metabolic stress (Levine, Hu et al. 2006) (Hupp and Walkinshaw 2007). The most widely studied p53 inhibitor, the MDM2 oncogene, is often over-produced in a range of cancers resulting in attenuation of the p53 response (Levine, Hu et al. 2006) (Arva, Gopen et al. 2005).

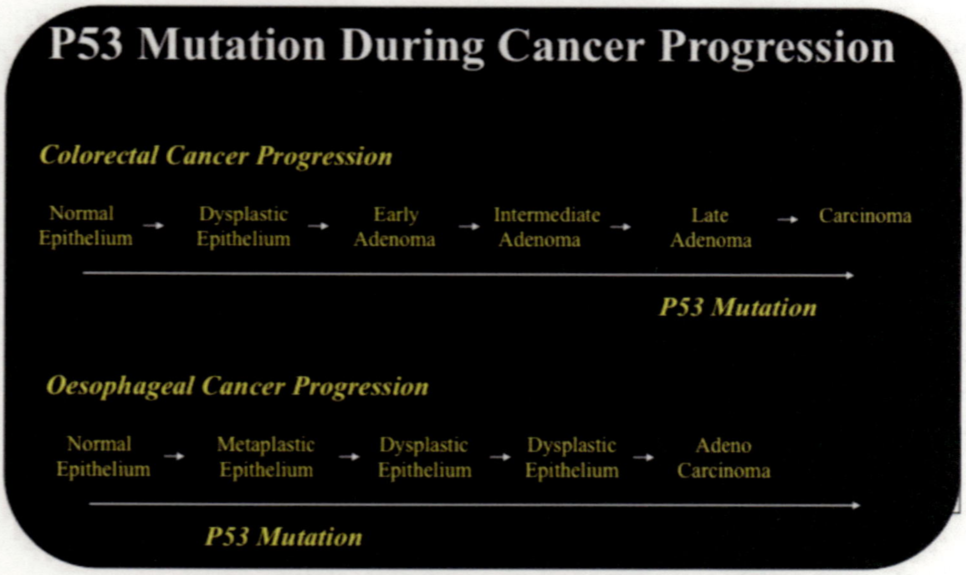

Fig. 3. **Model describing stage and tissue-specific mutation of the p53 gene in cancer progression.** Tissue morphology changes in the so-called cancer progression sequence has been categorized as metaplasia, dysplasia, adenoma, carcinoma, and metastasis. Key gene mutations occur at different stages in colorectal cancer and oesophageal cancer; colorectal cancer develops through mutations of APC in dysplasia, RAS in adenoma, and p53 in carcinoma. By contrast, oesophageal adenocarcinoma, that is linked in part to the DNA-damaging effects of acid and bile reflux, progresses through p16 and p53 mutation in metaplasia and through to RAS mutation in carcinoma. The unusual feature of oesophageal cancer is the very early selection of the p53 gene mutation very early in "progression" and highlights a novel opportunity to understand the environment-gene-proteome interactions in disease.

However, there is a need to develop novel p53 inhibitory screens in vertebrates, if not in human cancers, in order to expand our knowledge of cancer-causing gene pathways and to identify the proteome of novel and uncharacterized targets.
One approach to discover novel clinically relevant oncogenes that inhibit p53 would be to analyze key clinical tissue for gene products implicated in p53 silencing in human diseases using OMICs technologies; i.e. proteomics or transcriptomic methodologies. In order to identify potentially novel p53 inhibitors in clinical tissue, a clinical proteomics screen had previously been set up in a proliferative disease (Barrett's epithelium) which is an intermediate in the development of oesophageal adenocarcinoma. The notable feature of Barrett's epithelium is that selection pressures including acid and bile stresses are being placed on mutation of the p53 gene(Jankowski, Provenzale et al. 2002; Leedham, Preston et al. 2008) suggesting a relatively unique microenvironment for the identification of novel p53 modifiers (Hupp 2000; Darragh, Hunter et al. 2006; Little, Nelson et al. 2007). It is under this unique microenvironment that potentially novel pro-oncogenes might be identified. Accordingly, the proteomics approach to identifying a range of proteins upregulated in this proliferative tissue using clinically derived material identified a protein named Anterior Gradient-2 (AGR2) which was validated as a potent inhibitor of p53-dependent transcription(Yagui-Beltran, Craig et al. 2001; Pohler, Craig et al. 2004). AGR2 was originally identified as a potential secretory protein that is highly expressed in Xenopus eggs (Aberger, Weidinger et al. 1998). Apart from its function as a p53 inhibitor (Pohler, Craig et al. 2004), subsequent studies have shown a significant role for AGR2 in a range of biological pathways including cell migration, cellular transformation, metastasis (Liu, Rudland et al. 2005) (Wang, Hao et al. 2008), and limb regeneration in vertebrates (Kumar, Godwin et al. 2007). Clinical studies have also implicated the protein in inflammatory bowel disease (Zheng, Rosenstiel et al. 2006), hormone-dependent breast cancers (Zweitzig, Smirnov et al. 2007) (Mackay, Urruticoechea et al. 2007), and in predicting poor prognosis in prostate cancers (Zhang, Forootan et al. 2007). The molecular mechanisms underlying these wide-ranging biological pathways triggered by AGR2 are still not defined and as the AGR2 gene is confined to vertebrates, the AGR2 gene pathway cannot be analyzed and solved directly in genetic systems like yeast, flies, or worms. However, it remains important to determine what the interacting proteins-or Interactome-of AGR2 is in order to understand its role in development and cancer. One of the published binding proteins for AGR2 is the extracellular receptor linked to metastasis, C4.4A, possibly providing a therapeutic target for mAbs validation in AGR2-positive cancers.

3.2 Discovering novel Tamoxifen agonists using proteomics

Tamoxifen is one of the first generation smart therapies that can give rise to substantial improvements in disease management. However, tamoxifen has agonistic effects involving either intrinsic resistance or acquired resistance. This would indicate that there are factors differentially expressed in patients that confer tamoxifen resistance or that there are differences in tamoxifen induced proteins in patients that confer cancer cell growth. A number of transcriptomics approaches have been used to identify genes that are induced or suppressed by Tamoxifen that identify key rate-limiting stages of pro-oncogenicity. One of the most striking observations in Tamoxifen resistance is the suppression of the immune system regulatory factor IRF-1 and highlights again the important but under-studied link between suppression of the immune system and cancer development. However tantalizing the later data might be, this work was performed using cell lines and there is very little evaluation of Tamoxifen agonist targets using clinical tissue in conjunction with proteomics. The identification of proteins that are induced by Tamoxifen would identify potential targets for sensitization strategies. A very recent proteomics study was designed using clinical samples to search for differentially expressed proteins in tamoxifen resistant or tamoxifen-sensitive patients and identified a number of proteins that when expressed predict poor response, thus highlighting the power of proteome screens using well-defined clinical cancer samples to identify effector proteins of the disease (Umar, Kang et al. 2009).

3.3 Discovering clinically relevant pro-metastatic targets using proteomics

One of the key problems in cancer responses to treatment is not necessarily the initial response, but the relapsed or metastatic development. Thus, one approach to improve cancer treatments would be to not target an oncogene that is over-produced in cancers, but to target the proteins that have been specifically upregulated in the relapsed or invasive cancers. Although this is relatively difficult in all cancer types, it is possible in breast cancers where biopsies can be taken from original and invasive lymph node samples. The development of such clinical proteomics screens was recently published by Bouchal, Roumeliotis et al. 2009 iTRAQ-2DLC-MS/MS proteomic analysis has been used to identify proteins overproduced in metastatic tissue vs relapsed primary tissue from the same patient. This study revealed potential new biomarkers and therapeutic targets in metastatic breast cancer tissue that would not be possible to predict form other research approaches. From this screen one of the most up-regulated trans-membrane proteins was identified as IFITM1.

Interferon-induced transmembrane protein 1 (IFITM1), also known as 9–27, CD225, and Leu13, is a member of the interferon-induced transmembrane protein family. Its major role is as a component of a membrane complex that transduces antiproliferative and homotypic adhesion signals in lymphocytes (Lewin, Reid et al. 1991; Sato, Miller et al. 1997). The CD19 cell surface receptor complex regulates B lymphocyte development and function and is composed of at least four proteins; CD19, CD21 (CR2, complement receptor 2), CD81 (TSPAN-28) and IFITM1 (Sato, Miller et al. 1997). Aside from its physiological role it has been shown to promote cancer progression by enhancing cell migration and invasion in head and neck cancer and gastric cancer (Yang, Lee et al. 2005; Hatano, Kudo et al. 2008). IFITM1 knockdown has also been shown to inhibit proliferation, migration and invasion of glioma cells (Yu, Ng et al. 2010). Therapeutic monoclonal antibodies have been developed targeting the CD19 protein and have show efficacy in chronic lymphocyte leukemia (CLL) and related CD19(+) B-cell malignancies (Awan, Lapalombella et al. 2009). Since IFITM1 has been shown to form a receptor complex with CD19, targeting it with monoclonal antibodies could also prove beneficial.

3.4 Novel mAb therapeutics in cancer

Another example of a more sophisticated approaches using a combination of proteomics for target discovery in cancer tissue to novel mAb therapeutics stems from the pioneering work of Dario Neri's laboratory. Conventional chemotherapeutics work by targeting highly proliferating tissues such as cancer but also target those normal tissues which also proliferate such as endothelial cells. The idea that antibodies can target cancer tissues alone relies on identifying a target that is only expressed in the tumor or at very least at a threshold that wouldn't have massive side effects in normal tissue. A popular approach to identify such targets is to evaluate the differential expression of proteins in cancerous vs normal tissues but finding the appropriate technique which will give the most accurate results is difficult. Once method developed by Dario Neri is the biotinylation of proteins, this involves the in vivo perfusion of tumor baring animals or ex vivo perfusion of surgically resected human organs with reactive ester derivatives of biotin. The resulting biotinylated proteins can then be easily recovered using streptavidin followed by on-resin proteolyitic digestion and HPLC and finally mass spectrometry to identify proteins assessable in the circulatory system. This technique led to the identification of BST-2 as a novel target for antibody-based therapy (Schliemann, Roesli et al. 2010). Numerous proteomic techniques have been used over the years to discover new targets such as a phage display protocol where by mice are injected with a phage library and tissues excised and phage bound are identified (Pasqualini and Ruoslahti 1996). Direct analysis of tumor vs. non tumor vasculature via perfusion with colloidal silica beads (Jacobson, Schnitzer et al. 1992; Durr, Yu et al. 2004; Oh, Li et al. 2004). Finally a method of biotinylating proteins on the surface of endothelial cells or in the vasculature extra cellular matrix and subsequent proteomic analysis (Rybak, Ettorre et al. 2005; Roesli, Neri et al. 2006). Since tumors are continually proliferating they have a high demand for oxygen so require a very extensive vasculature system to supply their need. Targeting the tumor vasculature is an attractive approach to treat cancer and this technique has led to the identification of numerous potential targets present in tumor vasculature over normal vasculature.

Targeting the tumor neo-vasculature has been demonstrated by developing antibodies towards the EDA domain of fibronectin. This alternatively spliced extra-domain B (EDB) of fibronectin is one of the best characterized markers of angiogenesis and is essentially absent in all normal adult human tissue but is strongly expressed in the vasculature of most aggressive tumor types. Antibodies to this target have been shown to selectively localize to the tumor neo-vasculature in animal models and patients with cancer (Villa, Trachsel et al. 2008). Although these antibodies are not therapeutic themselves they are being used as carriers for other potent anti-tumor agents such as I^{131}, IL2 , interferon-α and TNF.

The ability to deliver cytokines, growth factors and other immunomodulators specifically to the tumor is a great advance in targeted therapeutics. Interferon-α is currently used in the clinic to treat some cancer types and exerts its anticancer effects either by direct action on the tumor or by indirect mechanisms effecting the patients immune system. The direct anti-tumor effects involve the inhibition of tumor cell proliferation, down regulation of oncogenes, up regulation of tumor suppressors and avtivating proapoptotic pathways. The immunostimulatory effects of interferon-α play a part in the indirect anticancer properties of interferon-α (Frey, Zivanovic et al. 2011). Interferon-α was the fisrt cytokine to to become approved for clinical use in 1986 in hairy cell leukemia and is widely used today for treatment of malignancies such as hepatitis c and metastatic melanoma and in combination with some anticancer drugs. One of the major limitations of interferon-α use is its short half-life and potent toxicity limiting the ability to increase dose. Using an antibody targeting the tumor vasculature and tagging it with interferon-α allows for specific tumor targeting with the cytokine, avoiding healthy tissue and without the high doses and subsequent toxicity of conventional interferon-α treatment. This potential new treatment could help further enhance current cancer treatments strategies (Frey, Zivanovic et al. 2011). The conjugation of bio-active agents such as IL-2 is a promising area in cancer treatment. There has been great success in conjugating the cytokine IL-2 to antibodies with an EDB-IL2 (L19-IL2) antibody currently in stage II clinical trials. L19-IL2 also shows high efficacy in lymphoma models active both as a monotherapy and very potent when used in combination with the anti-CD20 mAb rituximab (Schliemann, Palumbo et al. 2009).

4. Summary

The history of cancer research has shown us that highly inventive and innovative approaches like the use of model organisms such as bacteria to study fundamental mechanisms of DNA repair, the use of worms to study programmed cell death, and the use of yeast to study the cell cycle has identified fundamental hallmarks of cancers (Hanahan and Weinberg 2011). However, the by-pass of the immune system in human cancer development and the realization that many cancer genes are only expressed in vertebrates has placed more pressure on developing more physiological models to identify anti-cancer drug targets. We have reviewed here some of the key targets identified from exploiting our knowledge of the human physiology of cancer, the use of monoclonal therapeutics as a growing innovation in cancer treatment, and the use of mass spectrometry in conjunction with clinical approaches to develop more physiological therapeutic strategies.

5. References

Aberger, F., G. Weidinger, et al. (1998). "Anterior specification of embryonic ectoderm: the role of the Xenopus cement gland-specific gene XAG-2." Mech Dev 72(1-2): 115-30.

Aggarwal, S. (2010). "Targeted cancer therapies." Nat Rev Drug Discov 9(6): 427-8.

Arva, N. C., T. R. Gopen, et al. (2005). "A chromatin-associated and transcriptionally inactive p53-Mdm2 complex occurs in mdm2 SNP309 homozygous cells." J Biol Chem 280(29): 26776-87.

Awan, F. T., R. Lapalombella, et al. (2009). "CD19 targeting of chronic lymphocytic leukemia with a novel Fc-domain-engineered monoclonal antibody." Blood 115(6): 1204-13.

Bargou, R., E. Leo, et al. (2008). "Tumor regression in cancer patients by very low doses of a T cell-engaging antibody." Science 321(5891): 974-7.

Beck, A., T. Wurch, et al. (2010). "Strategies and challenges for the next generation of therapeutic antibodies." Nat Rev Immunol 10(5): 345-52.

Bouchal, P., Roumeliotis, T., Hrstka, R., Nenutil, R., Vojtesek, B., Garbis, S. D. 2009, Biomarker discovery in low-grade breast cancer using isobaric stable isotope tags and two-dimensional liquid chromatography-tandem mass spectrometry (iTRAQ-2DLC-MS/MS) based quantitative proteomic analysis J Proteome Res 8 362-73

Chang, J. C. (2007). "HER2 inhibition: from discovery to clinical practice." Clin Cancer Res 13(1): 1-3.

Collins, B. C., T. Y. Lau, et al. (2010). "Differential proteomics incorporating iTRAQ labeling and multi-dimensional separations." Methods Mol Biol 691: 369-83.

Cowden, C. J. and I. Paterson (1997). "Synthetic chemistry. Cancer drugs better than taxol?" Nature 387(6630): 238-9.

Darragh, J., M. Hunter, et al. (2006). "The Calcium Binding Domain of SEP53 is Required for Survival in Response to DCA-Mediated Stress." The FEBS Journal 273: 1930-1947.

Durr, E., J. Yu, et al. (2004). "Direct proteomic mapping of the lung microvascular endothelial cell surface in vivo and in cell culture." Nat Biotechnol 22(8): 985-92.

Easton, D. F., K. A. Pooley, et al. (2007). "Genome-wide association study identifies novel breast cancer susceptibility loci." Nature 447(7148): 1087-93.

Frey, K., A. Zivanovic, et al (2011).. "Antibody-based targeting of interferon-alpha to the tumor neovasculature: a critical evaluation." Integr Biol (Camb) 3(4): 468-78.

Frey, K., A. Zivanovic, et al. (2011). "Antibody-based targeting of interferon-alpha to the tumor neovasculature: a critical evaluation." Integr Biol (Camb) 3(4): 468-78.

Hanahan, D. and R. A. Weinberg (2000). "The hallmarks of cancer." Cell 100(1): 57-70.

Hanahan, D. and R. A. Weinberg (2011). "Hallmarks of cancer: the next generation." Cell 144(5): 646-74.

Hatano, H., Y. Kudo, et al. (2008). "IFN-induced transmembrane protein 1 promotes invasion at early stage of head and neck cancer progression." Clin Cancer Res 14(19): 6097-105.

Hrstka, R., R. Nenutil, et al. (2010). "The pro-metastatic protein anterior gradient-2 predicts poor prognosis in tamoxifen-treated breast cancers." Oncogene 29(34): 4838-47.

Hupp, T. R. (2000). "Development of physiological models to study stress protein responses." Methods Mol Biol 99: 465-83.

Hupp, T. R. and M. Walkinshaw (2007). "Multienzyme assembly of a p53 transcription complex." Nat Struct Mol Biol 14(10): 885-7.

Jacobson, B. S., J. E. Schnitzer, et al. (1992). "Isolation and partial characterization of the luminal plasmalemma of microvascular endothelium from rat lungs." Eur J Cell Biol 58(2): 296-306.

Jankowski, J. A., D. Provenzale, et al. (2002). "Esophageal adenocarcinoma arising from Barrett's metaplasia has regional variations in the west." Gastroenterology 122(2): 588-90.

Kerbel, R. S. (2006). "Antiangiogenic therapy: a universal chemosensitization strategy for cancer?" Science 312(5777): 1171-5.

Kim, Y. S., S. V. Alarcon, et al. (2009). "Update on Hsp90 inhibitors in clinical trial." Curr Top Med Chem 9(15): 1479-92.

King, C. R., M. H. Kraus, et al. (1985). "Amplification of a novel v-erbB-related gene in a human mammary carcinoma." Science 229(4717): 974-6.

Kumar, A., J. W. Godwin, et al. (2007). "Molecular basis for the nerve dependence of limb regeneration in an adult vertebrate." Science 318(5851): 772-7.

Lane, D. P., C. F. Cheok, et al. (2010). "Mdm2 and p53 are highly conserved from placozoans to man." Cell Cycle 9(3): 540-7.

Leedham, S. J., S. L. Preston, et al. (2008). "Individual crypt genetic heterogeneity and the origin of metaplastic glandular epithelium in human Barrett's oesophagus." Gut 57(8): 1041-8.

Levine, A. J., W. Hu, et al. (2006). "The P53 pathway: what questions remain to be explored?" Cell Death Differ.

Lewin, A. R., L. E. Reid, et al. (1991). "Molecular analysis of a human interferon-inducible gene family." Eur J Biochem 199(2): 417-23.

Little, T. J., L. Nelson, et al. (2007). "Adaptive evolution of a stress response protein." PLoS ONE 2(10): e1003.

Liu, D., P. S. Rudland, et al. (2005). "Human homologue of cement gland protein, a novel metastasis inducer associated with breast carcinomas." Cancer Res 65(9): 3796-805.

Mackay, A., A. Urruticoechea, et al. (2007). "Molecular response to aromatase inhibitor treatment in primary breast cancer." Breast Cancer Res 9(3): R37.

Maclaine, N. J. and T. R. Hupp (2009). "The regulation of p53 by phosphorylation: a model for how distinct signals integrate into the p53 pathway." Aging (Albany NY) 1(5): 490-502.

Medda, F., R. J. Russell, et al. (2009). "Novel cambinol analogs as sirtuin inhibitors: synthesis, biological evaluation, and rationalization of activity." J Med Chem 52(9): 2673-82.

Meijer, L., A. Borgne, et al. (1997). "Biochemical and cellular effects of roscovitine, a potent and selective inhibitor of the cyclin-dependent kinases cdc2, cdk2 and cdk5." Eur J Biochem 243(1-2): 527-36.

Nagorsen, D. and P. A. Baeuerle (2011). "Immunomodulatory therapy of cancer with T cell-engaging BiTE antibody blinatumomab." Exp Cell Res.

Oh, P., Y. Li, et al. (2004). "Subtractive proteomic mapping of the endothelial surface in lung and solid tumours for tissue-specific therapy." Nature 429(6992): 629-35.

Panchaud, A., A. Scherl, et al. (2009). "Precursor acquisition independent from ion count: how to dive deeper into the proteomics ocean." Anal Chem 81(15): 6481-8.

Pasqualini, R. and E. Ruoslahti (1996). "Organ targeting in vivo using phage display peptide libraries." Nature 380(6572): 364-6.

Pohler, E., A. L. Craig, et al. (2004). "The Barrett's antigen anterior gradient-2 silences the p53 transcriptional response to DNA damage." Mol Cell Proteomics 3(6): 534-47.

Rajagopalan, H., A. Bardelli, et al. (2002). "Tumorigenesis: RAF/RAS oncogenes and mismatch-repair status." Nature 418(6901): 934.

Roesli, C., D. Neri, et al. (2006). "In vivo protein biotinylation and sample preparation for the proteomic identification of organ- and disease-specific antigens accessible from the vasculature." Nat Protoc 1(1): 192-9.

Rule, S. (2011). "Velcade combinations in mantle cell lymphoma: are we learning anything?" Leuk Lymphoma 52(4): 545-7.

Rybak, J. N., A. Ettorre, et al. (2005). "In vivo protein biotinylation for identification of organ-specific antigens accessible from the vasculature." Nat Methods 2(4): 291-8.

Sato, S., A. S. Miller, et al. (1997). "Regulation of B lymphocyte development and activation by the CD19/CD21/CD81/Leu 13 complex requires the cytoplasmic domain of CD19." J Immunol 159(7): 3278-87.

Sawyers, C. L. (2007). "Cancer: mixing cocktails." Nature 449(7165): 993-6.

Schechter, A. L., D. F. Stern, et al. (1984). "The neu oncogene: an erb-B-related gene encoding a 185,000-Mr tumour antigen." Nature 312(5994): 513-6.

Schliemann, C., A. Palumbo, et al. (2009). "Complete eradication of human B-cell lymphoma xenografts using rituximab in combination with the immunocytokine L19-IL2." Blood 113(10): 2275-83.

Schliemann, C., C. Roesli, et al. (2010). "In vivo biotinylation of the vasculature in B-cell lymphoma identifies BST-2 as a target for antibody-based therapy." Blood 115(3): 736-44.

Slamon, D. J., G. M. Clark, et al. (1987). "Human breast cancer: correlation of relapse and survival with amplification of the HER-2/neu oncogene." Science 235(4785): 177-82.

Slamon, D. J., B. Leyland-Jones, et al. (2001). "Use of chemotherapy plus a monoclonal antibody against HER2 for metastatic breast cancer that overexpresses HER2." N Engl J Med 344(11): 783-92.

Swann, J. B. and M. J. Smyth (2007). "Immune surveillance of tumors." J Clin Invest 117(5): 1137-46.

Tai, W., R. Mahato, et al. (2010). "The role of HER2 in cancer therapy and targeted drug delivery." J Control Release 146(3): 264-75.

Thiry, A., J. M. Dogne, et al. (2006). "Targeting tumor-associated carbonic anhydrase IX in cancer therapy." Trends Pharmacol Sci 27(11): 566-73.

Umar, A., H. Kang, et al. (2009). "Identification of a putative protein profile associated with tamoxifen therapy resistance in breast cancer." Mol Cell Proteomics 8(6): 1278-94.

Vassilev, L. T., B. T. Vu, et al. (2004). "In vivo activation of the p53 pathway by small-molecule antagonists of MDM2." Science 303(5659): 844-8.

Villa, A., E. Trachsel, et al. (2008). "A high-affinity human monoclonal antibody specific to the alternatively spliced EDA domain of fibronectin efficiently targets tumor neo-vasculature in vivo." Int J Cancer 122(11): 2405-13.

Vousden, K. H. and D. P. Lane (2007). "p53 in health and disease." Nat Rev Mol Cell Biol 8(4): 275-83.

Vullo, D., A. Innocenti, et al. (2005). "Carbonic anhydrase inhibitors. Inhibition of the transmembrane isozyme XII with sulfonamides-a new target for the design of antitumor and antiglaucoma drugs?" Bioorg Med Chem Lett 15(4): 963-9.

Wang, S., J. Lu, et al. (2011). "Therapeutic potential and molecular mechanism of a novel, potent, non-peptide, Smac mimetic SM-164 in combination with TRAIL for cancer treatment." Mol Cancer Ther.

Wang, Z., Y. Hao, et al. (2008). "The adenocarcinoma-associated antigen, AGR2, promotes tumor growth, cell migration, and cellular transformation." Cancer Res 68(2): 492-7.

Weiner, L. M., R. Surana, et al. (2010). "Monoclonal antibodies: versatile platforms for cancer immunotherapy." Nat Rev Immunol 10(5): 317-27.

Yagui-Beltran, A., A. L. Craig, et al. (2001). "The human oesophageal squamous epithelium exhibits a novel type of heat shock protein response." Eur J Biochem 268(20): 5343-55.

Yang, Y., J. H. Lee, et al. (2005). "The interferon-inducible 9-27 gene modulates the susceptibility to natural killer cells and the invasiveness of gastric cancer cells." Cancer Lett 221(2): 191-200.

Yu, F., S. S. Ng, et al. (2010). "Knockdown of interferon-induced transmembrane protein 1 (IFITM1) inhibits proliferation, migration, and invasion of glioma cells." J Neurooncol.

Zatovicova, M., L. Jelenska, et al. (2010). "Carbonic anhydrase IX as an anticancer therapy target: preclinical evaluation of internalizing monoclonal antibody directed to catalytic domain." Curr Pharm Des 16(29): 3255-63.

Zhang, Y., S. S. Forootan, et al. (2007). "Increased expression of anterior gradient-2 is significantly associated with poor survival of prostate cancer patients." Prostate Cancer Prostatic Dis 10(3): 293-300.

Zheng, W., P. Rosenstiel, et al. (2006). "Evaluation of AGR2 and AGR3 as candidate genes for inflammatory bowel disease." Genes Immun 7(1): 11-8.

Zweitzig, D. R., D. A. Smirnov, et al. (2007). "Physiological stress induces the metastasis marker AGR2 in breast cancer cells." Mol Cell Biochem 306(1-2): 255-60.

10

MALDI-MSI and Ovarian Cancer Biomarkers

Rémi Longuespee[1], Charlotte Boyon[1,2], Olivier Kerdraon[3], Denis Vinatier[2], Isabelle Fournier[1], Robert Day[4] and Michel Salzet[1]

[1]*Université Nord de France, Laboratoire de Spectrométrie de Masse Biologique Fondamentale et Appliquée, Université de Lille 1, Cité Scientifique, Villeneuve d'Ascq*

[2]*Hôpital Jeanne de Flandre, service de Chirurgie Gynécologique, Lille*

[3]*Laboratoire d'Anatomie et de Cytologie Pathologiques, Lille*

[4]*Institut de pharmacologie de Sherbrooke, Université de Sherbrooke, Sherbrooke, Québec*

[1,2,3]*France*

[4]*Canada*

1. Introduction

Early diagnostic and disease management is one of the most important challenges facing modern medicine, which is particularly relevant in cancer. The lack of effective assays measuring multiple blood-based biomarkers is lacking in many types of cancer. Moreover, transforming a biomarker into a useful clinical diagnostic test is a complex process, which starts with identification, proceeds through validation, but also requires extensive performance testing metrics (i.e., sensitivity, specificity, positive and negative predictive values, false positive and false negative rates, inter-test reliability and test/retest reliability). Identification can be carried out by various means (gene arrays, purification procedures, proteomics), that focus on observed changes of the marker correlated with the disease progression, either in the tissue/tumor or in a body fluid. Many of these methodologies attempt to identify markers in a non-spatial context, for example in tissue extracts, which results in a higher likelihood of obtaining false positives, which are then discovered as such through further validation methods. To avoid these problems or to validate the potential biomarkers several approaches are used including the development of specific antibodies, using protein microarrays or including more refined techniques to include tissue laser dissection. The process is long, arduous and lacks predictive power. Additionally, these methods often require large amounts of material, such as would occur in studies of tumour tissues. Ideally, the direct detection of a protein within spatial context would provide the best chances of rapidly identifying a potential and useable biomarker. One of the most powerful mass spectrometry applications known to date, MALDI mass spectrometry imaging (MALDI-MSI) [1] does just that. This technology is a major new alternative that combines both biomarker identification and validation in a single step[1, 2]. It has recently successfully been used for *in situ* tracking of biomarkers, as predictors of cancer aggressiveness, and for improved therapeutic strategies[1,3-11]

2. MALDI Mass Spectrometry Imaging (MALDI-MSI)

Over these past ten years, important technical improvements in mass spectrometry instrumentation together with the growing importance of this method for compound identification had lead to the development of *direct analysis* of tissue samples. Mass spectrometry has become an analytical tool allowing identification of compounds directly from tissues without any extraction or separation and adding the essential and time saving spatial resolution to the analysis. Furthermore, in a single experiment, molecular information on hundreds of chemical or biological molecules can be retrieved. By automation of this method and powerful data processing, molecular maps are generated from single tissue sections. Another major advantage is the sensitivity of mass spectrometry instruments giving access to hundreds of compound molecular images after one set acquisition. Matrix-assisted laser desorption/ionization (MALDI) ion sources are well suited for this application as they can provide data on a range of biomolecular families ranging from small molecule drugs, peptides, proteins, oligonucleotides, sugars or lipids with a spatial resolution that approaches near cellular resolution. MALDI-imaging mass spectrometry (MALDI-MSI) was first introduced by Caprioli and coll.[12] but major improvements have been developed in by other groups seeking to improve sample preparations, instrumentation, image spatial resolution , as well as develop new fields of applications[2,12-14]. For example, MALDI-MSI technology has been used for biomarkers hunting, drug biodistribution tissue interactions in drug discovery as well as for the molecular diagnosis through biopsy analyses in pathology. The translational nature of this technology provides unique challenges and as yet unimagined opportunities that promise to transform the way disease is detected, treated, and managed.

Rather than focusing on genetic alterations that may lead to a particular disease, it is emerging that changes in protein expression patterns are the most accurate way to identify diseases in their early stages and to determine the most effective course of treatment. Indeed, genome sequences fails to provide certainty for post-translational modification events such as glycosylation, phosphorylation, acylation or partial proteolysis. One of the most common objectives in proteomics is the study of protein expression patterns (e.g., protein profiling) associated with diseases. Pathologies that cause changes in signal transduction pathways generally result in changes in specific cell phenotypes. Using MALDI-MSI in this context does not have knowledge prerequisite of the studied system due to the non-targeted nature of the analysis. Such data leads to the establishment of a classification of cell phenotypic changes at the molecular level and in this way can provide a better understanding of pathologies, can lead to new diagnostic biomarkers or even new therapeutic targets. The capacity of generating multidimensional pictures with a spatial resolution that can approach the cellular level, allows monitoring, in the same analysis, of the localization of drugs compounds and the changes in biomarkers expression[2].

In the context of the present discussion, there is a single clear advantage of MALDI_MSI, that is the spatial localization of identified compounds, that tremendously increases the predictive potential of which markers are most likely to be successful at the clinical level.

There are additional advantages to the MALDI-MSI approach for biomarker hunting. MALDI ion sources can identify a wide range of biomolecular families including small molecule drugs, peptides, proteins, sugars or lipids with a spatial resolutions that approaches the cellular level. Due to its high data acquisition, MALDI_MSI can permit the establishment of a classification of cell phenotypic changes at the molecular level, which can be used to complement histology techniques. The correlation between molecular images obtained by MALDI-MSI and the ones obtained by pathologists using classical histocytochemistry can be inclusive of all grades, stages, cancer types, and cell types. However, differently from classic histocytochemistry, MALDI-MSI allows identification at the molecular level, in each cell type. Combined with powerful multivariate analyses like the hierarchical classification and principal component analyses (PCA)[5], it is possible to identify biomarkers present in carcinoma region from one in a stromal area, from those in an interstitial region. Therefore, in a single analysis we can access multiple biomarkers present in a region of interest, characterize them *in situ*, without any tissue extraction. In regards to cancer tissues, which most often are high heterogeneous, the combination of MALDI_MSI and multivariate analyses are the most powerful and suited tools developed to date. Consequently, we propose that biomarkers uncovered using MALDI-MSI will be more clinically useful than those uncovered by standard methods, such as gene arrays or tissue extraction/fractionation, which lack spatial context. Other predictions also follow from this logic, as biomarkers are known for their potential roles in a disease's etiology. It therefore follows that they may well represent important therapeutic targets.

In the present chapter, we will focus on a single example, namely in ovarian, cancer, to establish the usefulness of MALDI MSI technology for tracking and validating new biomarkers.

3. Ovarian cancer

Ovarian cancer is the fourth leading cause of cancer death among women in Europe and the United States. Among biomarkers, cancer-antigen 125 (CA-125) is the most studied. CA-125 has a sensitivity of 80% and a specificity of 97% in epithelial cancer (stage III or IV, (**Table 1, Figure 1**)). However, its sensitivity is around 30% in stage I cancer, its increase is linked to

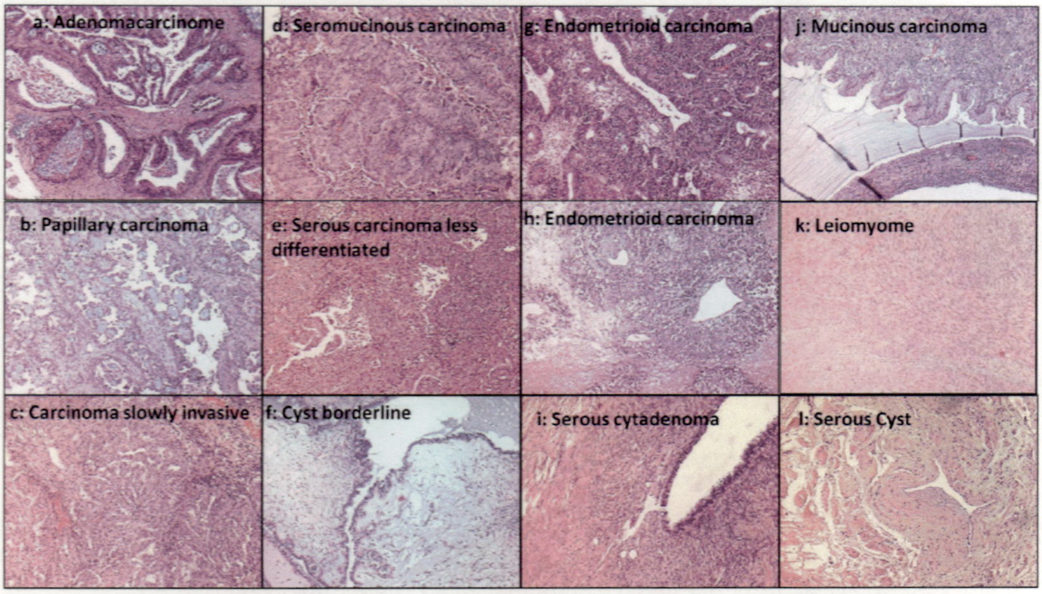

Fig. 1. Hematoxilin eosin staining of different type's of ovarian cancer and benign tissues.

several physiological phenomena and it is also detected in benign situations[15]. CA-125 is particularly useful for at-risk population diagnosis and following disease progression during therapeutic treatment. In this context, CA-125 is insufficient as a single biomarker for ovarian cancer diagnosis. The alternative is to identify additional biomarkers, using a proteomic strategy, that can better etablish the diagnosis and prognosis in regards to the tumor stage (**Table 2**)[16-24]. Presently, two strategies have been established. First has been the attempt to identify ovarian cancer markers in plasma SELDI-TOF profiling or chromatography coupled to mass spectrometry[17,25-30]. Second, has been the development of classic proteomic strategies using comparative 2D-gels and mass spectrometry[24,31-33] or using genomic methodologies (**Table 3**).

FIGO STAGE				
TNM	**FIGO**	**Description**	**Prevalence**	**% of survey after 5 years treatment**
TX		**Non evaluable primitive Tumor**		
T0		**No ovarian lesion**		
T1	**Stage I**	**Tumor limited to the ovary**	**25%**	
T1a	**Ia**	Unilateral, capsule intact, no ascite		80%
T1b	**Ib**	Bilateral, capsules intact, no ascite		75%
T1c	**Ic**	Limited to ovaries but presence of ascite		70%
T2	**Stage II**	**Tumor limited to the pelvis**	**11%**	
T2a	**IIa**	Extensions limited to the uterus and the ducts		60%
T2b	**IIb**	Extensions to the other pelvic issues		65%
T2c	**IIc**	Extensions to the other pelvic issues with ascites		65%
T3	**Stage III**	**Tumor limited to the abdomen**	**47%**	
T3a	**IIIa**	Peritoneal microscopic extension		40%
T3b	**IIIb**	Peritoneal implants less than 2 cm		25%
T3c	**IIIc-p**	Peritoneal implants more than 2cm		20%
N1	**IIIc-g**	**Lymphatic ganglia colonized: sub-pelvis, para-aortic and inguinal**		<10%
M1	**Stage IV**	**Metastasis at distance and pleural effusion**	**17%**	<10%

Table 1. Grading systems of epithelial carcinoma. FIGO 1995: Universal grading nomenclature.

Marker Name	Genomic	Proteomic	MALDI Imaging
Mesothelin-MUC16	99		
STAT3	99		
LPAAT-β (Lysophosphatidic acid acetyl transferase beta)	100		
Inhibin	101		
Kallikrein Family (9, 11, 13, 14)	102		5
Tu M2-PK	103		
c-MET	104-106		
MMP-2, MMP-9, MT1-MPP: Matrix metalloproteinase	107-109		5
EphA2	110-112		
PDEF (prostate-derived Ets factor)	63, 113		
IL-13	114		
MIF (Macrophage inhibiting factor)	63, 113		
NGAL (Neutrophil gelatinase-associated lipocalin)	115		5
CD46	116-118		
RCAS 1 (Receptor-binding cancer antigen expressed on SiSo cells)	64, 119		
Annexin 3	120		
Destrin	121, 122		
Cofilin-1		123	
GSTO1-1		121, 122	
IDHc		121, 122	
FK506 binding protein		124	
Leptin		125, 126	
Osteopontin		120	
insulin-like growth factor-II		127	
Prolactin		128	
78 kDa glucose-regulated protein		129	
Calreticulin		129	
Endoplasmic reticulum protein ERp29		129	
Endoplasmin		129	
Protein disulfideisomerase A3		129	
Actin, cytoplasmic 1		129	
Actin, cytoplasmic 2		129	
Macrophage capping protein		129	
Tropomyosin alpha 3 chain, alpha-4 chain		129	

Marker Name	Genomic	Proteomic	MALDI Imaging
Vimentin		129	5
Collagen alpha 1(VI) chain		129	
Dihydrolipoyllysineresidue succinyltransferase component of 2-oxoglutarate dehydrogenase		129	
Pyruvate dehydrogenase E1 component beta		129	
Superoxide dismutase [Cu-Zn]		129	
Chromobox protein homologue 5		129	
Lamin B1, B2		129	
14-3-3 protein		129	
Cathepsin B		129	
Heterogeneous nuclear ribonucleoprotein K		129	
Nucleophosmin		129	
Peroxiredoxin 2		129	
Prohibitin		129	
Receptor tyrosine-protein kinase erbB-3		129	
Fibrinogen gamma chain		129	
Splicing factor, arginine/serine-rich 5		129	
Elongation factor 1-beta		129	
Lysosomal protective protein		129	
Hemoglobin beta subunit		129	
Transitional endoplasmic reticulum ATPase		129	
Serum albumin		129	
Protein KIAA0586		129	
Similar to testis expressed sequence 13A		129	
SNRPF protein		129	
Fibrinogen gamma chain		129	
Transitional endoplasmic reticulum ATPase		129	
Heat shock 70 kDa protein 1, 60K protein		129	
Heterogeneous nuclear ribonucleoprotein K		129	
Keratin, type I cytoskeletal 7, 9, 18, 19 ?		129	5
Adenylosuccinate lyase		129	
Peroxiredoxin 2		129	
Glutathione *S*-transferase P		129	
Ras-related protein Rab-7		129	
Prohibitin		129	

Marker Name	Genomic	Proteomic	MALDI Imaging
Cathepsin B		129	
Heterogeneous nuclear ribonucleoprotein K		129	
Tumor protein D54		129	
Rho GDPdissociation inhibitor 1		129	
Annexin A2		129	
ATP synthase beta chain		129	
Heterogeneous nuclear ribonucleoprotein K		129	
Actin, cytoplasmic 1		129	
Heterogeneous nuclear ribonucleoprotein A/B		129	
Immunoprotease activator fragment 11 S			7
Mucin-9			5
Tetranectic			5
Urokinase plasminogen activator			5
Orosomucoid			5
S100-A2			5
S100-A11			5
Apolipoprotein A1			5
Transgelin			5
Prolargin			5
Lumican Precursor			5
Siderophilin			5
Alpha 1 antiprotease			5
Phosphatidyl Ethanolamine Binding Protein			5
Hemopexin			5
Profilin -1			5

Table 2. Biomarkers identified by genomic, classical proteomic or SELDI approaches.

Protein	Patient 1	Patient 2	Patient 3	Virus
VE2-HPV36	X		X	**HPV**
VE2-HPV39		X		**HPV**
VE6-HPV56			X	**HPV**
UL16-EBV	X	X	X	**EBV**
UL11-EBV	X	X	X	**EBV**

Table 3. Viral protein detected in patients tumor by NanoLC-IT MS/MS.

Our group has taken a different approach, attempting direct tissue analysis and peptide profiling followed by MALDI profiling and imaging[1,3-11,34-38]. Ovarian carcinomas (stages III and IV) and benign ovaries were directly analyzed by MALDI-TOF-MS after three different treatments for proteins, high hydrophobic proteins and peptides extraction. Hierarchical clustering based on principal component analysis (PCA) as well as PCA-Symbolic Discrimant Analysis (SDA)[34] was carried out using ClinProTools software to classify tissues. Principal component analysis was used in the unsupervised mode to differentiate tumors and healthy spectra based on their proteomic composition as determined by MALDI-MSI. These characterized proteins can be grouped into functional categories such as cell proliferation, immune response modulation, signaling to the cytoskeleton, and tumor progression[1,5,7,37].

4. Proteins involved in immune response modulation

Recent studies have shown that ovarian cancer-associated ascites may provide an immunosuppressive environment[39] **(Figure 2)**. A high CD4/CD8 ratio, which may indicate the presence of regulatory T-cells, is associated with poor outcomes. Recently, Clarke *et al.*[40] have validated in a cohort of 500 ovarian cancer patients that the presence of intraepithelial CD8+T-cells correlates with improved clinical outcomes for all stages of ovarian cancer. Curiel *et al.* demonstrated in 104 ovarian cancer patients that CD4+CD25+FoxP3+ Tregs suppress tumor-specific T-cell immunity and contribute to growth of the tumor *in vivo*[41]. These data point to a mechanism of immune suppression in ovarian cancer either by over-expression of Tregs or by the tumor itself by escaping the immune response by molecular mimicry or by escaping immunosurveillance[42,43]. Additional eveidence has reinforced the involvement of Tregs in ovarian cancer. CCL22, a protein secreted by dendritic cells and macrophages, highly expressed in tumor ascites is known to have a role in Treg cell migration in tumors[41]. Over-expression of the immunoregulatory enzyme indoleamine 2,3-dioxygenase (IDO) has also been demonstrated in ovarian cancer[44-47]. IDO suppresses the proliferation of effector T cells or natural killer cells and their killer functions[45,48]. In ovarian cancer, high IDO expression in tumor cells was correlated with a reduced number of tumor-infiltrating lymphocytes[44]. Reduced IL-2 and elevated TGF-β and IL-10 levels favor induced Tregs[49]. On the other hand, tumor cells escape the immune response by inducing peripheral mature DCs toinduce IL-10 CCR7+CD45RO+CD8+Tregs. Primary suppressive CCR7+CD45RO+CD8+ T cells are found in the tumor environment of patients with ovarian cancer[50]. Another way that tumor cells escape immunosurveillance is through the expression of Human Leukocyte antigen (HLA-G)[51,52,53{Sheu, 2007 #5782]. Recent studies have shown that the expression of HLA-G was detected in 22/33 (66.7%) primary tumor tissues, but was absent in normal ovarian tissues (P<0.01). Cytotoxicity studies showed that HLA-G expression dramatically inhibits cell lyses by NK-92 cells (P<0.01), which could be restored by the anti-HLA-G conformational mAb 87G (P<0.01). HLGA-G5 type has been detected in tumor and soluble form of HLA-G in ascites[54,55] and in the blood of patients[56]. HLA-G seems to be implicated in the immune response modulation through NKT cell inhibition[57]. In the tumor cells expressing a B7 costimulatory family molecule, B7H4 is known to inhibit antigen-dependent induction of T cell proliferation and activation. B7-H4 promotes the malignant transformation of epithelial cells by protecting them from apoptosis and seems to be expressed at an early stage of the tumor[58-60]. In the same way, tumor cells highly express the mesothelin-Mucin 16 (MUC16) which inhibits the formation of immune synapses between NK cells and ovarian tumor targets[61].

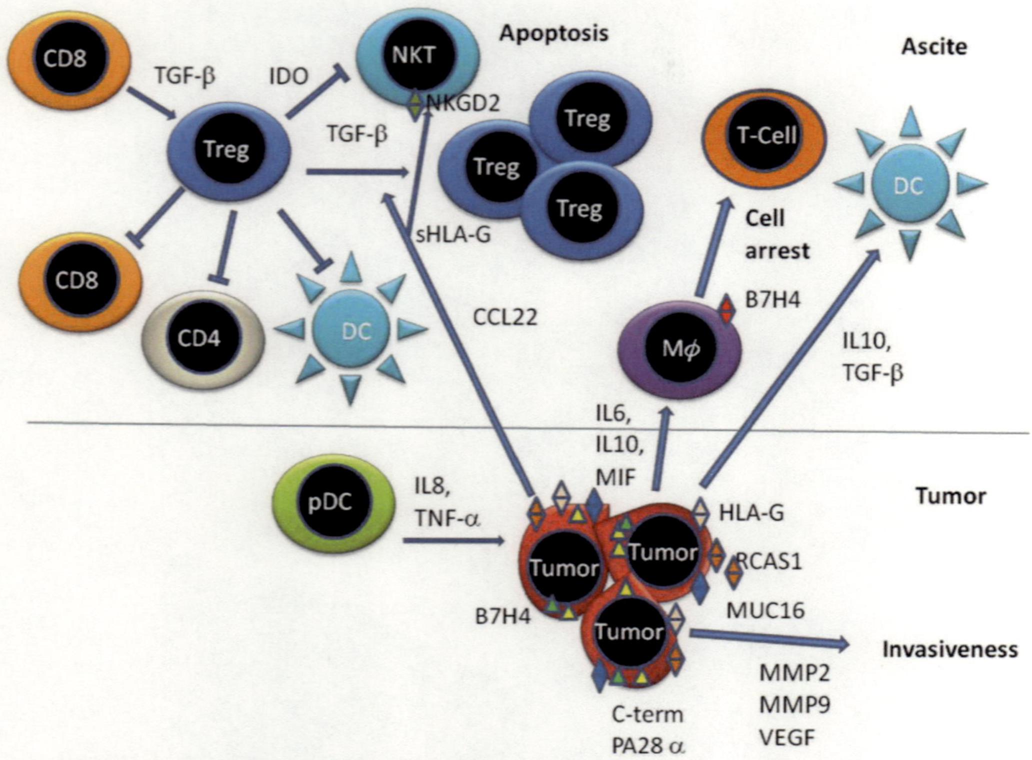

Fig. 2. Immune suppressive pathways in ovarian cancer.
Tregs are attracted to the tumor environment by CCL22 secreted by the tumor. Tregs inhibits CD4+, CD8+ via direct contact or by secretion of IL10 and TGF-β. NKT cells are inhibited by sHLA-G, MUC16, RCAS1 and MIF produced by the tumor and by IDO produced by Tregs. MIF acts through NKGD2 activation on NKT cells. The tumor environment expresses molecules that can convert functional APCs into dysfunctional ones. These dysfunctional APCs in turn stimulate Treg differentiation and expansion. The tumor produce IL6, IL8, pDcs are present in tumor environment and stimulate tumor growth by releasing TNF-α and IL8. IL6, IL10 are produced by Tregs and stimulate B7H4 expression in macrophages leading T-cell cycle arrest. IL10, TGF-b suppress APC function by inhibiting the expression of CD80, CD86.

Transcriptomic and proteomic studies perform at the level of the tumors confirm the active role of the tumor cells to escape the immune response. Transcriptomic studies have shown the over-expression of the macrophage migration inhibitory factor (MIF)[62,63], Receptor-binding cancer antigen expressed on SiSo cells[64] known to be implicated in lymphocytes apoptosis. MIF contributes to the inhibition of antitumoral CD8+ T and NK cells by down-regulation of NKG2D (NK cell receptor NK group 2D)[65].

From our MALDI-MSI studies, five factors involved in immune response modulation in mucinous tumors have been identified, namely a C-terminal fragment of the 11S immunoproteasome (Reg-alpha) (**Figure 3**), orosomucoid, apolipoprotein A1, hemopexin, and lumican which have also been detected in ascites[1,5,7,36,37].

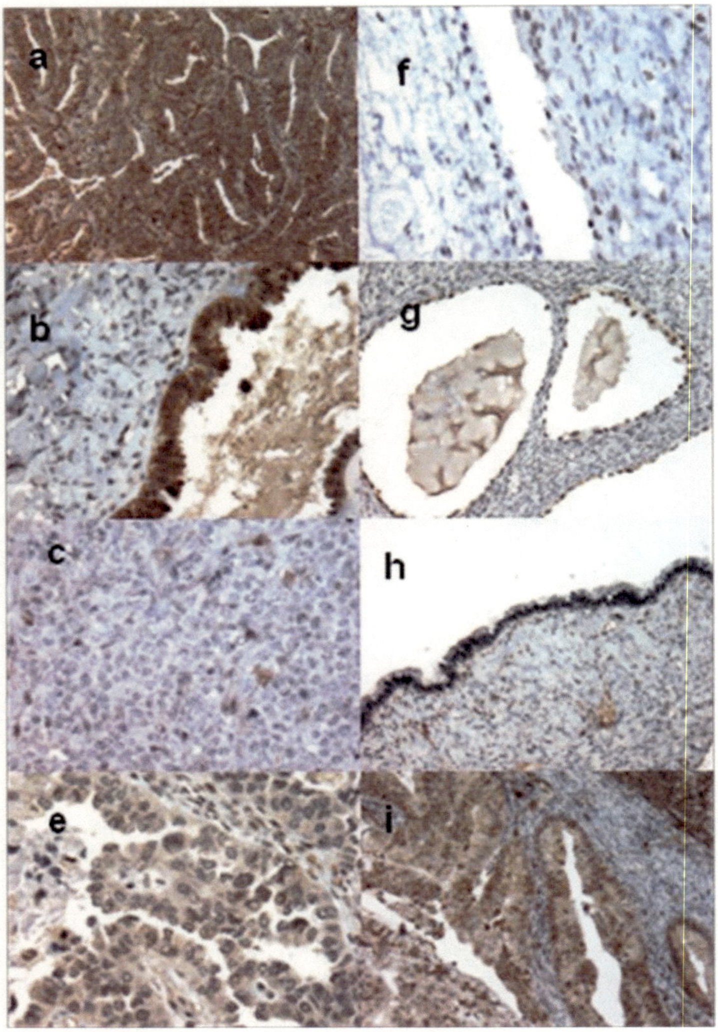

Fig. 3. Immunocytochemical studies with polyclonal antibody rose against the c-terminal part of Reg alpha.

a. Epithelial cells of immunolabeled differentiated endometrioid carcinoma
b. Epithelial cells of immunolabeled in carcinoma region
c. Cytoplasmic epithelial cells immunolabeling of nondifferentiated endometrioid carcinoma.
d. Epithelial cells of immunolabeled in clear cells adenocarcinoma (mesonephroma)
e. Nuclear epithelial cells immunolabeling of benign tumor
f. Nuclear epithelial cells immunolabeling of adenofibromatous tumor

PSME1 (proteasome activator complex subunit 1, 11S regulator complex [syn: PA28 alpha]) cleaved into the Reg-alpha fragment could lead to default self-antigen presentation[7]. PA28 is a regulatory complex associated with 20S proteasome that consists of 3 subunits: alpha, beta, and gamma[66]. Binding of the 11S regulator complex to the 20S proteasome does not depend on ATP hydrolysis and unlike the 19S regulatory subunit, the 11S regulator complex does not catalyze degradation of large proteins. Rather, it is responsible for MHC-class l antigen processing,[67-69] which is greatly improved by interferon gamma-induced expression of the alpha and beta subunits[70].

Several viral proteins that interact with these proteasome subunits have been reported, and may interfere with host anti-viral defenses, thereby contributing to cell transformation[71]. The manner in which they bind to the core particle via its subunits' C-terminal tails, and induce an α-ring conformational change to open the 20S gate, suggests a mechanism similar to that of the 19S particle[66]. No role in ovarian cancer has been demonstrated for the 11 S regulator complexes. Our data demonstrate a high level of expression of PA28 in carcinomas, especially in epithelial cells at stage III/ IV but also at early stages Ia (**Figure 4**).

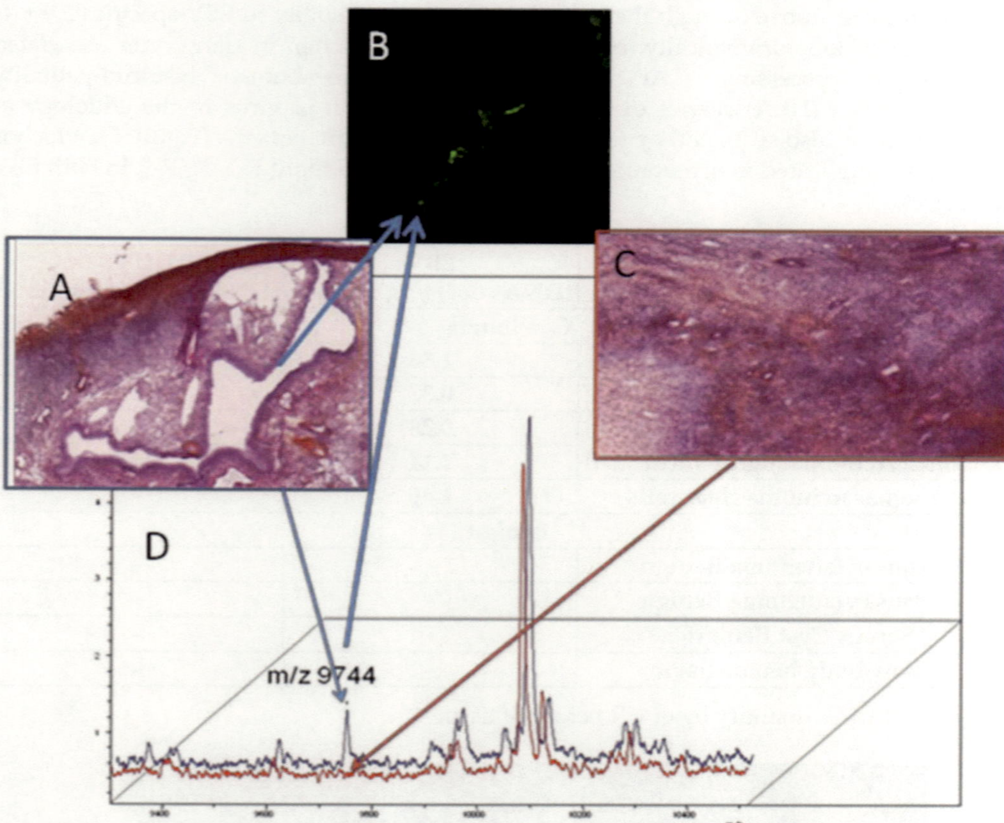

Fig. 4. C-terminal fragment of Reg alpha dectection in stage Ia of ovarian cancer.

a. Hematoxilin eosing staining of the carcinoma cell (acini)
b. Hematoxilin eosin staining of the benign region
c. Immunocytochemical studies with polyclonal antibody rose against the c-terminal part of Reg alpha
d. MALDI mass spectra obtained from carcinoma cell and from the benign region. The data point out the detection of the m/z of 9744 in carcinoma region in line with the immunocytochemical data.

The PA28 activator belongs to the antigen processing machinery (APM). Its alteration by cleavage in ovarian carcinomas may be a mechanism to evade immune recognition. Such a hypothesis has already been proposed for the case of APM chaperones such as TAP, LMP2, LMP10, and tapasin in colon carcinoma, small cell lung carcinoma, and pancreatic carcinoma cell lines. In fact, IFN-γ treatment of these carcinoma cell lines corrects the TAP, LMP, and tapasin deficiencies and enhances PA28 α, LMP7, calnexin and calreticulin expression, which is accompanied by increased levels of MHC class 1 antigens[72]. Recently, PSEM2 (proteasome activator complex subunit 2, PA28 Beta) has also been detected in ascites fluid, implicating its immune cell tolerance toward carcinoma cells and confirms the dysregulation of self-antigen processing in ovarian tumors[73]. Additionally, PA28 alpha seems to be a target for Epstein-Barr virus (EBV) and herpes virus (HV), as our proteomic and qPCR data indicates (**Tables 3 and 4**). Pudney and colleagues[74] have also shown that as EBV-infected cells move through the lytic cycle, their susceptibility to EBV-specific CD8+ T-cell recognition falls dramatically, concomitant with a reduction in transporter associated with antigen processing (TAP) function and surface human histocompatibility leukocyte antigen (HLA) class 1 expression. The implication of virus in the ethiology of ovarian cancer is also sustained by the over-expression of furin enzyme (Figure 5), which is known to be implicated in glycoprotein B cleavage through a motif R-X-K/R-R in both EBV and HV[75,76].

Tumor Type	EBV (DNA copies/ng tumors)	HHV6 (DNA copies/ng tumors)
	Carcinoma	
Serous adenocarcinoma	**1.56**	**0.82**
Mucous adenocarcinoma	**0.37**	**0.10**
Cytadenoma Carcinoma	**0.28**	**1.16**
Adenomacarcinoma highly infiltrated	**1.14**	**0.37**
Adenomacarcinoma clear cells	**1.46**	**-**
	Benign	
Fibrous cytadenoma Benign	**-**	**-**
Fibrous cytadenoma Benign	**-**	**-**
Serous Cyst Benign	**-**	**-**
Yellow body hemorrhagic	**-**	**-**

Table 4.Viral DNA quantify by qPCR per ng of tissue.

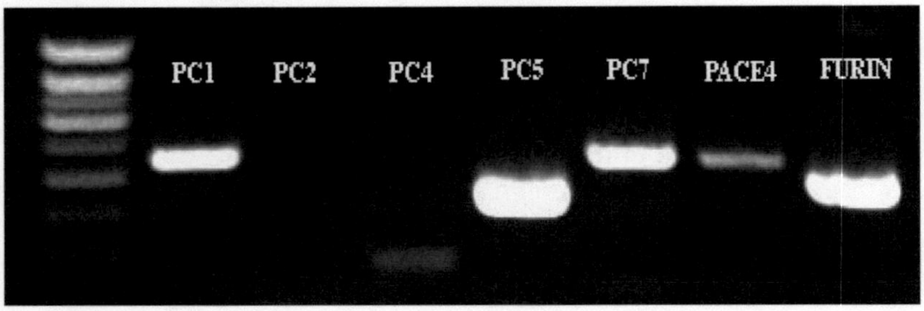

Fig. 5. RT-PCR amplification of prohormone convertase enzymes from serous stage III/IV carcinoma tissues.

Among the other four factors that might participate in the tolerance phenomenon by inhibiting immune activation, the acute phase protein, orosomucoid (ORM, also known as alpha1-acid glycoprotein or AGP), is normally increased in infection, inflammation, and cancer, and it seems to have immunosuppressive properties in ovarian carcinoma ascites through inhibition of IL-2 secretion by lymphocytes[77]. Similarly, apolipoprotein A1 has been detected in conjunction with transthyretin and transferrin in early-stage mucinous tumors[78]. ApoA-I is known to decrease expression of surface molecules such as CD1a, CD80, CD86, and HLA-DR in dendritic cells, and it stimulates the production of IL-10[79].

Interestingly, hemopexin has recently been demonstrated to reduce TNF α and IL-6 from macrophages during inflammation and limits TLR4 and TLR2 agonist-induced macrophage cytokine production[80]. We demonstrate that in SKOV-3 epithelial ovarian carcinoma cells, all TLRs are over-expressed with the exception of TLR9 and TLR10 (**Figure 6**). This is in line with the over-expression of lumican, which is a small LRR proteoglycan in the extracellular matrix. Along with other proteoglycans, such as decorin, biglycan, and prolargin, lumican is known to be over-expressed in breast cancer and to play a role in tumor progression[81,82]. However, as demonstrated for biglycan, which interacts with TLR2/4 on macrophages[83,84], we speculate that lumican is also involved in the activation of the inflammasome through TLR2/4 interaction. The activation of all danger-sensing receptors in carcinoma cells can be explained through the regulation of inflammation by carcinoma cells to facilitate tumor progression. In a sense, this implies that ovarian cancer cells act as "parasites" and use molecular mimicry[85] to escape the immune response, as they produce immunosuppressors to achieve tolerance (**Figure 7**).

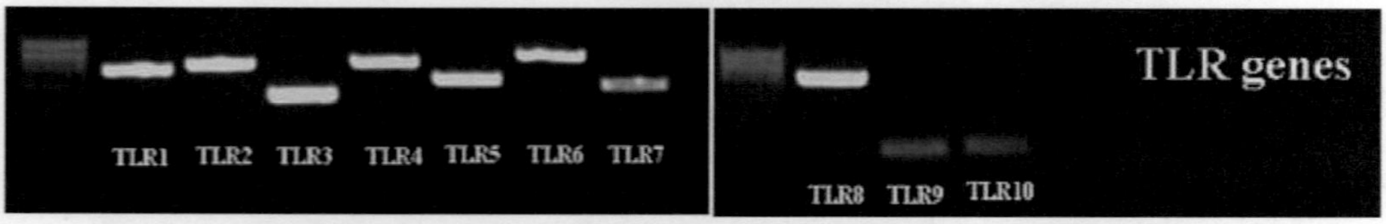

Fig. 6. RT-PCR amplification of Toll-like receptors from serous stage III/IV carcinoma tissues.

5. Proteins associated with cell proliferation

The S100 protein family has been previously detected in aggressive ovarian tumors[30]. In our study, we detected S100 A11 and S100 A12 proteins. S100 A11 has been detected in ovarian ascites[73]. S100 A11 (or calgizzarin) is known to regulate cell growth by inhibiting DNA synthesis[86,87]. S100 A12 is known to contribute to leukocyte migration in chronic inflammatory responses[88]. In conjunction with S100 proteins and cytoskeleton modifying proteins, we also detected expression of oviduct-specific glycoprotein (OGP, Mucin-9), a marker of normal oviductal epithelium. Our data are supportive of Woo and associates, who found that OGP is a tubal differentiation marker and may indicate early events in ovarian carcinogenesis. These data also support the hypothesis of oviduct ascini as the origin of serous ovarian carcinoma.

From immune components, stromal cell-derived factor-1 (SDF-1), the ligand of the CXCR4 receptor, is a CXC chemokine that induces proliferation in ovarian cancer cells by increasing the phosphorylation and activation of extracellular signal-regulated kinases (ERK)1/2, which in turn is correlated to epidermal growth factor (EGF) receptor transactivation.

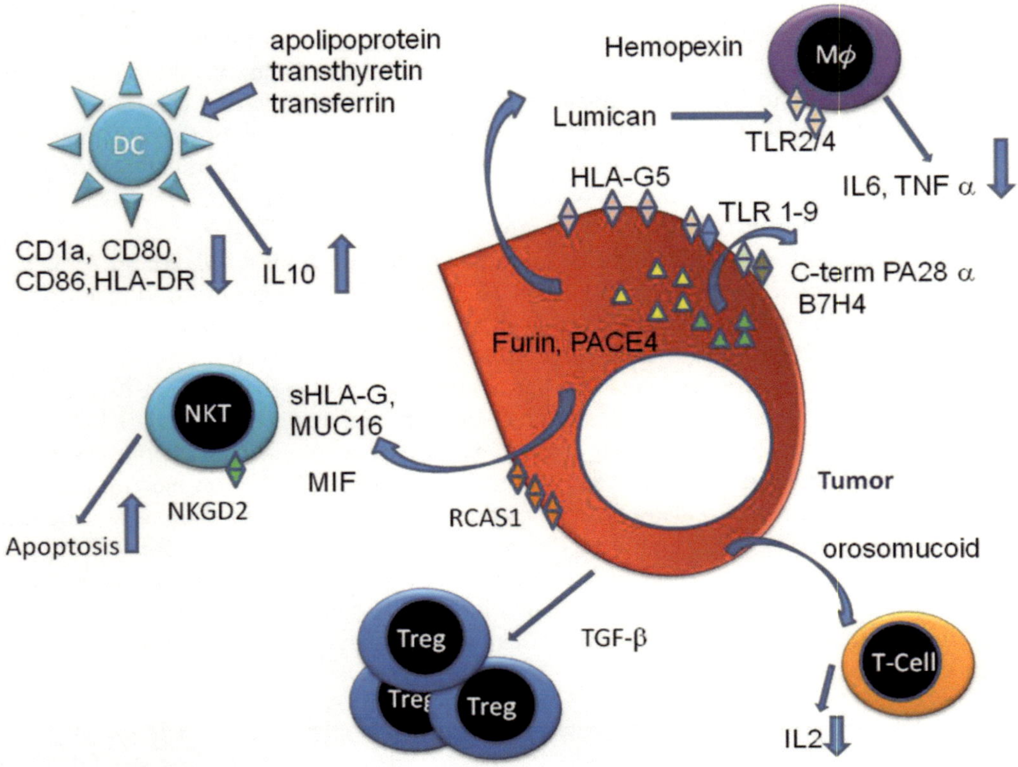

Fig. 7. Tumor cell factors production for escaping immune response.
Apolipoprotein A1 has been detected in conjunction with transthyretin and transferrin in early-stage mucinous tumors. Lumican, which is a small LRR proteoglycan in the extracellular matrix is known to be overexpressed in breast cancer and to play a role in tumor progression. ApoA-I is known to decrease expression of surface molecules such as CD1a, CD80, CD86, and HLA-DR in dendritic cells, and it stimulates the production of IL-10 hemopexin has recently been demonstrated to reduce TNF and IL-6 from macrophages during inflammation, and it limits TLR4 and TLR2 agonist-induced macrophage cytokine production. Orosomucoid have immunosuppressive properties in ovarian carcinoma ascites through inhibition of IL-2 secretion by lymphocytes. The tumor environment expresses molecules that can convert functional APCs into dysfunctional ones. These dysfunctional APCs in turn stimulate Treg differentiation and expansion. The tumor produces IL6, IL8, MUC18, MIF, RCAS1, sHLA-G exerting negative effects on the T-Cells. PA28 activator belongs to the antigen processing machinery (APM). Its alteration by cleavage by (furin, PACE4) in ovarian carcinomas participates in a mechanism to evade immune recognition.

Similarly, TGF-β produced by Treg cells stimulates tumor cell proliferation and increases matrix metalloproteinase's (MMP) production and enhances invasiveness of ovarian cancer cells[89-93]. In ovarian cancer, IL7 acts as a growth factor, like in breast cancer, and has been found in ascites and plasma[39,94,95]. pDcs are also present in tumor environment and stimulate tumor growth by releasing TNF-α and IL8. The sum of these data reflect that cytokines exert pleiotropic effects in ovarian cancer and exert a major role in tumor proliferation.

6. Signaling to the cytoskeleton

Several candidate proteins, including profilin-1, cofilin-1, vimentin, and cytokeratin 19 are involved in the intracellular signaling to the cytoskeleton. Changes in cell phenotype, such as the conversion of epithelial cells to mesenchymal cells, are integral not only to embryonic development but also to cancer invasion and metastasis. Cells undergoing the epithelial-mesenchymal transition (EMT) lose their epithelial morphology, reorganize their cytoskeleton, and acquire a motile phenotype through the up- and down-regulation of several molecules, including tight and adherent junction proteins and mesenchymal markers. TGF-β has been described to induce EMT in ovarian adenosarcoma cells[96]. (**Figure 8A**)

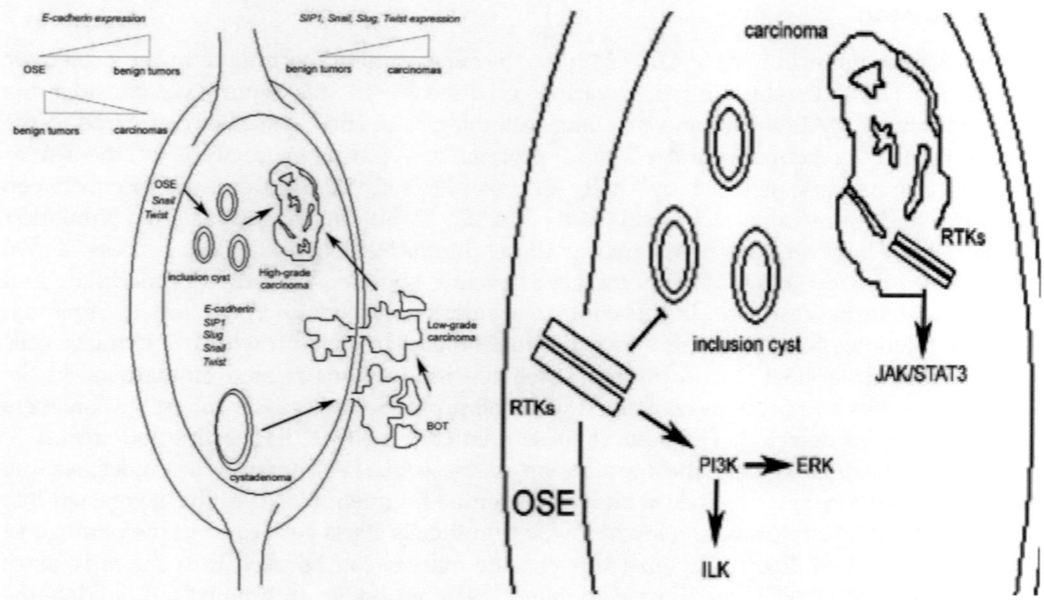

Figure 8.

A: Schematic illustration of E-cadherin, SIP1, Snail, Slug and Twist during ovarian progression. In this model, epithelial ovarian tumors have been classified into two broad categories: type I tumors including low-grade serous carcinomas, mucinous, endometrioid, and clear cells carcinomas seem to develop from their precursors, namely borderline ovarian tumors (BOTs), in a stepwise manner; type II including high-grade serous malignancies develop from the OSE or inclusion cysts without a common precursor.OSE cells covering the ovarian surface do not express E-cadherin but are positive for Snail and Twist expression. As depicted, E-cadherin expression changes during ovarian cancer progression showing an inverse correlation compared to SIP1, Snail, Slug and Twist expression[93].

B: A simplified overview of signalling network regulating EGF-induced EMT. In OSE cells, activation of the EGF receptor tyrosine kinases (RTKs) by EGF results in activation of the phosphatidylinositol 3-kinase (PI3K), which activates ILK and ERK pathways. EGF treated OSE cells display a molecular signature characteristic of EMT and are less likely to undergo a conversion in inclusion cysts.JAK/STAT3 pathway is required to induce EMT in ovarian cancer cells. Ovarian cancer cells that undergo EMT lose the expression of E-cadherin and NGAL and show an increased motility.

In the human lung adenocarcinoma cell line A549, this differentiation is accompanied by modification in the expression of several cytoskeleton proteins including β-actin, cofilin 1, moesin, filamin A and B, heat-shock protein beta-1, transgelin-2, S100 A11, and calpactin. These changes presumably increase migratory and invasive abilities[97]. We recently demonstrated that treatment of the ovarian cancer cell line SKOV-3 with TGF-β (10 ng/mL, 24 h) increases the expression of cofilin and profilin-1 at mRNA and protein level, and modifies its cytoskeletal organization as assessed by confocal microscopy analysis[98]. After binding to its receptor, TGF-β stimulates the reorganization of the actin cytoskeleton and triggers the formation of stress fibers and cellular protrusions[98] (**Figure 8B**).

7. Conclusion

A decade after its inception, MALDI-MSI has become a unique technique in the proteomic arsenal for biomarker hunting in a variety of diseases. In this report, we consider the contributions of MALDI-MSI and profiling technologies to clinical studies compared to the ones obtained by genomic and classical proteomic. A stringent analysis of the list of potential biomarkers detected by three technologies reflects little convergence between genomic and proteomic (classical and MALDI MSI) investigations by biomarker comparison. However, when integrating theses biomarkers in biological process, a real convergence can be shown. What emerges is picture showing how tumors modulate and escape the immune response. In this context, several biomarkers can be detected. Similarly, immune tolerance forced by the tumor production and interaction with the immune cells also revealed, in ascites and in plasma, some specific immune related biomarkers. In the same way, genes and proteins associated with cell proliferation, cell migration, invasiveness and EMT can be detected. The sum of these data confirm that diagnostics and treatment efficacy can be followed by the modulation of these markers. One of the most exciting finding is based on data obtained with the C-terminal fragment of Reg-alpha, suggested that self modulation mechanism developed by the tumor cells starts very early in the pathogenic process. Antibodies directed against this specific marker can be used to track early stage tumor cells. MALDI-MSI can be used to detect these antibodies in tumors and validate the therapeutic strategy.

A decade after its inception, MALDI-MSI has become a unique technique in the proteomic arsenal for biomarker hunting. At this stage of development, it is important to ask whether we can consider this technique to be sufficiently developed for routine use in a clinical setting or an indispensable technology used in translational research. In this report, we have considered the contributions of MALDI-MSI and profiling technologies for clinical studies, outlining new directions that are required to align these technologies with the objectives of clinical proteomics.

8. Acknowledgements

Supported by grants from Agence Nationale de la Recherche (ANR PCV to IF), Institut du Cancer (INCA to IF), Institut de Recherche en Santé du Canada (ISRC to MS & RD), the Ministère du Développement Économique de l'Innovation et de l'Exportation (MDEIE to R.D), the Fond de la recherche en santé du Québec (FRSQ to R.D) and the Région Nord-Pas de Calais (to RL). R.D. is a member of the Centre de Recherche Clinique Etienne-Le Bel (Sherbrooke, Qc, Canada)

9. References

[1] Franck, J.; Arafah, K.; Elayed, M.; Bonnel, D.; Vergara, D.; Jacquet, A.; Vinatier, D.; Wisztorski, M.; Day, R.; Fournier, I.; Salzet, M., MALDI imaging mass spectrometry: state of the art technology in clinical proteomics. *Mol Cell Proteomics* 2009, *8* (9), 2023-33.

[2] Fournier, I.; Wisztorski, M.; Salzet, M., Tissue imaging using MALDI-MS: a new frontier of histopathology proteomics. *Expert Rev Proteomics* 2008, *5* (3), 413-24.

[3] Amstalden van Hove, E. R.; Blackwell, T. R.; Klinkert, I.; Eijkel, G. B.; Heeren, R. M.; Glunde, K., Multimodal mass spectrometric imaging of small molecules reveals distinct spatio-molecular signatures in differentially metastatic breast tumor models. *Cancer Res 70* (22), 9012-21.

[4] Drake, R. R.; Cazares, L. H.; Jones, E. E.; Fuller, T. W.; Semmes, O. J.; Laronga, C., Challenges to Developing Proteomic-Based Breast Cancer Diagnostics. *OMICS*.

[5] El Ayed, M.; Bonnel, D.; Longuespee, R.; Castelier, C.; Franck, J.; Vergara, D.; Desmons, A.; Tasiemski, A.; Kenani, A.; Vinatier, D.; Day, R.; Fournier, I.; Salzet, M., MALDI imaging mass spectrometry in ovarian cancer for tracking, identifying, and validating biomarkers. *Med Sci Monit* 2010, *16* (8), BR233-45.

[6] Gustafsson, J. O.; Oehler, M. K.; Ruszkiewicz, A.; McColl, S. R.; Hoffmann, P., MALDI Imaging Mass Spectrometry (MALDI-IMS)-Application of Spatial Proteomics for Ovarian Cancer Classification and Diagnosis. *Int J Mol Sci 12* (1), 773-94.

[7] Lemaire, R.; Menguellet, S. A.; Stauber, J.; Marchaudon, V.; Lucot, J. P.; Collinet, P.; Farine, M. O.; Vinatier, D.; Day, R.; Ducoroy, P.; Salzet, M.; Fournier, I., Specific MALDI imaging and profiling for biomarker hunting and validation: fragment of the 11S proteasome activator complex, Reg alpha fragment, is a new potential ovary cancer biomarker. *J Proteome Res* 2007, *6* (11), 4127-34.

[8] Schwamborn, K.; Caprioli, R. M., MALDI imaging mass spectrometry--painting molecular pictures. *Mol Oncol 4* (6), 529-38.

[9] Schwamborn, K.; Caprioli, R. M., Molecular imaging by mass spectrometry--looking beyond classical histology. *Nat Rev Cancer 10* (9), 639-46.

[10] Schwamborn, K.; Krieg, R. C.; Jirak, P.; Ott, G.; Knuchel, R.; Rosenwald, A.; Wellmann, A., Application of MALDI imaging for the diagnosis of classical Hodgkin lymphoma. *J Cancer Res Clin Oncol 136* (11), 1651-5.

[11] Schwamborn, K.; Krieg, R. C.; Uhlig, S.; Ikenberg, H.; Wellmann, A., MALDI imaging as a specific diagnostic tool for routine cervical cytology specimens. *Int J Mol Med 27* (3), 417-21.

[12] Caprioli, R. M.; Farmer, T. B.; Gile, J., Molecular imaging of biological samples: localization of peptides and proteins using MALDI-TOF MS. *Anal Chem* 1997, *69* (23), 4751-60.

[13] McDonnell, L. A.; Heeren, R. M., Imaging mass spectrometry. *Mass Spectrom Rev* 2007, *26* (4), 606-43.

[14] Wisztorski, M.; Lemaire, R.; Stauber, J.; Menguelet, S. A.; Croix, D.; Mathe, O. J.; Day, R.; Salzet, M.; Fournier, I., New developments in MALDI imaging for pathology proteomic studies. *Curr Pharm Des* 2007, *13* (32), 3317-24.

[15] Lambaudie, E.; Collinet, P.; Vinatier, D., [Ovarian cancers and CA 125 in 2006]. *Gynecol Obstet Fertil* 2006, *34* (3), 254-7.

[16] Edwards, B. K.; Brown, M. L.; Wingo, P. A.; Howe, H. L.; Ward, E.; Ries, L. A.; Schrag, D.; Jamison, P. M.; Jemal, A.; Wu, X. C.; Friedman, C.; Harlan, L.; Warren, J.; Anderson, R. N.; Pickle, L. W., Annual report to the nation on the status of cancer, 1975-2002, featuring population-based trends in cancer treatment. *J Natl Cancer Inst* 2005, *97* (19), 1407-27.

[17] Ardekani, A. M.; Liotta, L. A.; Petricoin, E. F., 3rd, Clinical potential of proteomics in the diagnosis of ovarian cancer. *Expert Rev Mol Diagn* 2002, *2* (4), 312-20.

[18] Bandera, C. A.; Tsui, H. W.; Mok, S. C.; Tsui, F. W., Expression of cytokines and receptors in normal, immortalized, and malignant ovarian epithelial cell lines. *Anticancer Res* 2003, *23* (4), 3151-7.

[19] Conrads, T. P.; Fusaro, V. A.; Ross, S.; Johann, D.; Rajapakse, V.; Hitt, B. A.; Steinberg, S. M.; Kohn, E. C.; Fishman, D. A.; Whitely, G.; Barrett, J. C.; Liotta, L. A.; Petricoin, E. F., 3rd; Veenstra, T. D., High-resolution serum proteomic features for ovarian cancer detection. *Endocr Relat Cancer* 2004, *11* (2), 163-78.

[20] Conrads, T. P.; Zhou, M.; Petricoin, E. F., 3rd; Liotta, L.; Veenstra, T. D., Cancer diagnosis using proteomic patterns. *Expert Rev Mol Diagn* 2003, *3* (4), 411-20.

[21] Fields, M. M.; Chevlen, E., Ovarian cancer screening: a look at the evidence. *Clin J Oncol Nurs* 2006, *10* (1), 77-81.

[22] Johann, D. J., Jr.; McGuigan, M. D.; Patel, A. R.; Tomov, S.; Ross, S.; Conrads, T. P.; Veenstra, T. D.; Fishman, D. A.; Whiteley, G. R.; Petricoin, E. F., 3rd; Liotta, L. A., Clinical proteomics and biomarker discovery. *Ann N Y Acad Sci* 2004, *1022*, 295-305.

[23] Kohn, E. C.; Mills, G. B.; Liotta, L., Promising directions for the diagnosis and management of gynecological cancers. *Int J Gynaecol Obstet* 2003, *83 Suppl 1*, 203-9.

[24] Rapkiewicz, A. V.; Espina, V.; Petricoin, E. F., 3rd; Liotta, L. A., Biomarkers of ovarian tumours. *Eur J Cancer* 2004, *40* (17), 2604-12.

[25] Petricoin, E. F.; Ardekani, A. M.; Hitt, B. A.; Levine, P. J.; Fusaro, V. A.; Steinberg, S. M.; Mills, G. B.; Simone, C.; Fishman, D. A.; Kohn, E. C.; Liotta, L. A., Use of proteomic patterns in serum to identify ovarian cancer. *Lancet* 2002, *359* (9306), 572-7.

[26] Bergen, H. R., 3rd; Vasmatzis, G.; Cliby, W. A.; Johnson, K. L.; Oberg, A. L.; Muddiman, D. C., Discovery of ovarian cancer biomarkers in serum using NanoLC electrospray ionization TOF and FT-ICR mass spectrometry. *Dis Markers* 2003, *19* (4-5), 239-49.

[27] Diamandis, E. P., Proteomic patterns in serum and identification of ovarian cancer. *Lancet* 2002, *360* (9327), 170; author reply 170-1.

[28] Engwegen, J. Y.; Gast, M. C.; Schellens, J. H.; Beijnen, J. H., Clinical proteomics: searching for better tumour markers with SELDI-TOF mass spectrometry. *Trends Pharmacol Sci* 2006, *27* (5), 251-9.

[29] Fung, E. T.; Yip, T. T.; Lomas, L.; Wang, Z.; Yip, C.; Meng, X. Y.; Lin, S.; Zhang, F.; Zhang, Z.; Chan, D. W.; Weinberger, S. R., Classification of cancer types by measuring variants of host response proteins using SELDI serum assays. *Int J Cancer* 2005, *115* (5), 783-9.

[30] Kikuchi, N.; Horiuchi, A.; Osada, R.; Imai, T.; Wang, C.; Chen, X.; Konishi, I., Nuclear expression of S100A4 is associated with aggressive behavior of epithelial ovarian carcinoma: an important autocrine/paracrine factor in tumor progression. *Cancer Sci* 2006, *97* (10), 1061-9.

[31] Rai, A. J.; Zhang, Z.; Rosenzweig, J.; Shih Ie, M.; Pham, T.; Fung, E. T.; Sokoll, L. J.; Chan, D. W., Proteomic approaches to tumor marker discovery. *Arch Pathol Lab Med* 2002, *126* (12), 1518-26.

[32] Xiao, Z.; Prieto, D.; Conrads, T. P.; Veenstra, T. D.; Issaq, H. J., Proteomic patterns: their potential for disease diagnosis. *Mol Cell Endocrinol* 2005, *230* (1-2), 95-106.

[33] Zhu, Y.; Wu, R.; Sangha, N.; Yoo, C.; Cho, K. R.; Shedden, K. A.; Katabuchi, H.; Lubman, D. M., Classifications of ovarian cancer tissues by proteomic patterns. *Proteomics* 2006, *6* (21), 5846-56.

[34] Bonnel, D., Longuespee, R, Frank, J, Roudbaraki, M, Gosset, P, Day, R, Salzet, M, Fournier I, Principal Component Analysis-Symbolic Discriminant Analyses (PCA-SDA) for Biomarkers Hunting and Validation Through on Tissue Bottom-up or In Source Decay in MALDI-MSI: Application to prostate cancer. *Anal Bioanal Chem* 2011, *In press*.

[35] D'Anjou, F., Routhier, S., Perreault, J.P., Lati,l A., Bonnel, D., Fournier, I., Salzet, M., Day, R., Molecular validation of PACE4 as a target in prostate cancer. *Translational Oncology* 2011.

[36] Franck, J.; Longuespee, R.; Wisztorski, M.; Van Remoortere, A.; Van Zeijl, R.; Deelder, A.; Salzet, M.; McDonnell, L.; Fournier, I., MALDI mass spectrometry imaging of proteins exceeding 30,000 daltons. *Med Sci Monit 16* (9), BR293-9.

[37] Lemaire, R., Lucot,J.P.,Collinet,P.,Vinatier,D.,Tabet,J.C.,Salzet,M.,Fournier, I., New developments in direct analyses by MALDI mass spectrometry for study ovarian cancer. *Mol Cell Proteomics* 2005, *4*, S305-S308.

[38] Stauber, J., Lemaire, R., Wisztorski, M., Ait-Menguellet, S., Lucot, J.P., Vinatier, D., Desmons, A., Deschamps, M., Proess, G., Rudolf, I., Salzet, M., Fournier, I. , New developments in MALDI imaging mass spectrometry for pathological proteomic studies; Introduction to a novel concept, the specific MALDI imaging. *Mol Cell Proteomics* 2006, *5*, S247-S249.

[39] Giuntoli, R. L., 2nd; Webb, T. J.; Zoso, A.; Rogers, O.; Diaz-Montes, T. P.; Bristow, R. E.; Oelke, M., Ovarian cancer-associated ascites demonstrates altered immune environment: implications for antitumor immunity. *Anticancer Res* 2009, *29* (8), 2875-84.

[40] Clarke, B.; Tinker, A. V.; Lee, C. H.; Subramanian, S.; van de Rijn, M.; Turbin, D.; Kalloger, S.; Han, G.; Ceballos, K.; Cadungog, M. G.; Huntsman, D. G.; Coukos, G.; Gilks, C. B., Intraepithelial T cells and prognosis in ovarian carcinoma: novel associations with stage, tumor type, and BRCA1 loss. *Mod Pathol* 2009, *22* (3), 393-402.

[41] Curiel, T. J.; Coukos, G.; Zou, L.; Alvarez, X.; Cheng, P.; Mottram, P.; Evdemon-Hogan, M.; Conejo-Garcia, J. R.; Zhang, L.; Burow, M.; Zhu, Y.; Wei, S.; Kryczek, I.; Daniel, B.; Gordon, A.; Myers, L.; Lackner, A.; Disis, M. L.; Knutson, K. L.; Chen, L.; Zou, W., Specific recruitment of regulatory T cells in ovarian carcinoma fosters immune privilege and predicts reduced survival. *Nat Med* 2004, *10* (9), 942-9.

[42] Preston, C. C.; Goode, E. L.; Hartmann, L. C.; Kalli, K. R.; Knutson, K. L., Immunity and immune suppression in human ovarian cancer. *Immunotherapy 3* (4), 539-56.

[43] Yigit, R.; Massuger, L. F.; Figdor, C. G.; Torensma, R., Ovarian cancer creates a suppressive microenvironment to escape immune elimination. *Gynecol Oncol 117* (2), 366-72.

[44] Nonaka, H.; Saga, Y.; Fujiwara, H.; Akimoto, H.; Yamada, A.; Kagawa, S.; Takei, Y.; Machida, S.; Takikawa, O.; Suzuki, M., Indoleamine 2,3-dioxygenase promotes peritoneal dissemination of ovarian cancer through inhibition of natural killercell function and angiogenesis promotion. *Int J Oncol 38* (1), 113-20.

[45] Ino, K., Indoleamine 2,3-dioxygenase and immune tolerance in ovarian cancer. *Curr Opin Obstet Gynecol 23* (1), 13-8.

[46] Inaba, T.; Ino, K.; Kajiyama, H.; Yamamoto, E.; Shibata, K.; Nawa, A.; Nagasaka, T.; Akimoto, H.; Takikawa, O.; Kikkawa, F., Role of the immunosuppressive enzyme indoleamine 2,3-dioxygenase in the progression of ovarian carcinoma. *Gynecol Oncol* 2009, *115* (2), 185-92.

[47] Okamoto, A.; Nikaido, T.; Ochiai, K.; Takakura, S.; Saito, M.; Aoki, Y.; Ishii, N.; Yanaihara, N.; Yamada, K.; Takikawa, O.; Kawaguchi, R.; Isonishi, S.; Tanaka, T.; Urashima, M., Indoleamine 2,3-dioxygenase serves as a marker of poor prognosis in gene expression profiles of serous ovarian cancer cells. *Clin Cancer Res* 2005, *11* (16), 6030-9.

[48] Nelson, B. H., IDO and outcomes in ovarian cancer. *Gynecol Oncol* 2009, *115* (2), 179-80.

[49] Loercher, A. E.; Nash, M. A.; Kavanagh, J. J.; Platsoucas, C. D.; Freedman, R. S., Identification of an IL-10-producing HLA-DR-negative monocyte subset in the malignant ascites of patients with ovarian carcinoma that inhibits cytokine protein expression and proliferation of autologous T cells. *J Immunol* 1999, *163* (11), 6251-60.

[50] Wei, S.; Kryczek, I.; Zou, L.; Daniel, B.; Cheng, P.; Mottram, P.; Curiel, T.; Lange, A.; Zou, W., Plasmacytoid dendritic cells induce CD8+ regulatory T cells in human ovarian carcinoma. *Cancer Res* 2005, *65* (12), 5020-6.

[51] Jung, Y. W.; Kim, Y. T.; Kim, S. W.; Kim, S.; Kim, J. H.; Cho, N. H.; Kim, J. W., Correlation of human leukocyte antigen-G (HLA-G) expression and disease progression in epithelial ovarian cancer. *Reprod Sci* 2009, *16* (11), 1103-11.

[52] Menier, C.; Prevot, S.; Carosella, E. D.; Rouas-Freiss, N., Human leukocyte antigen-G is expressed in advanced-stage ovarian carcinoma of high-grade histology. *Hum Immunol* 2009, *70* (12), 1006-9.

[53] Sheu, J. J.; Shih Ie, M., Clinical and biological significance of HLA-G expression in ovarian cancer. *Semin Cancer Biol* 2007, *17* (6), 436-43.

[54] Rebmann, V.; Regel, J.; Stolke, D.; Grosse-Wilde, H., Secretion of sHLA-G molecules in malignancies. *Semin Cancer Biol* 2003, *13* (5), 371-7.

[55] Singer, G.; Rebmann, V.; Chen, Y. C.; Liu, H. T.; Ali, S. Z.; Reinsberg, J.; McMaster, M. T.; Pfeiffer, K.; Chan, D. W.; Wardelmann, E.; Grosse-Wilde, H.; Cheng, C. C.; Kurman, R. J.; Shih Ie, M., HLA-G is a potential tumor marker in malignant ascites. *Clin Cancer Res* 2003, *9* (12), 4460-4.

[56] Mach, P.; Blecharz, P.; Basta, P.; Marianowski, P.; Skret-Magierlo, J.; Kojs, Z.; Grabiec, M.; Wicherek, L., Differences in the soluble HLA-G blood serum concentration levels in patients with ovarian cancer and ovarian and deep endometriosis. *Am J Reprod Immunol 63* (5), 387-95.

[57] Lin, A.; Yan, W. H.; Xu, H. H.; Gan, M. F.; Cai, J. F.; Zhu, M.; Zhou, M. Y., HLA-G expression in human ovarian carcinoma counteracts NK cell function. *Ann Oncol* 2007, *18* (11), 1804-9.

[58] Simon, I.; Katsaros, D.; Rigault de la Longrais, I.; Massobrio, M.; Scorilas, A.; Kim, N. W.; Sarno, M. J.; Wolfert, R. L.; Diamandis, E. P., B7-H4 is over-expressed in early-

stage ovarian cancer and is independent of CA125 expression. *Gynecol Oncol* 2007, *106* (2), 334-41.

[59] Simon, I.; Liu, Y.; Krall, K. L.; Urban, N.; Wolfert, R. L.; Kim, N. W.; McIntosh, M. W., Evaluation of the novel serum markers B7-H4, Spondin 2, and DcR3 for diagnosis and early detection of ovarian cancer. *Gynecol Oncol* 2007, *106* (1), 112-8.

[60] Simon, I.; Zhuo, S.; Corral, L.; Diamandis, E. P.; Sarno, M. J.; Wolfert, R. L.; Kim, N. W., B7-h4 is a novel membrane-bound protein and a candidate serum and tissue biomarker for ovarian cancer. *Cancer Res* 2006, *66* (3), 1570-5.

[61] Gubbels, J. A.; Felder, M.; Horibata, S.; Belisle, J. A.; Kapur, A.; Holden, H.; Petrie, S.; Migneault, M.; Rancourt, C.; Connor, J. P.; Patankar, M. S., MUC16 provides immune protection by inhibiting synapse formation between NK and ovarian tumor cells. *Mol Cancer 9*, 11.

[62] Krockenberger, M.; Dombrowski, Y.; Weidler, C.; Ossadnik, M.; Honig, A.; Hausler, S.; Voigt, H.; Becker, J. C.; Leng, L.; Steinle, A.; Weller, M.; Bucala, R.; Dietl, J.; Wischhusen, J., Macrophage migration inhibitory factor contributes to the immune escape of ovarian cancer by down-regulating NKG2D. *J Immunol* 2008, *180* (11), 7338-48.

[63] Agarwal, R.; Whang, D. H.; Alvero, A. B.; Visintin, I.; Lai, Y.; Segal, E. A.; Schwartz, P.; Ward, D.; Rutherford, T.; Mor, G., Macrophage migration inhibitory factor expression in ovarian cancer. *Am J Obstet Gynecol* 2007, *196* (4), 348 e1-5.

[64] Sonoda, K.; Miyamoto, S.; Yotsumoto, F.; Yagi, H.; Nakashima, M.; Watanabe, T.; Nakano, H., Clinical significance of RCAS1 as a biomarker of ovarian cancer. *Oncol Rep* 2007, *17* (3), 623-8.

[65] McGilvray, R. W.; Eagle, R. A.; Rolland, P.; Jafferji, I.; Trowsdale, J.; Durrant, L. G., ULBP2 and RAET1E NKG2D ligands are independent predictors of poor prognosis in ovarian cancer patients. *Int J Cancer 127* (6), 1412-20.

[66] Yang, Y.; Fruh, K.; Ahn, K.; Peterson, P. A., In vivo assembly of the proteasomal complexes, implications for antigen processing. *J Biol Chem* 1995, *270* (46), 27687-94.

[67] Kloetzel, P. M., The proteasome system: a neglected tool for improvement of novel therapeutic strategies? *Gene Ther* 1998, *5* (10), 1297-8.

[68] Rivett, A. J.; Gardner, R. C., Proteasome inhibitors: from in vitro uses to clinical trials. *J Pept Sci* 2000, *6* (9), 478-88.

[69] Rotem-Yehudar, R.; Groettrup, M.; Soza, A.; Kloetzel, P. M.; Ehrlich, R., LMP-associated proteolytic activities and TAP-dependent peptide transport for class 1 MHC molecules are suppressed in cell lines transformed by the highly oncogenic adenovirus 12. *J Exp Med* 1996, *183* (2), 499-514.

[70] Kuckelkorn, U.; Ruppert, T.; Strehl, B.; Jungblut, P. R.; Zimny-Arndt, U.; Lamer, S.; Prinz, I.; Drung, I.; Kloetzel, P. M.; Kaufmann, S. H.; Steinhoff, U., Link between organ-specific antigen processing by 20S proteasomes and CD8(+) T cell-mediated autoimmunity. *J Exp Med* 2002, *195* (8), 983-90.

[71] Regad, T.; Saib, A.; Lallemand-Breitenbach, V.; Pandolfi, P. P.; de The, H.; Chelbi-Alix, M. K., PML mediates the interferon-induced antiviral state against a complex retrovirus via its association with the viral transactivator. *EMBO J* 2001, *20* (13), 3495-505.

[72] Delp, K.; Momburg, F.; Hilmes, C.; Huber, C.; Seliger, B., Functional deficiencies of components of the MHC class I antigen pathway in human tumors of epithelial origin. *Bone Marrow Transplant* 2000, *25 Suppl 2*, S88-95.

[73] Gortzak-Uzan, L.; Ignatchenko, A.; Evangelou, A. I.; Agochiya, M.; Brown, K. A.; St Onge, P.; Kireeva, I.; Schmitt-Ulms, G.; Brown, T. J.; Murphy, J.; Rosen, B.; Shaw, P.; Jurisica, I.; Kislinger, T., A proteome resource of ovarian cancer ascites: integrated proteomic and bioinformatic analyses to identify putative biomarkers. *J Proteome Res* 2008, *7* (1), 339-51.

[74] Pudney, V. A.; Leese, A. M.; Rickinson, A. B.; Hislop, A. D., CD8+ immunodominance among Epstein-Barr virus lytic cycle antigens directly reflects the efficiency of antigen presentation in lytically infected cells. *J Exp Med* 2005, *201* (3), 349-60.

[75] Sorem, J.; Jardetzky, T. S.; Longnecker, R., Cleavage and secretion of Epstein-Barr virus glycoprotein 42 promote membrane fusion with B lymphocytes. *J Virol* 2009, *83* (13), 6664-72.

[76] Sorem, J.; Longnecker, R., Cleavage of Epstein-Barr virus glycoprotein B is required for full function in cell-cell fusion with both epithelial and B cells. *J Gen Virol* 2009, *90* (Pt 3), 591-5.

[77] Elg, S. A.; Mayer, A. R.; Carson, L. F.; Twiggs, L. B.; Hill, R. B.; Ramakrishnan, S., Alpha-1 acid glycoprotein is an immunosuppressive factor found in ascites from ovaria carcinoma. *Cancer* 1997, *80* (8), 1448-56.

[78] Nosov, V.; Su, F.; Amneus, M.; Birrer, M.; Robins, T.; Kotlerman, J.; Reddy, S.; Farias-Eisner, R., Validation of serum biomarkers for detection of early-stage ovarian cancer. *Am J Obstet Gynecol* 2009, *200* (6), 639 e1-5.

[79] Kim, K. D.; Lim, H. Y.; Lee, H. G.; Yoon, D. Y.; Choe, Y. K.; Choi, I.; Paik, S. G.; Kim, Y. S.; Yang, Y.; Lim, J. S., Apolipoprotein A-I induces IL-10 and PGE2 production in human monocytes and inhibits dendritic cell differentiation and maturation. *Biochem Biophys Res Commun* 2005, *338* (2), 1126-36.

[80] Liang, X.; Lin, T.; Sun, G.; Beasley-Topliffe, L.; Cavaillon, J. M.; Warren, H. S., Hemopexin down-regulates LPS-induced proinflammatory cytokines from macrophages. *J Leukoc Biol* 2009, *86* (2), 229-35.

[81] Leygue, E.; Snell, L.; Dotzlaw, H.; Hole, K.; Hiller-Hitchcock, T.; Roughley, P. J.; Watson, P. H.; Murphy, L. C., Expression of lumican in human breast carcinoma. *Cancer Res* 1998, *58* (7), 1348-52.

[82] Leygue, E.; Snell, L.; Dotzlaw, H.; Troup, S.; Hiller-Hitchcock, T.; Murphy, L. C.; Roughley, P. J.; Watson, P. H., Lumican and decorin are differentially expressed in human breast carcinoma. *J Pathol* 2000, *192* (3), 313-20.

[83] Babelova, A.; Moreth, K.; Tsalastra-Greul, W.; Zeng-Brouwers, J.; Eickelberg, O.; Young, M. F.; Bruckner, P.; Pfeilschifter, J.; Schaefer, R. M.; Groene, H. J.; Schaefer, L., Biglycan: A danger signal that activates the NLRP3 inflammasome via toll-like and P2X receptors. *J Biol Chem* 2009.

[84] Schaefer, L.; Babelova, A.; Kiss, E.; Hausser, H. J.; Baliova, M.; Krzyzankova, M.; Marsche, G.; Young, M. F.; Mihalik, D.; Gotte, M.; Malle, E.; Schaefer, R. M.; Grone, H. J., The matrix component biglycan is proinflammatory and signals through Toll-like receptors 4 and 2 in macrophages. *J Clin Invest* 2005, *115* (8), 2223-33.

[85] Salzet, M.; Capron, A.; Stefano, G. B., Molecular crosstalk in host-parasite relationships: schistosome- and leech-host interactions. *Parasitol Today* 2000, *16* (12), 536-40.

[86] Makino, E.; Sakaguchi, M.; Iwatsuki, K.; Huh, N. H., Introduction of an N-terminal peptide of S100C/A11 into human cells induces apoptotic cell death. *J Mol Med* 2004, *82* (9), 612-20.

[87] Sakaguchi, M.; Miyazaki, M.; Sonegawa, H.; Kashiwagi, M.; Ohba, M.; Kuroki, T.; Namba, M.; Huh, N. H., PKCalpha mediates TGFbeta-induced growth inhibition of human keratinocytes via phosphorylation of S100C/A11. *J Cell Biol* 2004, *164* (7), 979-84.

[88] Yang, Z.; Tao, T.; Raftery, M. J.; Youssef, P.; Di Girolamo, N.; Geczy, C. L., Proinflammatory properties of the human S100 protein S100A12. *J Leukoc Biol* 2001, *69* (6), 986-94.

[89] Do, T. V.; Kubba, L. A.; Du, H.; Sturgis, C. D.; Woodruff, T. K., Transforming growth factor-beta1, transforming growth factor-beta2, and transforming growth factor-beta3 enhance ovarian cancer metastatic potential by inducing a Smad3-dependent epithelial-to-mesenchymal transition. *Mol Cancer Res* 2008, *6* (5), 695-705.

[90] Rodriguez, G. C.; Haisley, C.; Hurteau, J.; Moser, T. L.; Whitaker, R.; Bast, R. C., Jr.; Stack, M. S., Regulation of invasion of epithelial ovarian cancer by transforming growth factor-beta. *Gynecol Oncol* 2001, *80* (2), 245-53.

[91] Sood, A. K.; Fletcher, M. S.; Coffin, J. E.; Yang, M.; Seftor, E. A.; Gruman, L. M.; Gershenson, D. M.; Hendrix, M. J., Functional role of matrix metalloproteinases in ovarian tumor cell plasticity. *Am J Obstet Gynecol* 2004, *190* (4), 899-909.

[92] Sood, A. K.; Seftor, E. A.; Fletcher, M. S.; Gardner, L. M.; Heidger, P. M.; Buller, R. E.; Seftor, R. E.; Hendrix, M. J., Molecular determinants of ovarian cancer plasticity. *Am J Pathol* 2001, *158* (4), 1279-88.

[93] Vergara, D.; Merlot, B.; Lucot, J. P.; Collinet, P.; Vinatier, D.; Fournier, I.; Salzet, M., Epithelial-mesenchymal transition in ovarian cancer. *Cancer Lett* 2009.

[94] Xie, X.; Ye, D.; Chen, H.; Lu, W.; Cheng, B.; Zhong, H., Interleukin-7 and suppression of local peritoneal immunity in ovarian carcinoma. *Int J Gynaecol Obstet* 2004, *85* (2), 151-8.

[95] Lambeck, A. J.; Crijns, A. P.; Leffers, N.; Sluiter, W. J.; ten Hoor, K. A.; Braid, M.; van der Zee, A. G.; Daemen, T.; Nijman, H. W.; Kast, W. M., Serum cytokine profiling as a diagnostic and prognostic tool in ovarian cancer: a potential role for interleukin 7. *Clin Cancer Res* 2007, *13* (8), 2385-91.

[96] Kitagawa, K.; Murata, A.; Matsuura, N.; Tohya, K.; Takaichi, S.; Monden, M.; Inoue, M., Epithelial-mesenchymal transformation of a newly established cell line from ovarian adenosarcoma by transforming growth factor-beta1. *Int J Cancer* 1996, *66* (1), 91-7.

[97] Keshamouni, V. G.; Michailidis, G.; Grasso, C. S.; Anthwal, S.; Strahler, J. R.; Walker, A.; Arenberg, D. A.; Reddy, R. C.; Akulapalli, S.; Thannickal, V. J.; Standiford, T. J.; Andrews, P. C.; Omenn, G. S., Differential protein expression profiling by iTRAQ-2DLC-MS/MS of lung cancer cells undergoing epithelial-mesenchymal transition reveals a migratory/invasive phenotype. *J Proteome Res* 2006, *5* (5), 1143-54.

[98] Vergara, D.; Merlot, B.; Lucot, J. P.; Collinet, P.; Vinatier, D.; Fournier, I.; Salzet, M., Epithelial-mesenchymal transition in ovarian cancer. *Cancer Lett 291* (1), 59-66.

[99] Tinelli, A.; Vergara, D.; Martignago, R.; Leo, G.; Malvasi, A.; Tinelli, R.; Marsigliante, S.; Maffia, M.; Lorusso, V., Ovarian cancer biomarkers: a focus on genomic and proteomic findings. *Curr Genomics* 2007, *8* (5), 335-42.

[100] Diefenbach, C. S.; Soslow, R. A.; Iasonos, A.; Linkov, I.; Hedvat, C.; Bonham, L.; Singer, J.; Barakat, R. R.; Aghajanian, C.; Dupont, J., Lysophosphatidic acid acyltransferase-beta (LPAAT-beta) is highly expressed in advanced ovarian cancer and is associated with aggressive histology and poor survival. *Cancer* 2006, *107* (7), 1511-9.

[101] Kim, H.; Watkinson, J.; Varadan, V.; Anastassiou, D., Multi-cancer computational analysis reveals invasion-associated variant of desmoplastic reaction involving INHBA, THBS2 and COL11A1. *BMC Med Genomics* 3, 51.

[102] Oikonomopoulou, K.; Batruch, I.; Smith, C. R.; Soosaipillai, A.; Diamandis, E. P.; Hollenberg, M. D., Functional proteomics of kallikrein-related peptidases in ovarian cancer ascites fluid. *Biol Chem 391* (4), 381-90.

[103] Ahmed, A. S.; Dew, T.; Lawton, F. G.; Papadopoulos, A. J.; Devaja, O.; Raju, K. S.; Sherwood, R. A., Tumour M2-PK as a predictor of surgical outcome in ovarian cancer, a prospective cohort study. *Eur J Gynaecol Oncol* 2007, *28* (2), 103-8.

[104] Ayhan, A.; Ertunc, D.; Tok, E. C., Expression of the c-Met in advanced epithelial ovarian cancer and its prognostic significance. *Int J Gynecol Cancer* 2005, *15* (4), 618-23.

[105] Tang, M. K.; Zhou, H. Y.; Yam, J. W.; Wong, A. S., c-Met overexpression contributes to the acquired apoptotic resistance of nonadherent ovarian cancer cells through a cross talk mediated by phosphatidylinositol 3-kinase and extracellular signal-regulated kinase 1/2. *Neoplasia 12* (2), 128-38.

[106] Zhou, H. Y.; Pon, Y. L.; Wong, A. S., HGF/MET signaling in ovarian cancer. *Curr Mol Med* 2008, *8* (6), 469-80.

[107] Coffelt, S. B.; Marini, F. C.; Watson, K.; Zwezdaryk, K. J.; Dembinski, J. L.; LaMarca, H. L.; Tomchuck, S. L.; Honer zu Bentrup, K.; Danka, E. S.; Henkle, S. L.; Scandurro, A. B., The pro-inflammatory peptide LL-37 promotes ovarian tumor progression through recruitment of multipotent mesenchymal stromal cells. *Proc Natl Acad Sci U S A* 2009, *106* (10), 3806-11.

[108] Kenny, H. A.; Lengyel, E., MMP-2 functions as an early response protein in ovarian cancer metastasis. *Cell Cycle* 2009, *8* (5), 683-8.

[109] Zohny, S. F.; Fayed, S. T., Clinical utility of circulating matrix metalloproteinase-7 (MMP-7), CC chemokine ligand 18 (CCL18) and CC chemokine ligand 11 (CCL11) as markers for diagnosis of epithelial ovarian cancer. *Med Oncol 27* (4), 1246-53.

[110] Landen, C. N.; Kinch, M. S.; Sood, A. K., EphA2 as a target for ovarian cancer therapy. *Expert Opin Ther Targets* 2005, *9* (6), 1179-87.

[111] Lu, C.; Shahzad, M. M.; Wang, H.; Landen, C. N.; Kim, S. W.; Allen, J.; Nick, A. M.; Jennings, N.; Kinch, M. S.; Bar-Eli, M.; Sood, A. K., EphA2 overexpression promotes ovarian cancer growth. *Cancer Biol Ther* 2008, *7* (7), 1098-103.

[112] Thaker, P. H.; Deavers, M.; Celestino, J.; Thornton, A.; Fletcher, M. S.; Landen, C. N.; Kinch, M. S.; Kiener, P. A.; Sood, A. K., EphA2 expression is associated with aggressive features in ovarian carcinoma. *Clin Cancer Res* 2004, *10* (15), 5145-50.

[113] Kobel, M.; Kalloger, S. E.; Boyd, N.; McKinney, S.; Mehl, E.; Palmer, C.; Leung, S.; Bowen, N. J.; Ionescu, D. N.; Rajput, A.; Prentice, L. M.; Miller, D.; Santos, J.; Swenerton, K.; Gilks, C. B.; Huntsman, D., Ovarian carcinoma subtypes are different diseases: implications for biomarker studies. *PLoS Med* 2008, *5* (12), e232.

[114] Ripley, D.; Shoup, B.; Majewski, A.; Chegini, N., Differential expression of interleukins IL-13 and IL-15 in normal ovarian tissue and ovarian carcinomas. *Gynecol Oncol* 2004, *92* (3), 761-8.

[115] Lim, R.; Ahmed, N.; Borregaard, N.; Riley, C.; Wafai, R.; Thompson, E. W.; Quinn, M. A.; Rice, G. E., Neutrophil gelatinase-associated lipocalin (NGAL) an early-screening biomarker for ovarian cancer: NGAL is associated with epidermal growth factor-induced epithelio-mesenchymal transition. *Int J Cancer* 2007, *120* (11), 2426-34.

[116] Bjorge, L.; Hakulinen, J.; Vintermyr, O. K.; Jarva, H.; Jensen, T. S.; Iversen, O. E.; Meri, S., Ascitic complement system in ovarian cancer. *Br J Cancer* 2005, *92* (5), 895-905.

[117] Fischer, D. C.; Noack, K.; Runnebaum, I. B.; Watermann, D. O.; Kieback, D. G.; Stamm, S.; Stickeler, E., Expression of splicing factors in human ovarian cancer. *Oncol Rep* 2004, *11* (5), 1085-90.

[118] Surowiak, P.; Materna, V.; Maciejczyk, A.; Kaplenko, I.; Spaczynski, M.; Dietel, M.; Lage, H.; Zabel, M., CD46 expression is indicative of shorter revival-free survival for ovarian cancer patients. *Anticancer Res* 2006, *26* (6C), 4943-8.

[119] Rousseau, J.; Tetu, B.; Caron, D.; Malenfant, P.; Cattaruzzi, P.; Audette, M.; Doillon, C.; Tremblay, J. P.; Guerette, B., RCAS1 is associated with ductal breast cancer progression. *Biochem Biophys Res Commun* 2002, *293* (5), 1544-9.

[120] Tilli, T. M.; Franco, V. F.; Robbs, B. K.; Wanderley, J. L.; de Azevedo da Silva, F. R.; de Mello, K. D.; Viola, J. P.; Weber, G. F.; Gimba, E. R., Osteopontin-c Splicing Isoform Contributes to Ovarian Cancer Progression. *Mol Cancer Res.*

[121] Yan, X. D.; Pan, L. Y., [Proteomic analysis of human ovarian cancer cell lines and their platinum-resistant clones]. *Zhonghua Fu Chan Ke Za Zhi* 2006, *41* (9), 584-7.

[122] Yan, X. D.; Pan, L. Y.; Yuan, Y.; Lang, J. H.; Mao, N., Identification of platinum-resistance associated proteins through proteomic analysis of human ovarian cancer cells and their platinum-resistant sublines. *J Proteome Res* 2007, *6* (2), 772-80.

[123] Nishimura, S.; Tsuda, H.; Kataoka, F.; Arao, T.; Nomura, H.; Chiyoda, T.; Susumu, N.; Nishio, K.; Aoki, D., Overexpression of cofilin 1 can predict progression-free survival in patients with epithelial ovarian cancer receiving standard therapy. *Hum Pathol.*

[124] Jones, M. B.; Krutzsch, H.; Shu, H.; Zhao, Y.; Liotta, L. A.; Kohn, E. C.; Petricoin, E. F., 3rd, Proteomic analysis and identification of new biomarkers and therapeutic targets for invasive ovarian cancer. *Proteomics* 2002, *2* (1), 76-84.

[125] Alper, T.; Kahraman, H.; Cetinkaya, M. B.; Yanik, F.; Akcay, G.; Bedir, A.; Malatyalioglu, E.; Kokcu, A., Serum leptin and body composition in polycystic ovarian syndrome. *Ann Saudi Med* 2004, *24* (1), 9-12.

[126] Erturk, E.; Tuncel, E., Polycystic ovarian disease and serum leptin levels? *Fertil Steril* 2003, *80* (4), 1068-9; author reply 1069-70.

[127] Qian, B.; Katsaros, D.; Lu, L.; Canuto, E. M.; Benedetto, C.; Beeghly-Fadiel, A.; Yu, H., IGF-II promoter specific methylation and expression in epithelial ovarian cancer and their associations with disease characteristics. *Oncol Rep 25* (1), 203-13.

[128] Park, E. K.; Johnson, A. R.; Yates, D. H.; Thomas, P. S., Evaluation of ovarian cancer biomarkers in subjects with benign asbestos-related pleural diseases. *Clin Chem Lab Med 49* (1), 147-50.

[129] Bengtsson, S.; Krogh, M.; Szigyarto, C. A.; Uhlen, M.; Schedvins, K.; Silfversward, C.; Linder, S.; Auer, G.; Alaiya, A.; James, P., Large-scale proteomics analysis of human ovarian cancer for biomarkers. *J Proteome Res* 2007, *6* (4), 1440-50.

11

Computational Strategies in Cancer Drug Discovery

Gabriela Mustata Wilson[1] and Yagmur Muftuoglu[2]
[1]*Health Services and Health Administration, College of Nursing and Health Professions, University of Southern Indiana, Evansville*
[2]*Department of Pharmacology, Yale University, New Haven*
USA

1. Introduction

Over the last 40 years since "the war on cancer" began, cancer death rates have been significantly declining. Major advances in molecular and cellular biology have led to several breakthroughs in the field of cancer research. One of the most important advances in this area was probably the identification of genes that are closely involved in cancer initiation, progression, invasion, and angiogenesis, particularly those that cause cancer, those that suppress it, and those that promote or inhibit programmed cell death (apoptosis). As a result, the rates of new diagnoses and the rates of death from all cancers combined continue to decline. The National Cancer Institute's Cancer Trends Report for 2009/2010 highlights the fact that the four most common cancers – of the prostate, breast, lung, and colorectal, specifically – have dropped considerably in the past few years (National Cancer Institute - Cancer Trends Progress Report - 2009/2010).

Toward the study and treatment of such cancers, there are 680 genes, 545 proteins and 3 RNAs associated with 102 different types of cancer that have been identified to date (National Cancer Institute - Cancer Trends Progress Report - 2009/2010). Targeting these, a total of 1370 drugs, out of which 1056 are small molecules and 314 are biologics, are either in preclinical or clinical trials or are already FDA approved (National Cancer Institute - Cancer

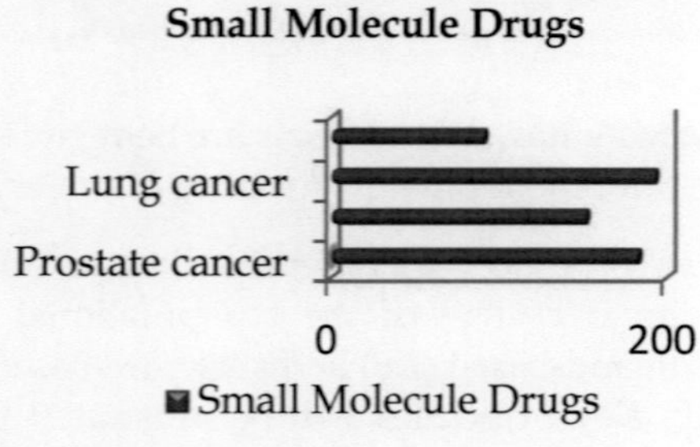

Fig. 1. Small molecule drugs developed for the four most common cancers: prostate, breast, lung, and colorectal.

Trends Progress Report - 2009/2010). As shown in Fig.1, the number of small molecule drugs developed for the four most common cancers mentioned earlier is rather impressive. This dramatic resurgence reflects not only our increasing understanding of the genes and pathways that are responsible for the initiation and progress of cancer, but also the fact that we now have access to a much more powerful range of drug discovery technologies.

The development of new anticancer drugs proves to be a very intricate, costly, and time-consuming process. The advancement and broad application of experimental methods hold enormous promise as foundations for the rapid discovery of new anticancer therapeutics. Towards this goal, computer-aided drug discovery is becoming increasingly important, given the advantage that much less investment in technology, resources, and time is required. Due to the dramatic increase of information available on genomics, small-molecules, and protein structures, computational tools are now being integrated at almost every stage in the discovery and development pipeline for drug discovery (see Fig.2).

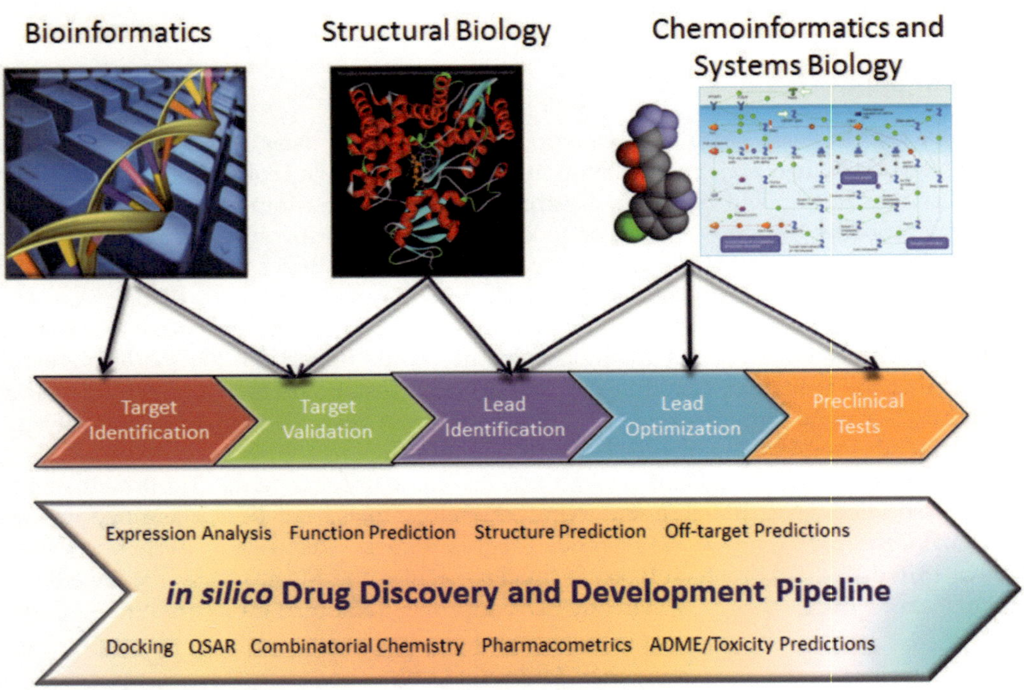

Fig. 2. Schematic diagram showing how *in silico* tools are being integrated at almost every stage in the discovery and development pipeline for drug discovery.

Acknowledging that the area of cancer therapeutics is a complex and time-consuming process, this chapter gives an overview of the computational methodologies used for rational drug design, such as ligand-based (LB) and structure-based (SB) approaches, as well as systems biology modeling. Key principles will be illustrated through case studies that explore the field of anticancer drug design to demonstrate that research advances, with the aid of *in silico* drug design and computational systems biology, have the potential to create novel anticancer drugs that will give hope to millions of cancer patients.

2. Computational strategies

The application of computational tools to drug discovery, including cancer research, has grown steadily for the past couple of years. *In silico* drug design consists of a collection of tools that help to make rational decisions at the different steps of the drug discovery process, such as the identification of a biomolecular target of therapeutical interest, the selection or the design of new lead compounds, and their modification to obtain better affinities, as well as pharmacokinetic and pharmacodynamic properties.

2.1 Structure-based approaches

The first step in developing a drug is to find a small molecule that will bind to a target protein and alter its biological functions. Target structure availability provides a good starting point for modeling target-ligand interactions using structure-based (SB) approaches (Anderson 2003; Gane and Dean 2000; Klebe 2000). Efficacious computational approaches may release the heavy burdens traditionally placed on experimental work. The goals of such methods include identifying effective modifications of existing lead compounds, as well as discovering novel lead compounds (*de novo* design). In recent years, several cases of successful applications of structure-based drug design have been reported (Combs 2007; Coumar et al. 2009; Khan et al. 2010; van Montfort and Workman 2009). Given the three-dimensional structure of a target molecule, chemical compounds having potentially high affinity for this target can be designed rationally with the aid of computational methods. Based on a binding site-derived pharmacophore model, a pattern of putative interaction sites, the results consist of a collection of virtual ligands complementary to a three-dimensional structure of the binding pocket.

A successful example of structure-based pharmacophore modeling can be found in the identification of PUMA inhibitors (Mustata et al. 2011). PUMA, the p53 upregulated modulator of apoptosis, is induced by a wide range of apoptotic stimuli through both p53-dependent and -independent mechanisms. This cancer treatment target is central in mitochondria-mediated cell death by interacting with all known antiapoptotic Bcl-2 family members (Yu and Zhang 2009). Over the years, it has become increasingly apparent that apoptosis acts as a barrier against oncogenesis. Deregulated apoptosis contributes to tumor formation, tumor progression, and impaired responsiveness to anticancer therapies, and recent studies suggest that the function of PUMA is compromised in cancer cells (Yu and Zhang 2009).

Based on the binding of BH3-only proteins with Bcl-2-like proteins, a number of approaches have been used to identify small molecules that can modulate these interactions and, therefore, inhibit apoptosis. Most of the efforts have focused on the development of Bcl-2 family inhibitors that mimic the actions of the proapoptotic BH3 domains (Cory and Adams 2002; Fesik 2005). A number of such compounds have been identified through a variety of methods, including computational modeling, structure-based design, and high-throughput screening of natural product and synthetic libraries (Zhang et al. 2007). Most notably, this approach led to the development of a potent and specific Bcl-2/Bcl-XL small-molecule inhibitor called ABT-737. Derivatives of ABT-737 are being tested in clinical trials, and several have already demonstrated effective antitumor effects in preclinical models (Bruncko et al. 2007). ABT-737 has extremely high affinity for Bcl-XL, Bcl-2 and Bcl-w, with a dissociation constant (Ki) below 1nM for each of them, but it binds poorly to Mcl-1 and A1 (Oltersdorf et al. 2005). Consequently, ABT and its analogs are found to induce apoptosis in a variety of cancer cells with overexpression of Bcl-XL and Bcl-2 in cell culture and in mice.

Motivated by the success of ABT-737 and derivatives, Mustata et al. (Mustata et al. 2011) used a structure-based approach to identify small molecular BH3 decoys or inhibitors that mimic the conserved bind surface (interactions) provided by the Bcl-2 like proteins to sequester PUMA, and therefore prevent its binding to Bcl-2-like proteins, thereby preventing apoptosis. The authors used the 3D structure of PUMA BH3 domain in complex with Mcl-1, a member of the pro-survival Bcl2-family (Day et al. 2008), to visualize and derive the most relevant protein-protein interactions and also to determine if these interactions are conserved among other Bcl-2 family members. They identified two conserved salt bridges (between Arg142 (PUMA BH3) - Asp237 (human Mcl-1) and Asp146 (PUMA BH3) – Arg244 (human Mcl-1)) and one conserved hydrophobic interaction (Leu141 (PUMA BH3) – Phe251 (human Mcl-1)).

These interactions were 'translated' into pharmacophoric features, resulting in a structure-based pharmacophore model. The model was used to screen ZINC8.0 database, which resulted in 48 hits from which they selected the 13 most promising based on *in silico* ADME/Toxicity profiling and favorable binding energies. *In vitro* and *in vivo* biological analyses concluded that ten of these inhibited PUMA-induced apoptosis at 25 μM, and eight of these inhibited PUMA-induced growth suppression in DLD1 cells using an adenovirus expressing PUMA. It was also found that, in HCT116 cells deficient in cyclin-dependent kinase (CDK) inhibitor p21 (p21-KO cells), three unreported compounds outside of the 13 originally purchased reduced PUMA-induced apoptosis and growth suppression in a significant manner when all three were added at 25 μM 15 minutes following irradiation. In this way, the authors of this study were able to identify a handful of PUMA inhibitors that displayed inhibitory activity *in vitro* and antiapoptotic activity in several relevant cell lines through the generation of an SB pharmacophore model.

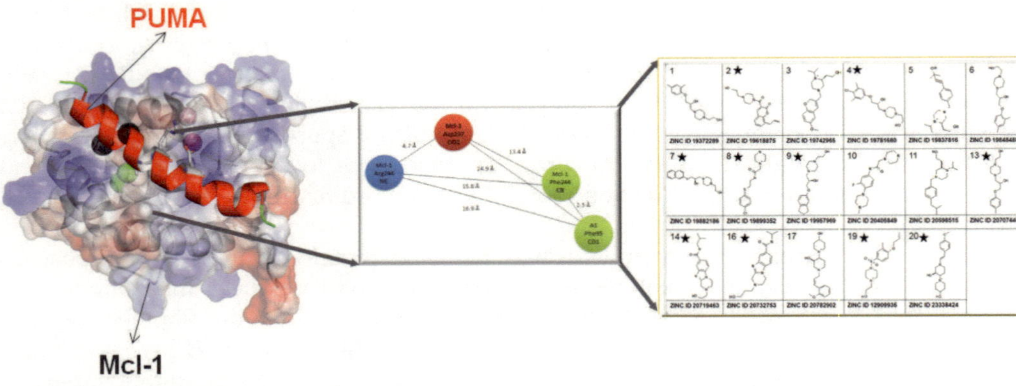

Fig. 3. Computational strategy employed towards the identification of PUMA-Bcl-2 disruptors. The complex between MPUMA and one of the Bcl2 proteins, Mcl1, is represented on the left side. The two-dimensional pharmacophore is represented in the middle, together with the inter-residue distances. Key conserved interactions derived from sequence and structural data include an Asp-Arg salt-bridge interaction (PUMA Asp146.$O_{\delta 1}$ with MCl-1 Arg244.N_ε and A-1 Arg88.N_ε, blue feature), an Arg-Asp salt-bridge interaction (PUMA Arg142.NH_1 with MCl-1 Asp237.$O_{\delta 2}$, red feature), and a Leu-Phe hydrophobic interaction (PUMA Leu141.$C_{\delta 1}$ with MCl-1 Phe251.C_β and A1 Phe95.$C_{\delta 1}$, green features). The structures of the 20 small-molecule candidates are shown on the right.

2.2 Ligand-based approaches

The information gained from structure-based studies provides a good starting point for optimizing select ligands using ligand-based approaches. Ligand-based drug design exploits information about known active compounds (and possibly about inactive compounds, as well) to discover new actives (Stahura and Bajorath 2005). Ligand-based approaches rely on the central similarity-property principal, which states that similar molecules should exhibit similar properties (Johnson and Maggiora 1990). Therefore, the activity prediction of a compound or a set of compounds will be done based on the similarity or distance to a set of reference ligands with known bioactivity to a protein target (Rognan 2007). Different types of two- and three-dimensional molecular descriptors, features, and substructures in combination with a variety of classification schemes – such as recursive partitioning, Bayesian statistics, neural networks, or other machine-learning methods – have been used for this purpose.

Pharmacophore-based virtual screening can be viewed as the intersection between structure-based and ligand-based approaches, as either the protein structure or known ligands can be used as references to build the models (i.e. receptor-based pharmacophore and ligand-based pharmacophore). One advantage of similarity searching over a pharmacophore-based search is that it does not require a set of structurally unrelated compounds of similar biological activity to derive a model. Thus, similarity-based virtual screening has proven very convenient, as it is computationally inexpensive and requires relatively less information (Sheridan and Kearsley 2002).

For similarity searching, even one active molecule can be used to search a database for related compounds. It mostly uses 2D descriptors, also called topological descriptors, which are derived from the connectivity table of the molecule and take into account distances among atoms in terms of number of bonds in the shortest path between them. The most commonly used descriptors are topological fingerprints (Hert et al. 2004), which encode the presence or absence of substructural fragments in molecules in a binary fingerprint without taking into account the number of occurrences of the feature.

These fingerprints can be pre-calculated and compared, usually by means of their Tanimoto distance, in a very fast and efficient manner to any reference set. The encoded substructures can either be a predefined list common to all sets of molecules analyzed or a list that depends on the analyzed set, in which all the encountered substructures up to a certain path length are considered. Contrary to similarity searching, pharmacophore searching has perhaps proven the most widely applied virtual screening method in terms of novel lead discovery, with hit rates for selected data sets of 1 to 20% (Good et al. 2000). Conversely, substructure-based fingerprints methods provide poorer scaffold hopping, as they are based in common substructure searching.

An interesting example of small-molecules designed using a ligand-based approach is the case of tubulin inhibitors (Chiang et al. 2009). Tubulin polymerization, an essential component of cell cycle progression and cell division, represents an important target in anticancer therapy. Several antimitotic agents – like vinblastine and colchicine – have already been discovered and are clinically used, despite often low bioavailability, significant toxicity, rapid acquired resistance, and the resulting overexpression of drug-resistant pumps that eject these antimitotic inhibitors from the cell. However, due to these unfavorable properties, researchers have devoted substantial effort to discover new agents with more tolerable and effective properties, especially since it is believed that antimitotic agents could work to diminish blood supply to cancerous tumors. The authors of this study based their model generation on a set of 21 indole-derivatives synthesized originally (Liou et al. 2006) for potential tubulin inhibition by this research group and used structure-activity relationship (SAR) analysis to drive it. These compounds were chosen such that their inhibitory half-maximal concentration (IC_{50}) values spanned over three orders of magnitude, from 1.2 nM to 6 µM (Liou et al. 2006).

Based on the chemical similarities of these compounds, the authors selected four common pharmacophoric features, including a hydrogen bond donor (HBD), a hydrogen bond acceptor (HBA), hydrophobic group (HY), and a hydrophobic aromatic group (HYA). They also used the HypoRefine feature to generate excluded volumes (EX) in an attempt to separate inactive compounds from active ones (Fig. 4). Following validation of their most significant pharmacophore hypothesis, the authors then used the hypothesis to screen both the ChemDiv database and an in-house database of approximately 130,000 compounds. Although the authors do not report the resulting number of hits, they note that the top 1000 hits were then made subject to visual inspection, ruling out all but 142 of them.

These compounds were then biologically tested using the human oral squamous carcinoma KB cell line. From among these 142 biologically tested compounds, four, shown in Fig. 4, were found to inhibit the KB cell line with IC_{50}values of 187 nM, 2.0 µM, 3.0 µM, and 5.7 µM, respectively. The most potent compound in this set of four active molecules was also found to inhibit the proliferation of other cancer cell lines like MCF-7, NCI-H460, and SF-268, giving IC_{50}values of 236 nM, 285 nM, and 319 nM.

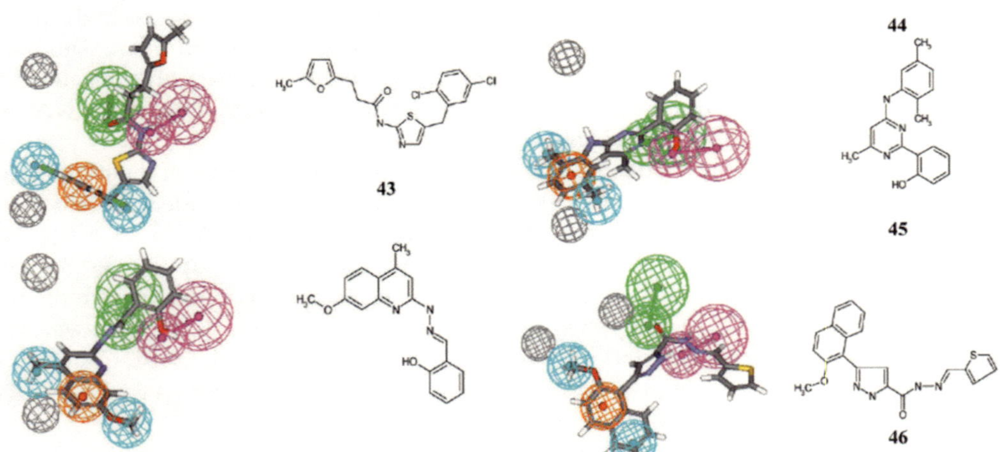

Fig. 4. The mapping configuration of four hit compounds found to inhibit the KB cell line onto the pharmacophore model along with their chemical structures. The pharmacophore model is represented by the colored spheres: HBD (magenta), HBA (green), HY (cyan), HYA (dark orange), and EX (black). Reprinted from the Journal of Medicinal Chemistry, 2009, 52, 4221-4233, Copyright 2009 American Chemical Society.

Another example of an LB approach is the development of a 3-dimensional pharmacophore model generated utilizing a set of known inhibitors of c-Myc-Max heterodimer formation (Mustata et al. 2009). c-Myc is a member of the basic helix-loop-helix leucine zipper protein family (bHLH-ZIP). Dimerization with another bHLH-ZIP protein, Max, controls biological functions like apoptosis, transcriptional activation, and cellular transformation. Inhibition of the interactions between these two important proteins therefore represents yet another means for potential cancer treatment. This is especially true since deregulation of the c-Myc oncogene is a hallmark of cancer-related abnormalities leading to especially aggressive tumors in the cervix, colon, lung, breast, and hematopoietic organs (Nesbit et al. 1998).

Previously, the authors of this study showed through nuclear magnetic resonance (NMR) studies that inhibitors of the c-Myc-Max dimerization function by binding to the inherently disordered c-Myc protein, altering its structure and making it incapable of dimerization with the Max protein (Hammoudeh et al. 2009).

For this study, they aimed to develop an LB model based on previous work in an effort to discover new classes of potential c-Myc-Max inhibitors. The authors made use of the Genetic Algorithm with Linear Assignment for Hypermolecular Alignment of Datasets (GALAHAD) in SYBYL 8.0 software (Shepphird and Clark 2006) to develop a ligand-based pharmacophore model that takes into account ligand flexibility, steric overlaps, and strain energies. Model generation was based on a set of six c-Myc-Max inhibitors that these authors had previously reported - composed of the original compound, which they called 10058-F4, and five compounds derived from it - and gave 20 pharmacophore model hypotheses. The model that received the best overall score was found to contain two hydrophobic features, two acceptor atoms, and one donor atom; this is shown in Fig.5.

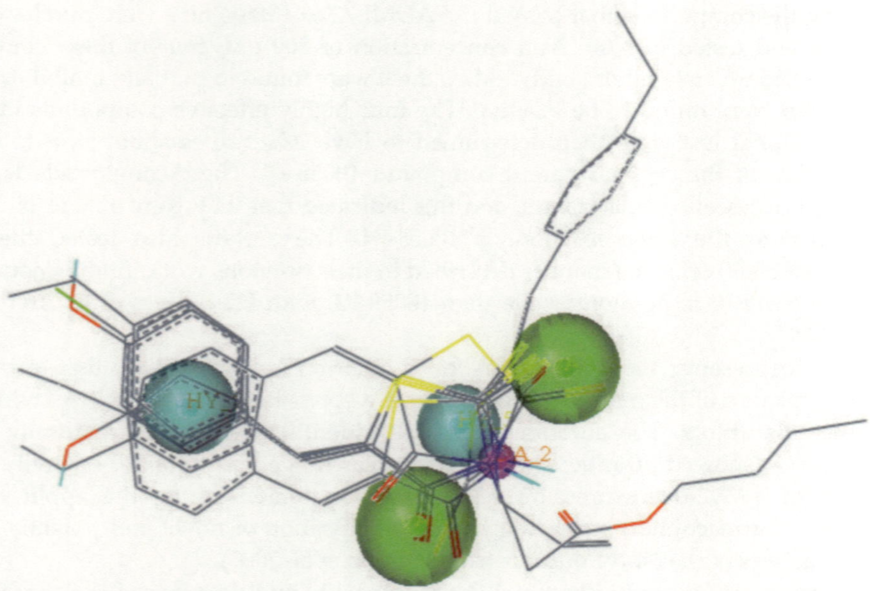

Fig. 5. GALAHAD model obtained from six compounds in the biological data. It includes two hydrophobes (light blue), one donor atom (purple), and two acceptor atoms (green)., and the sphere sizes indicate query tolerances.

By making use of two inactive analogues of the original compound, 10058-F4, the authors of this study were also able to refine the highest-scoring pharmacophore model generated through their work. This was accomplished using the Tuplets function in SYBYL 8.0 (Shepphird and Clark 2006) software. The refined LB model was then tested using a set of ten compounds composed of four inactive analogues of the original compound 10058-F4 and the six compounds described above. This validation step resulted in one false negative, one false positive, and eight correct identifications.

The refined and validated LB model was then used to screen the set of approximately five million drug-like compounds of the ZINC 7.0 database, resulting in 15,822 hits, which amounts to about 0.31% of the ZINC 7.0 drug-like molecule database. Since the Tanimoto score of this set was found to be 0.50, it was determined that it was, indeed, composed of structurally-diverse molecules based on similar biological activity data referenced by this study.

The 100 top-ranking compounds among the 15,822 hits that resulted from the database screening were then tested by adsorption, distribution, metabolism, excretion, and toxicity (ADME/Tox) analyses using ADME Boxes version 4.0 software (Mustata et al. 2009) in an attempt to rationally devonvolute the extensive hit-list. The highest-ranking 30 compounds that passed the ADME/Tox filtering steps were then analyzed for their predicted probability of being an inhibitor of or metabolite for the cytochrome P450 isoform CYP3A4. The authors rationalized that this was necessary since the original compound 10058-F4 was previously found to be extensively metabolized, resulting in rapid clearance, and that the CYP3A4 is believed to metabolize more than 50% of drugs in the human body.

From among the compounds that passed the ADME/Tox filters, nine were purchased from ChemBridge and tested *in vitro*. At a concentration of 200 µM, four of these compounds were found to completely inhibit c-Myc-Max, three were found to partially inhibit it, and the remaining two were found to be inactive. The four highly effective compounds identified through this initial test were then determined to have IC_{50} values about two- to ten-fold lower than that of the original parent compound 10058-F4. These compounds were also tested using fluorescence polarization, and this indicated that they were able to bind to the c-Myc protein at the same location as 10058-F4. The authors also tested these four compounds in HL60 cells in a manner described in their previous work, finding compounds 5360134 and 6370870 to be more active than 10058-F4, with IC_{50} values of 23, 16.7, and 35 µM, respectively.

This study respresents the first report of a pharmacophore model that provides a hypothetical picture of the main chemical features responsible for the activity of c-Myc-Max heterodimer disruptors. The authors successfully identified a set of structurally diverse compounds that showed affinities in the micromolar range and inhibitory activity against the growth of c-Myc-overexpressing cells, therefore demonstrating the applicability of ligand-based pharmacophore modeling to the identification of novel and potentially more puissant inhibitors of the c-Myc oncoprotein (Mustata et al. 2009).

The same group also recently identified the binding site and determined the conformation by which the parental compound, 10058-F4, binds c-Myc and stabilizes the intrinsically disordered monomer over the highly ordered c-Myc-Max heterodimer (Follis et al. 2008; Follis et al. 2009). Docking of the top two newly identified Myc-Max heterodimer disruptors revealed similar binding mode to the 10058-F4 parental compound (Fig.5), centered around residues 402-412 (Follis et al. 2008; Follis et al. 2009). This information should allow the authors to define the major structural determinants of affinity/specificity.

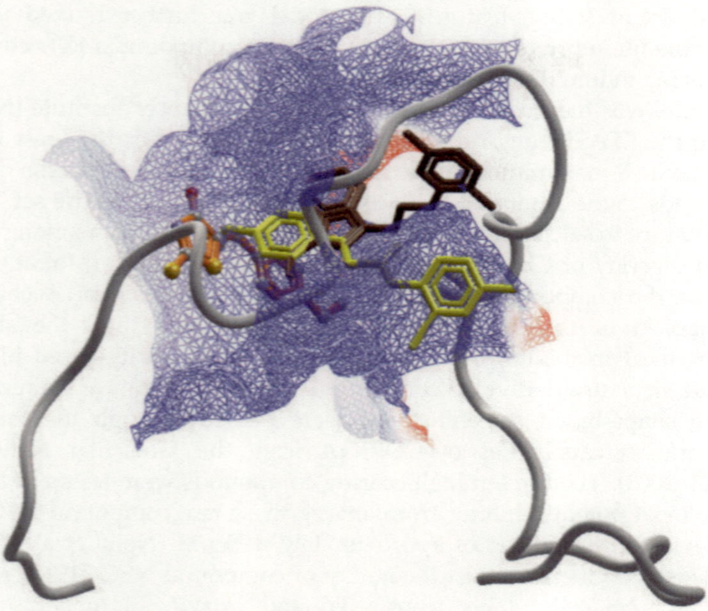

Fig. 6. Docking of the two most active compounds, 5360134 and 6370870, to the c-Myc fragment that binds the parenteral compound 10058-F4. The electrostatic interaction surface at the binding site region is displayed and colored red for negative charge and blue for positive charge. Docking simulations were performed using Molegro Virtual Docker, taking into account side chain flexibility for all residues (Thomsen and Christensen 2006).

Another successful example of LBDD is the targeting of I Kappa B Kinase β (Noha et al. 2011). The NF-κB signaling pathway, which is activated by tumor necrosis factor-α (TNF-α), stimulates through a complex signaling cascade that leads to the transcription of proinflammatory target genes, including I kappa B kinase β (IKK-β), the expression of which may promote tumor growth in the human body. As a result, IKK-β, a key player in this pathway, represents yet another potential target for the treatment of cancer, in addition to inflammation . Since previous attempts at molecular docking that have used the active site of homology models for IKK-β were riddled with uncertainty due to the lack of an accurate three-dimensional X-ray crystal structure (Noha et al. 2011) the authors of this study decided to use LB pharmacophore modeling to identify new compounds with affinity to IKK-β.

The LB pharmacophore model for this study was based on a set of five compounds with high activity (i.e. IC_{50} values of 100 nM or less) and at least a several-fold difference in selectivity for IKK-β over IKK-α in an attempt to develop an IKK-β inhibitor-specific pharmacophore model. Pharmacophore model hypotheses were built using the "HipHop algorithm" of the Catalyst 4.11 (Patel et al. 2002) software built into the DiscoveryStudio 2.1 package. The highest-ranking LB model hypothesis was iteratively refined with shape constraints and exclusion volume spheres (XVOLs) using the "refinement algorithm" available in DiscoveryStudio as "steric refinement with excluded volumes" based on two biologically inactive compounds from the literature. The final LB model contained one hydrogen-bond acceptor (HBA), one hydrophobic (H), one aromatic ring (RA), and two

hydrogen-bond donor (HBD) features. The model was further refined using a dataset extracted from the literature of 44 biologically inactive compounds, 128 active compounds, and 12,775 diverse random decoy compounds.
The refined model was then used to screen the National Cancer Institute (NCI) compound database using the "FAST" algorithm on DiscoveryStudio with the "fast flexible" search function to generate a maximum of 100 conformations per molecule in the database. Out of 247041 compounds in the database, 1860, comprising 0.8% of the entire set, were identified as hits. In an attempt to select for the most relevant compounds from among these extensive hits, the Rapid Overlay of Chemical Structures (ROCs) algorithm (Moffat et al. 2008) was used to analyze the compounds extracted from the NCI database. A combined scoring function, composed of the ROCS "color force field" score and the shape Tanimoto coefficient, was used in this form of three-dimensional similarity-based hit ranking. Two very active and structurally-diverse compounds from the literature training dataset were chosen for the shape-based screening and were passed through the three-dimensional geometry generation capabilities of CORINA from the Molecular Networks program (Sadowski et al. 2003). The top ten high-scoring compounds were tested *in vitro*, and it was found that the most potent inhibitor from among these ten, compound NSC 719177, could inhibit IKK-β with an IC_{50} value of approximately 6.95 μM (Noha et al. 2011). Cell-based analyses were also conducted to test the ability of compound NSC 719177 to inhibit NF-κB activation in HEK293 cells stably transfected and carrying a luciferase reporter gene activated by a promoter composed of multiple copies of the NF-κB response element. Compound NSC 719177 was found to have a cell-based assay IC_{50} value of approximately 5.85 μM and exhibited dose-dependent activity in inhibiting TNF-α-induced luciferase activity. Therefore, Noha and colleagues (Noha et al. 2011) were able to demonstrate the successful application of ligand-based approaches to the identification of low micromolar inhibitors against IKK-β.

2.3 Combined structure-based and ligand-based approaches

The studies discussed earlier are only a few, and by no mean the most, representative examples for cancer research. Nevertheless, it is clear that structure-based and ligand-based drug design approaches have a great impact on the discovery of anticancer drugs, and the combination provided by these complementary computational methods are even more valuable. One recent example of how both methods could be integrated in cancer research is the development of a "merged" pharmacophore model for aromatase reported by Muftuoglu and Mustata (Muftuoglu and Mustata 2010) toward the identification of better breast cancer drugs.
Excluding cancers of the skin, breast cancer is the most frequently diagnosed cancer in women (2011) and ranks second as a cause of cancer death (after lung cancer). Currently, one of eight American women has the chance of having invasive breast cancer some time during her life. Approximately two-thirds of breast cancer tumors are hormone dependent, requiring estrogens to grow (Brueggemeier et al. 2005). One approach in treating hormone-dependent cancer is to interfere with endogenous hormone production. Aromatase has always been considered the most promising target for the endocrine treatment of breast cancer (Meunier et al. 2004; Meunier et al. 2004) because, by inhibiting the aromatase enzyme, the estrogen production is decreased and the tumor growth stopped or reduced.
The recent study reported by Muftuoglu and Mustata (Muftuoglu and Mustata 2010) is the first study aimed to develop a pharmacophore model, based on both ligand and structural

information, to screen for new classes of effective AIs. The model developed was generated through a merging of a ligand-based model and a structure-based model.

The structure-based pharmacophore model was generated using the recent X-ray structure deposited in the Protein Data Bank (PDB) [pdb code: 3EQM] (Ghosh et al. 2009), which contains the chemical features important for androstenedione–enzyme interaction, while the LB model was developed from the most comprehensive list of non-steroidal aromatase inhibitors. Development of the final model, named the Merged Model (see Fig.7), required a database of both active AIs and inactive compounds for use in the training and testing sets, in addition to structural information based on the X-ray crystal structure of aromatase. As such, two test sets were created: a training set, to develop the LB model, and a test set, to validate the LB, SB, and Merged Models. The training set was composed of 20 of the most active AIs found in the literature.

The test set, on the other hand was composed of 36 slightly less active AIs and nine inactive compounds, also found in the literature. Both sets, however, represented a collection of structurally very diverse compounds. The LB model, as shown in Fig.7, was generated using the Conformation Import function and the PCHD scheme from the Pharmacophore Elucidation function in MOE (Chemical Computing Group 2008), and resulted in four pharmacophoric features: two hydrophobic/aromatic groups, one hydrogen bond acceptor, and one hydrogen bond acceptor projection. In addition, an SB model was also generated based on the x-ray crystal structure of aromatase using LigandScout software (Wolber and Langer 2005), which included excluded volume areas to reflect possible steric hindrances. The resulting SB model, shown in Fig.7, was composed of three chemical features - one hydrophobic/aromatic group and one hydrogen bond acceptor - in addition to 11 excluded volume spheres. The two models, LB and SB, were then merged into one, named the "Merged Model" (see Fig.7) to capture both types of information (i.e., known active and inactive inhibitors as well as the structure of the enzyme).

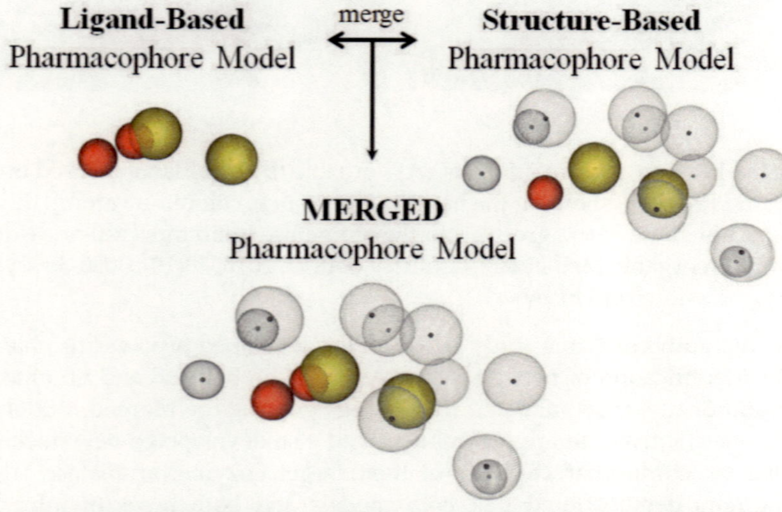

Fig. 7. Schematic diagram depicting the general methodology for the development of the Merged Model based off of the original SB and LB models. Hydrophobic groups are shown as light yellow spheres, hydrogen-bond acceptors are shown as red spheres, and excluded volumes are shown as gray spheres.

All three models were also computationally validated using the active and inactive compounds of the test set. In the end, it was found that the LB model is more discriminating than the SB Model, while the SB Model performs better in identifying active inhibitors. The Merged Model, however, was found to combine the strengths of each, proving superior to both original models. The authors of this study, therefore, would choose the Merged Model for screening of virtual libraries, although this piece of their work is not yet published.

The authors do, however, discuss another area of analysis they pursued - virtual docking - by explaining the theory behind a three-stage process that focuses in on the most stable binding conformation for a ligand based on optimization and individualized pose selection. Stage One governs the entry of the ligand into the binding pocket, where all AIs are believed to bind and some are experimentally proven to be binding. Stage Two allows for the prediction of each ligand's coordinating heteroatom, since it is known that non-steroidal AIs bind in the active site of aromatase by heteroatom coordination as the sixth ligand to the iron atom of the aromatase heme moiety. And lastly, Stage Three refines the binding conformation predictions made in Stage Two. The authors of this study refer to this new method as Refined Virtual Docking and implement the protocol for two aromatase inhibitors (Fig.8).

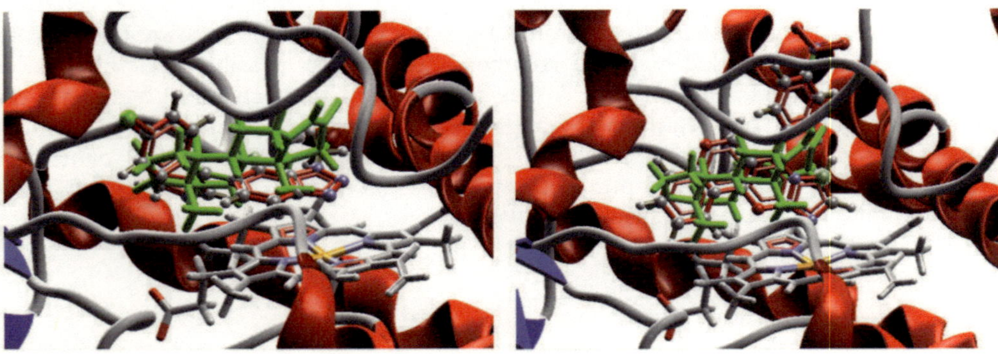

A. B.

Fig. 8. Predicted binding conformations of (A) vorozole (B) 3-imidazolyl based on the Refined Docking Protocol, showing the heme moiety (stick, colored by atom), the preferred adrostenedione substrate (stick, green), and the aromatase inhibitors (ball-and-stick). Reprinted from Bioorganic Medicinal Chemistry Letters, 2010, 20(10), 3050-3064 , Copyright (2010), with permission from Elsevier.

In summary, the authors of this study successfully developed a powerful pharmacophore model for the identification of new classes of AI based on both LB and SB pharmacophore modeling. Additionally, they validated the models, proving the Merged Model to be more powerful and specific than the original models, and also developed a new docking protocol specific to the structural characteristics of their target enzyme, aromatase. Through this study, the authors demonstrated that both models and both types of information (i.e., known active and inactive inhibitors as well as the structure of the target enzyme) are essential to the development of a successful pharmacophore model, and subsequently, to the identification of novel, potent, highly specific, and potentially less toxic aromatase inhibitors.

2.4 Computational systems biology

Systems Biology is directly applicable in the medical sciences, as the ability to therapeutically target complex diseases such as cancer will be greatly improved by a global understanding of the unified signaling and regulatory network that integrates all environmental signals into a net outcome or phenotype. One example of such application is the identification of new uses for existing molecular targets through a systems biology analysis of the differences between normal and diseased samples. A second example can be found in the elucidation of complex signaling relationships or network analysis, which would allow for targeting of the most appropriate region of a signaling cascade for the development of more efficient and safe therapeutic agents. This could be achieved through studies that characterize perturbations of the biological system caused by small molecules, including existing therapeutic agents. The information gained through such studies could be extremely valuable since it would enable us to discriminate between cellular changes associated with therapeutic benefits and cellular changes associated with side-effects.

A dynamic model of such a network could be adapted to describe its changes in the context of a disease, for example by incorporating genetic mutations as changes in the node states or in interactions. The model would be able to predict the phenotypes associated with mutations and their combination with diverse environmental signals, and it would provide strategies for reversing a diseased phenotype into a healthy one. This emerging understanding would enable fundamental advances in cancer treatment by allowing clinicians to prescribe treatments specifically targeted to individuals and their present conditions. Treatments then may be tailored so that the least invasive intervention yields the greatest system-wide benefit, maximizes the body's self-healing abilities, and minimizes side effects. In this way, linking molecular characterizations to clinical phenotypes in a causal manner will be a key challenge of systems medicine, and several promising steps have already been made in this direction.

For example, such a methodology can be applied to prostate cancer, one of the most frequent malignancies and the second-leading cause of cancer mortality in North American males (Jemal et al. 2009). Although prostate cancer rates are progressing slowly, there are cases in which tumors behave aggressively, resulting in poor prognosis and eventually in the death of the patient. Disruptions in the balance of the insulin-like growth factor (IGF) axis and downstream signaling proteins have been attributed a critical role in the establishment and maintenance of the transformed phenotype in prostate cancer.

A recent study performed by Vellaichamy and collaborators from University of Michigan together with GeneGo, Inc. (Vellaichamy et al. 2010) demonstrates in a very elegant manner how computational systems biology approaches can be applied to better understand the biology and biochemistry of prostate cancer in order to establish new prognostic markers and to detect cellular functions suitable for therapeutic interference. These authors applied a topological scoring approach to investigate the response of LNCap prostate cancer cells, a well-studied model system for prostate cancer progression, to treatment with synthetic androgen (R1881). Their computational method combines disease- or condition-specific, high-throughput molecular data with the global network of protein interactions to identify nodes which occupy significant network positions with respect to differentially expressed genes or proteins in the molecular dataset.

Using such analysis, they were able to identify individual signaling cascades leading to the top transcriptional regulators revealing that PI3K signaling is supported by consistently high topological scores derived from both proteomics and microarray datasets. Fig.9 shows this cascade in the context of IGF signaling, with the PI3K cascade highlighted by the red line, where all of the elements that achieve high topological scores with respect to both sets are marked by red boxes. Through this study, the authors determined the central role of this pathway in regulating events that follow androgen treatment: through inhibition of GSK3 kinase and its ability to phosphorylate c-Myc and cyclin D (Fig.9).

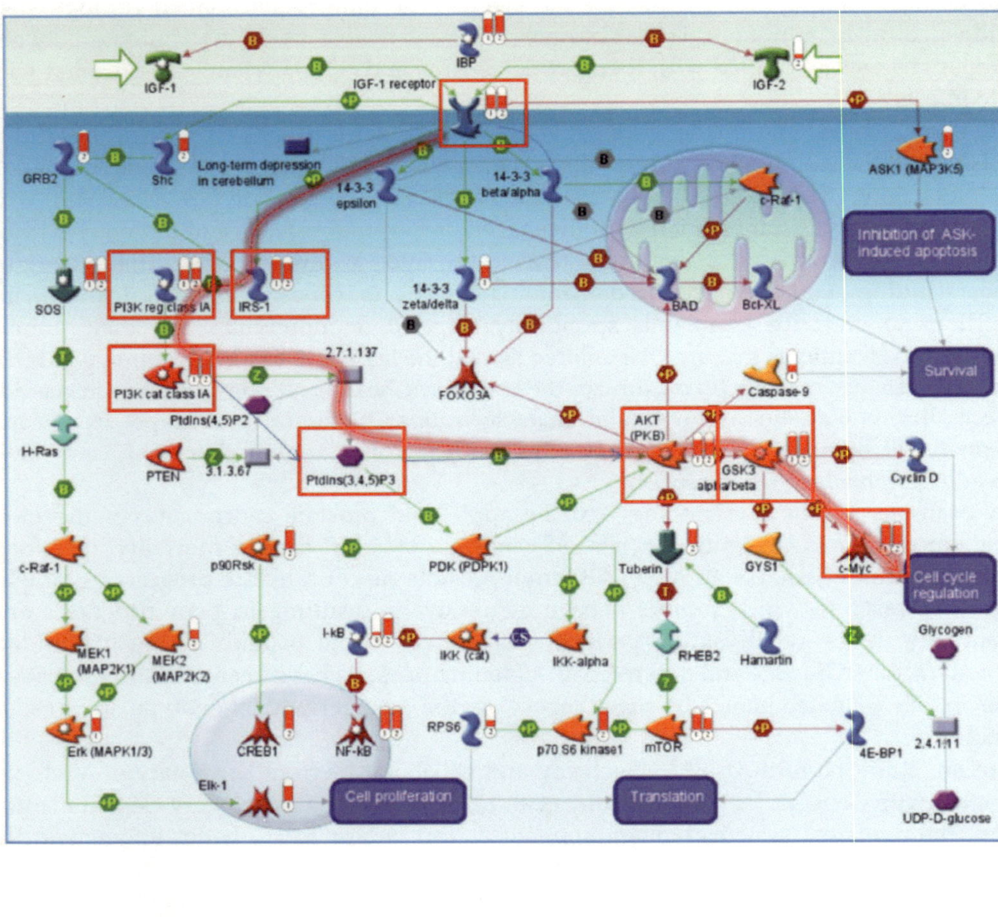

Fig. 9. Map for IGF signaling showing topologically significant genes identified from microarrays and iTRAQ proteomics. Red level in the "thermometers" represents relative rank (percentile) of a protein in the corresponding list of topologically significant proteins. Red boxes and highlighted path illustrate signaling cascade with strongest support from both sets. Adapted from Vellaichamy et al., PLoS One (2010), vol 5 (6), 1-10 with permission fromPloS ONE.

3. Conclusions

Undoubtedly, computational approaches have had a major impact on the design of anticancer drugs and drug candidates over the years and have provided fruitful insights into cancer in general. Nevertheless, to be useful to a biologist or a physician, computational models generated using these approaches should produce useful predictions that match experimental results, allow experiments to be performed *in silico* to save time and cost, and facilitate the understanding of how a system or process works. In that sense, computational approaches have room for improvement in all of the major areas: virtual screening techniques, ADME/Toxicity predictions, and ligand docking protocols.

The optimization of these techniques can be represented by its own theoretical feedback signaling system: the biology informs the computational approaches, which, in turn, inform the biology, and so on, creating immense room for both fundamental breakthroughs and incredible application-based advancements. The field is continuously evolving and challenges still remain, but we expect to see accelerated activity in this area as compounds continue to move through clinical trials and as the science and technology continue to develop. We hope this chapter will stimulate researchers to adopt and apply computational tools to the discovery of future cancer drugs.

4. References

National Cancer Institute - Cancer Trends Progress Report - 2009/2010.

MetaDrug, GeneGo Inc., St. Joseph, MI, http://www.genego.com

Anderson AC (2003) The process of structure-based drug design. Chem Biol 10: 787-797

Gane PJ and Dean PM (2000) Recent advances in structure-based rational drug design. Curr Opin Struct Biol 10: 401-404

Klebe G (2000) Recent developments in structure-based drug design. J Mol Med 78: 269-281

Combs AP (2007) Structure-based drug design of new leads for phosphatase research. IDrugs 10: 112-115

Coumar MS, Leou JS, Shukla P, Wu JS, Dixit AK, Lin WH, Chang CY, Lien TW, Tan UK, Chen CH, Hsu JT, Chao YS, Wu SY, and Hsieh HP (2009) Structure-based drug design of novel Aurora kinase A inhibitors: structural basis for potency and specificity. J Med Chem 52: 1050-1062

Khan A, Prakash A, Kumar D, Rawat A, Srivastava R, and Srivastava R (2010) Virtual screening and pharmacophore studies for ftase inhibitors using Indian plant anticancer compounds database. Bioinformation 5: 62-66

van Montfort RL and Workman P (2009) Structure-based design of molecular cancer therapeutics. Trends Biotechnol 27: 315-328

Mustata G, Li M, Zevola N, Bakan A, Zhang L, Epperly M, Greenberger JS, Yu J, and Bahar I (2011) Development of small-molecule PUMA inhibitors for mitigating radiation-induced cell death. Curr Top Med Chem 11: 281-290

Yu J and Zhang L (2009) PUMA, a potent killer with or without p53. Oncogene 27: S71-S83

Cory S and Adams JM (2002) The Bcl2 family: regulators of the cellular life-or-death switch. Nat Rev Cancer 2: 647-656

Fesik SW (2005) Promoting apoptosis as a strategy for cancer drug discovery. Nat Rev Cancer 5: 876-885

Zhang L, Ming L, and Yu J (2007) BH3 mimetics to improve cancer therapy; mechanisms and examples. Drug Resist Updat 10: 207-217

Bruncko M, Oost TK, Belli BA, Ding H, Joseph MK, Kunzer A, Martineau D, McClellan WJ, Mitten M, Ng SC, Nimmer PM, Oltersdorf T, Park CM, Petros AM, Shoemaker AR, Song X, Wang X, Wendt MD, Zhang H, Fesik SW, Rosenberg SH, and Elmore SW (2007) Studies leading to potent, dual inhibitors of Bcl-2 and Bcl-xL. J Med Chem 50: 641-662

Oltersdorf T, Elmore SW, Shoemaker AR, Armstrong RC, Augeri DJ, Belli BA, Bruncko M, Deckwerth TL, Dinges J, Hajduk PJ, Joseph MK, Kitada S, Korsmeyer SJ, Kunzer AR, Letai A, Li C, Mitten MJ, Nettesheim DG, Ng S, Nimmer PM, O'Connor JM, Oleksijew A, Petros AM, Reed JC, Shen W, Tahir SK, Thompson CB, Tomaselli KJ, Wang B, Wendt MD, Zhang H, Fesik SW, and Rosenberg SH (2005) An inhibitor of Bcl-2 family proteins induces regression of solid tumours. Nature 435: 677-681

Day CL, Smits C, Fan FC, Lee EF, Fairlie WD, and Hinds MG (2008) Structure of the BH3 domains from the p53-inducible BH3-only proteins Noxa and Puma in complex with Mcl-1. J Mol Biol 380: 958-971

Stahura FL and Bajorath J (2005) New methodologies for ligand-based virtual screening. Curr Pharm Des 11: 1189-1202

Johnson M and Maggiora G (1990) Concepts and applications of molecular similarity. John Wiley & Sons, Inc., New York,

Rognan D (2007) Chemogenomic approaches to rational drug design. Br J Pharmacol 152: 38-52

Sheridan RP and Kearsley SK (2002) Why do we need so many chemical similarity search methods? Drug Discov Today 7: 903-911

Hert J, Willett P, Wilton DJ, Acklin P, Azzaoui K, Jacoby E, and Schuffenhauer A (2004) Comparison of fingerprint-based methods for virtual screening using multiple bioactive reference structures. J Chem Inf Comput Sci 44: 1177-1185

Good AC, Krystek SR, and Mason JS (2000) High-throughput and virtual screening: core lead discovery technologies move towards integration. Drug Discov Today 5: 61-69

Chiang YK, Kuo CC, Wu YS, Chen CT, Coumar MS, Wu JS, Hsieh HP, Chang CY, Jseng HY, Wu MH, Leou JS, Song JS, Chang JY, Lyu PC, Chao YS, and Wu SY (2009) Generation of ligand-based pharmacophore model and virtual screening for identification of novel tubulin inhibitors with potent anticancer activity. J Med Chem 52: 4221-4233

Liou JP, Mahindroo N, Chang CW, Guo FM, Lee SW, Tan UK, Yeh TK, Kuo CC, Chang YW, Lu PH, Tung YS, Lin KT, Chang JY, and Hsieh HP (2006) Structure-activity relationship studies of 3-aroylindoles as potent antimitotic agents. ChemMedChem 1: 1106-1118

Mustata G, Follis AV, Hammoudeh DI, Metallo SJ, Wang H, Prochownik EV, Lazo JS, and Bahar I (2009) Discovery of novel Myc-Max heterodimer disruptors with a three-dimensional pharmacophore model. J Med Chem 52: 1247-1250

Nesbit CE, Grove LE, Yin X, and Prochownik EV (1998) Differential apoptotic behaviors of c-myc, N-myc, and L-myc oncoproteins. Cell Growth Differ 9: 731-741

Hammoudeh DI, Follis AV, Prochownik EV, and Metallo SJ (2009) Multiple independent binding sites for small-molecule inhibitors on the oncoprotein c-Myc. J Am Chem Soc 131: 7390-7401

Shepphird JK and Clark RD (2006) A marriage made in torsional space: using GALAHAD models to drive pharmacophore multiplet searches. J Comput Aided Mol Des 20: 763-771

Follis AV, Hammoudeh DI, Wang H, Prochownik EV, and Metallo SJ (2008) Structural rationale for the coupled binding and unfolding of the c-Myc oncoprotein by small molecules. Chem Biol 15: 1149-1155

Follis AV, Hammoudeh DI, Daab AT, and Metallo SJ (2009) Small-molecule perturbation of competing interactions between c-Myc and Max. Bioorg Med Chem Lett 19: 807-810

Thomsen R and Christensen MH (2006) MolDock: a new technique for high-accuracy molecular docking. J Med Chem 49: 3315-3321

Noha SM, Atanasov AG, Schuster D, Markt P, Fakhrudin N, Heiss EH, Schrammel O, Rollinger JM, Stuppner H, Dirsch VM, and Wolber G (2011) Discovery of a novel IKK-beta inhibitor by ligand-based virtual screening techniques. Bioorg Med Chem Lett 21: 577-583

Patel Y, Gillet VJ, Bravi G, and Leach AR (2002) A comparison of the pharmacophore identification programs: Catalyst, DISCO and GASP. J Comput Aided Mol Des 16: 653-681

Moffat K, Gillet VJ, Whittle M, Bravi G, and Leach AR (2008) A comparison of field-based similarity searching methods: CatShape, FBSS, and ROCS. J Chem Inf Model 48: 719-729

Sadowski J, Schwab C, and Gasteiger J (2003) CORINA: 3D Structure Generator.

Muftuoglu Y and Mustata G (2010) Pharmacophore modeling strategies for the development of novel nonsteroidal inhibitors of human aromatase (CYP19). Bioorg Med Chem Lett 20: 3050-3064

Brueggemeier RW, Hackett JC, and az-Cruz ES (2005) Aromatase inhibitors in the treatment of breast cancer. Endocr Rev 26: 331-345

Meunier B, de Visser SP, and Shaik S (2004) Mechanism of oxidation reactions catalyzed by cytochrome p450 enzymes. Chem Rev 104: 3947-3980

Meunier B, de Visser SP, and Shaik S (2004) Mechanism of oxidation reactions catalyzed by cytochrome p450 enzymes. Chem Rev 104: 3947-3980

Ghosh D, Griswold J, Erman M, and Pangborn W (2009) Structural basis for androgen specificity and oestrogen synthesis in human aromatase. Nature 457: 219-223

Chemical Computing Group (2008) MOE.

Wolber G and Langer T (2005) LigandScout: 3-D pharmacophores derived from protein-bound ligands and their use as virtual screening filters. J Chem Inf Model 45: 160-169

Jemal A, Siegel R, Ward E, Hao Y, Xu J, and Thun MJ (2009) Cancer statistics, 2009. CA Cancer J Clin 59: 225-249

Vellaichamy A, Dezso Z, JeBailey L, Chinnaiyan AM, Sreekumar A, Nesvizhskii AI, Omenn GS, and Bugrim A (2010) "Topological significance" analysis of gene expression and proteomic profiles from prostate cancer cells reveals key mechanisms of androgen response. PLoS One 5: e10936

12

Science and Affordability of Cancer Drugs and Radiotherapy in the World - Win-Win Scenarios

Ahmed Elzawawy
President of ICEDOC & ICEDOC's Experts in Cancer without Borders,
Co-President of SEMCO, Port Said,
Egypt

1. Introduction

In the real world, there is an important step before seeing the effects and the outcome of cancer treatment. This step is to see that treatment become accessible and affordable for cancer patients. The rapidly increasing of costs of novel cancer drugs and radiation therapy equipment doesn`t commensurate with the slowly improvement of outcome. Thus, each advance in treatment, the magnitude of the increase in the cost of treatment exceeded the magnitude of improvement of efficacy. (Schrag, 2004). Pharmaceutical companies are developing costly novel cancer drugs that are marketed in the USA, Western Europe, and Japan with fewer markets and opportunities in Low and Middle Income Countries (LMICs). By the year 2020, among the 20 million new cancer cases, 70% will be located in the countries that have collectively, just 5% of the global cancer control resources. (Ferlay et al, 2010, Porter et al., 1999 & Stewart & Kleihues, 2003). At present, it is roughly estimated that at least half of cancer patients in the world have no access to cancer therapy. This situation is particularly marked –with variability – in LMICs. The problem is particularly tragic for Radiotherapy in sub- Saharan Africa where only 5% of cancer patients have access to radiotherapy (Elzawawy, 2008, Porter et, 1999). However, there are also variable proportions of cancer patients in high income countries like the USA who have difficulties in obtaining expensive cancer drug treatment and radiotherapy. (Bach, 2007 & Malin, 2010). There is no indication that the costs of these drugs will diminish in the future in the USA (Meropol & Schulman, 2007).

In the next decade, with the expected increase of numbers of cancer patients particularly in LMICs and with the increasing costs of treatment with novel drugs and radiation therapy particularly in LMICs, then, this situation would be aggravated and it could present more difficulties for all stakeholders; cancer patients, oncologists, health policy makers and governments, manufactures of cancer drugs and radiotherapy equipment and economists. This could cause difficulties for the wheel of advances in treatment and science and in marketing of innovation. Hence, a pressing need emerges for scientific initiatives. One of the recent scientific initiatives, in which most of representatives of the key international organizations are sharing in its meetings and development, is The Win-Win Scientific initiative that was proposed first by ICEDOC's Experts in Cancer without borders on December 2007. (ICEDOC is The International Campaign for Establishment and Development of Oncology Centers. www.icedoc.org). Breast Cancer is the most frequent malignancy among females with about 1.4 million cases annually in the world. Multiple treatment modalities and drugs are used in its management (Ferlay et al, 2010 & Stewart & Kleihues, 2003). The present chapter focuses on updating the exploration of examples of the published and ongoing scientific researches and approaches that could lead to resource sparing and cost effective radiotherapy, chemotherapy and hormonal treatment of breast cancer as a model that could be expanded to other cancers in the world. Despite of all difficult challenges and the expected increase of problems of affordability and marketing of increasingly expensive cancer treatment, we aim at developing win-win scientifically based initiative and scenarios in which the interests of the main stakeholders are really considered. We stress on the notions of not compromising the overall outcome of treatment and to pay attention to the ways of its assessment in different parts of the world. North-North, North-South and South-South scientific collaboration are warranted in order that more cancer patients in the world would have access to cost effective treatment tailored to realistic conditions of each community.

2. Resource sparing in radiotherapy for breast cancer

2.1 Postoperative – post mastectomy and post lumpectomy – radiotherapy of breast cancer

2.1.1 Altered fraction schedules

2.1.1.1 Shorten fractionation for postoperative radiotherapy (Hypofractionation)

An example is The UK standardization of breast radiotherapy (START) randomized trial B. Between 1999 and 2001, 2215 women with early breast cancer (pT1-3a pN0-1 M0) at 23 centers in the UK were randomly assigned after primary surgery to receive 50 Gy in 25 fractions of 20 Gy over 5 weeks or 40 Gy in 15 fractions of 267 Gy over 3 weeks. Women were eligible for the trial if they were aged over 18 years, did not have an immediate reconstruction, and were available for follow-up. Randomization method was computer generated and was not blinded. The protocol specified principal endpoints were local-regional tumor relapse, defined as reappearance of cancer at irradiated sites, late normal tissue effects, and quality of life. Analysis was by intention to treat. This study is registered as an International Standard Randomized Controlled Trial, number ISRCTN59368779. The study showed that the radiation schedule delivering 40 Gy in 15 fractions offer rates of local-regional relapse and adverse effects at least as favorable as the standard of 50 Gy in 25 fractions (The START Trialists' Group, 2008). However, it is critical to realize that the late effects produced by RT are strongly related to dose per fraction. Therefore, higher dose per fraction increases the susceptibility of normal tissues to RT. It is for this reason that the data on late lung and cardiac morbidity and survival rates is very important when hypofractionated regimens are employed in breast cancer. The Oxford meta-analysis has reported that RT reduced the annual mortality from breast cancer by 13% but increased the annual mortality rate from other causes by 21%. Also, this increase was due primarily to an excess number of deaths from cardiovascular causes (Early Breast Cancer Trialists' Collaborative Group, 2000). By radiobiological rationale, hypofractionation has the potential for worsening cardiovascular side effects. Furthermore, the cardiac side effects take up to 15 years to manifest completely after treatment and persist well beyond this period (Munshi A. 2007). The hypofractionation in post mastectomy or lumpectomy radiotherapy has not been applied in the vast majority of centers in the world. This strategy will however be watched with keen interest since it has the potential to drastically reduce treatment times and has important financial implications. (Munshi, 2009). There is a midway solution that could be also reasonable particularly for LMICs; the fractionation of 45 Gy in 18 fractions –used in Port Said, Egypt- which is adopted from the fractionations practiced successfully along years since the seventieth in many French centers (Sarrazin et al., 1989)

2.1.1.2 Accelerated partial breast irradiation (APBI)

Although hailed as a paradigm shift, the breast conservative treatment that emerged in the 1980s was in fact an extension of the Halstedian concept, wherein whole-breast irradiation (WBI) compensated for the limited surgery. Observations that 80-90% of breast recurrences after breast conservative surgery and WBI occur in the tumor bed questions the need for protracted elective WBI, and provides the rationale for accelerated-partial-breast irradiation (APBI) of small cancers without adverse features predisposing to multicenteric recurrence. APBI would mark a paradigm shift and a major advance in treatment. This would allow many more women to opt for breast conservation, resolve the dilemmas regarding chemotherapy and radiotherapy sequencing and perhaps would be more cost effective. (Sarin, 2005). Several techniques including multicatheter interstitial brachytherapy, intracavitary brachytherapy, intraoperative radiation therapy, and 3D conformal external beam radiation therapy have been proposed, and each of them has its own advantages and drawbacks. Although APBI is increasingly used in the United States and Europe, and the short-term results are promising, its equivalence with whole breast radiation therapy is not fully established. In addition, because the average breast size in some countries like Japan is considerably smaller than in the West world, the application of APBI to Japanese patients is technically more challenging. At this point, APBI is still an investigational treatment in Japan, and the optimal method of radiation delivery as well as its long-term efficacy and safety should be clarified in clinical trials (Mitsumori & Hiraoka, 2008). Our point of view is that in LMICs, breast cancer cases are usually more advanced than in the West and the price of machines would be expensive. However, we suggest thinking about the manufacture of a low cost 50 KV Radiotherapy machines adapted for the use in some middle income countries and that could be used for some other indications too.

2.1.1.3 Concurrent boost radiotherapy (CBRT) during the course of whole-breast radiotherapy (WBRT)

It implies giving boost radiotherapy concurrently during the course of WBRT itself instead of giving it sequentially after WBRT. There are different ways to deliver CBRT. A study was done to shorten the relatively long duration of treatment by delivering a concomitant boost (CB) to the tumor bed on Saturdays (Jalali et al., 2007). Thirty patients with locally advanced breast cancers suitable for breast conservation following neoadjuvant doxorubicin / epirubicin chemotherapy (CAF/CEF) were accrued in the study. Conventional RT (CRT) to the whole breast was delivered 5 days a week to a dose of 50 Gy, using 6-10 MV photons. In addition, an electron boost to the tumor bed was delivered every Saturday (12.5 Gy/5 fractions, weekly fraction on Saturday). With this, the entire RT treatment was completed in 5 weeks instead of the usual 6 weeks. All patients completed RT within the stipulated time with no grade IV skin toxicity in either group. CB did not significantly affect the global cosmetic results as compared with the CRT group at the end of 3 years (P=0.23). In another study, 52 patients with early-stage node-negative breast cancer were enrolled. The RT dose to the whole breast was 40.5 Gy in 2.7 Gy/fraction with a CB of 4.5 Gy in 0.3 Gy/fraction. With this, the entire RT treatment was completed in 3 weeks No acute Clinical toxicity criteria (CTC) grade III or IV and no late soft tissue toxicity were noted. The cosmetic results observed were good to excellent. (Chadha et al., 2007). These studies demonstrate that giving a CB during whole-breast RT is a viable resource-sparing option and does not lead to any detriment in local control and cosmetic outcome. (Munshi. 2009)

2.1.2 Less number of radiation fields

Since systemic adjuvant therapy is given to most patients today, the traditional radiotherapy technique has been modified, many authors no longer recommended that patients who have undergone complete or level I/II axillary dissections should receive full axillary radiotherapy since survival is not improved and the risk of lymhoedema is increased. Also, the isolated internal mammary chain failure is rare even when radiotherapy is not given (Truong et al., 2004). However, still areas of controvert exist regarding irradiation of the regional lymph nodes (Axillary, supraclavicular and internal mammary lymph nodes). The Applied Radiation Biology and Radiotherapy (ARBR) Section of the Division of Human Health, International Atomic Energy Agency (IAEA), pays great attention to resource sparing strategies in cancer radiotherapy. One of the on-going important multicentre randomized studies is about resource sparing in breast cancer treatment. It is started in the year 2007. This study is comparing irradiation of the chest-wall only versus irradiation of the chest-wall and the supraclavicular field in patients who underwent a mastectomy. In addition, the ARBR Section is conducting clinical trials in cervical cancer, oesophagus, lung, rectal, glioblastoma multiforme, nasopharyngeal cancer and painful bone metastasis.

2.2 Palliative radiotherapy of painful bone metastasis

2.2.1 Single versus multiple fractions

Radiotherapy remains the main modality of management for symptomatic bone metastases. The goal of radiotherapy in such cases is to provide pain relief and optimization of quality of life (QoL) with minimal displacement, discomfort, hospitalization, morbidity for patients and minimal cost and time commitment as well. Performance status and degree of systemic disease must be considered prior to treatment. (Janjan et al., 2009 & Fairchild & Stephen, 2011). Approximately 25 randomized clinical trials and three meta-analysis have demonstrated equivalency of single and multiple fraction radiotherapy for bone relief from uncomplicated bone metastases. Other advantages of single fraction include decreased cost and lower risk of acute effects (Chow et al., 2007). The single fraction is preferred when examining the cost utility, but there is higher rate of retreatment associated with single-fraction radiotherapy (Van den Hout et al, 2003). In a randomized clinical trial with two palliative radiotherapy regimens 8 Gy/I fraction versus 30 Gy/10 fractions, the overall responses were 75% and 86% successively while the rate of re-treatment were 28% and 2% successively. (Foro et al, 2008). Similar results were obtained from a prospective randomized multi centeric trial in which the total number of patients was 376. The rate of re-treatment (15%) was also higher in the group of Single 8 fraction than the rate of retreatment (4%) in the group treated with 30 Gy/10 Fractions. (Kaasa et al. 2006). However, most authors recommend multiple fractionations for primary treatment of complicated bone metastases for which there is no surgical option, or for postoperative treatment. The goals of postoperative radiation therapy are to decrease pain, promote healing and minimize the risk of progression (Fairchild & Stephen, 2011).

It is worthwhile to note that the treatment of asymptomatic bone metastases may deferred unless the patient is at risk of a serious adverse outcome such as spinal cord compression or impending pathological fracture (Janjan et al., 2009).

2.2.2 Half-body irradiation

Retrospective and prospective phase I and II studies suggest that single dose (6-8 Gy) hemibody irradiation provides pain relief in 70-80% of patients with multiple sites painful metastases. Studies also report decreased opioid use and need for localized external beam radiotherapy. Patients should be premedicated with intravenous fluid, antiemetics, corticosteroids and analgesics in case pain flare. Sequential treatment of both upper and lower Hemibody Irradiation requires a 6 weeks gap for recovery of myelosuppresion. (Fairchild & Stephen, 2011)

2.2.3 The follow up of radiotherapy of bone metastases

According to the International bone metastases consensus working party recommendation, the determination of response is clinical, thus biochemical or imaging studies -with subsequent costs- are not routinely required in follow up. (Chow et al., 2002).

2.3 General measures

These could be done by the local professionals and health authorities or in consultation with regional and/or international institutions and organizations particularly The International Atomic Energy Agency (IAEA) and its Applied Radiation Biology and Radiotherapy Section (ARBR) and The Program of Action for Cancer Therapy (PACT). These include:

2.3.1 General strategic planning of radiotherapy facilities in developing countries

In a Consultation to the World Health Organization, a global strategy for Radiotherapy was proposed. It considered different local parameters including the Gross National Product GNP per Capita that categorized countries in the world into 4 groups (Levels). Accordingly series of three tier radiotherapy service was proposed, with internet-based intercommunication strategy (Porter et al., 1999). One of the interesting proposal that goes with the three tier system is the creation of an integrated three-tier radiotherapy service, which consists of primary, secondary, and tertiary radiotherapy centres in developing countries—coordinated through a teleradiotherapy network. Such a network could be cost effective, help to bridge the gap, and give all patients access to the state-of-the-art technology in radiotherapy (Datta & Rajasekar, 2004). The Breast Health Global Initiative (BHGI), suggested four levels for availability breast cancer management; Basic, Limited, Enhanced and Maximal (Anderson et al., 2006, Anderson & Cazap, 2009 & Bese et al., 2008).

2.3.2 Practical modifications of the system of work in radiotherapy departments

These are in order treat more numbers of patients, like to increase the hour work of cobalt machines in developing countries, the increase the number of fractions a week from 5 to be 6 fractions in certain applications (Overgaard et al., 2006), the reduction of Machine down-time in many developing country institutions that is mainly due to problems of maintenance and lack of culture of local regular preventive maintenance (Bhadrasain, 2005). In our view, we emphasizes on **the** importance of programs that should developed in order to assure that most of the problems of down-time of machines would be fixed in the soonest as possible by the local teams either solely or and with prompt telecommunication with manufcturer maintenance staff.

2.3.3 Professional training

Customized and regular updating training are recommended for the local medical and technical staff and maintainers (Bhadrasain, 2005 &Porter et al., 1999). This because the local staff -and not the sophistication in machines- are the back bone of resource sparing and successful cost effective treatment for more number of patients.

2.4 Future directions regarding radiotherapy

From the above cited points and examples, and by rough estimation, and without additional high resources, the number of breast cancer patients treated by the present existing facilities of radiotherapy could be nearly doubled particularly in middle income countries. This could increase the cost-effectiveness of radiotherapy in the world and hopefully would be a stimulus for increasing facilities of radiotherapy in the world.
It is estimated that at least 5,000 additional radiotherapy machines are presently needed worldwide and, by 2015, at least 10,000 radiotherapy machines may be needed to meet growing treatment demand. It is estimated that during the upcoming 20-year,it is estimated that 100 million cancer victims in the developing countries will require radiotherapy, for cure or the relief of symptoms such as pain and bleeding. Sadly, only 20-25% of patients in developing countries that need radiotherapy can access it today, and the situation will only worsen in the future unless steps are taken to address it (Bhadrasain, 2005 & Yip, 2011).
In a recent study done in the US, only 77.6% of breast cancer patients received RT among the 135 patients undergoing mastectomy with strong indications. One of the causes of not receiving radiotherapy is the socio-economic condition (Jagsi et al.,2010). Hence, even in the US there are disparities in access to radiotherapy, but, surely it is not comparable with the situation in LMICs. In well-developed countries today, around one-half of the cancer patients require radiotherapy. In developing countries, however, an even greater proportion require radiotherapy due to the location and relatively advanced stages at presentation of many common cancers, which precludes adequate treatment by surgery alone (Bhadrasain, 2005 & Porter et al. 1999). Contrary to belief, radiotherapy is a cost-effective and not that expensive, it is salient to note that the cost of one military jet would represents the entire costs of radiotherapy for a country in some of parts of the world (Porter et. al. 1999).
Developing countries should evolve their own evidence-based guidelines and cost sparing in cancer treatment. For example, chemo-radiation of solid tumors in the nutritionally deprived patient may not accrue the same level of benefit as seen in the literature from affluent countries Clinical trials conducted in developing countries can most appropriately address these important questions in a scientifically robust manner. Ideas for such studies are always welcomed, even from individuals. Clinical investigators from developing countries are the key to appropriately addressing those challenges, by the rational utilization of radiotherapy and allied technologies - both new and old (Bhadrasain, 2005). Furthermore, The PACT/IAEA has formed recently an Advisory Group for Increasing Access to Radiation Therapy in Developing Countries (AGaRT), that includes international experts from organizations, national representatives and in collaboration with manufactures. ICEDOC is represented in this promising effort of PACT that -hopefully- if the international will, science and the interests of stakeholders including the manufacturers

come together in a win-win environment to achieve feasible objectives, then, it could be a turning point in the history of affordability of Radiotherapy of cancer in many underserved regions in the world.

3. Cost sparing in Breast Cancer Systemic Therapy (BCST)

In reviewing the current literature, we provide examples of innovative ideas, evidence-based approaches, and ongoing efforts that could decrease costs of BCST without compromising outcomes.

3.1 Relatively recent and expensive drugs

3.1.1 Evidence based cost effective indications of drugs

An example is the limitation of the use of Trastuzumab in breast cancer to women with non-metastatic disease and known HER2/neu positive status (Yarney et al., 2008). Limiting the use of Trastuzumab to women with ERBB2 positive status is cost effective measure, even with the additional associated cost of the test (de Sousa & Bines, 2009). Nevertheless, in the United States, a recent study revealed that up to 20% of patients receiving Trastuzumab were never tested nor had any documentation of a positive test result (Phillips et al, 2009).

3.1.2 Shorter course of treatment

An example is the shorter course of trastuzumab. The optimal duration of adjuvant trastuzumab therapy remains undetermined. There are trials in progress comparing 52 weeks of trastuzumab with 9 weeks, 3 months and 6 months. The FinHer (Finland Herceptin) study indicated that a 9-week period of trastuzumab administration is effective in women with HER2/neu-positive breast cancer. This means saving of around 80-90% of the cost of longer course (Joensuu et al., 2009). This is in addition to less total time of hospitalization, less risks of cardiac toxicities due to trastuzumab and less cost of the subsequent supportive treatment due to longer courses.

3.1.3 Pharmacokinetic studies to lower the dose by changing regimen of infusion

This is based on application of the pharmacological information and how the drug is transformed to its active ingredient in the body. An example is the low dose, prolonged infusion of gemcitabine. Hence, the habitual dose of 1000-1250 mg/m^2 for one patient could be enough for 4-5 patients. Phase I–II trials of low dose gemcitabine in prolonged infusion (of 250 mg and 180 mg/m2 for 6 and 24 h, respectively) and its comparable results in responding solid cancers like non-small cell lung cancer, breast, pancreas, and bladder cancers are encouraging. The explanation lies in the saturation of the enzyme deoxcytidine kinase needed for conversion of gemcitabine into its active form gemcitabine triphosphate, which occurs after short conventional infusion and leaves most of the drug unmetabolized (Zwitter et. al, 2005 & Khaled et al, 2008).

3.1.4 Dugs interactions and pharmacokinetic based studies

Lapatinib is an oral dual tyrosine kinase inhibitor of both epidermal growth factor receptor and *ERBB2*, approved for advanced *ERBB2*-positive breast cancer after failure of trastuzumab treatment. Pharmacokinetic-based studies include the example that showed that lapatinib taken orally with food and beverage containing CYP3A such as grapefruit juice, and not on an empty stomach as stated on the label, results in increased plasma levels and could reduce the dose and costs of lapatinib by 80%. Hence, for this expensive drug the habitual dose for one patient which is around 1250-1500 mg per day, could be enough for five patients, in addition to save cost of treatment of diarrhea due to lapatinib. It was suggested that the diarrhea is caused by the unabsorbed drug in the gut (Ratain and Cohen, 2007). Pharmacokinetic studies that pursue ways to enhance bioavailability of agents could markedly decrease the required doses and subsequent cost of treatment. Strategies include the support of clinical trial processes to pursue evidence to support less costly and optimal therapeutic efficacy outcomes (Elzawawy, 2008 & 2009).

3.1.5 Interrupted courses

Potential research questions include the interrupted courses of Aromatase inhibitors (AI) that probably would be also effective as continuous therapy after prior Tamoxifen and/or AI treatment. The hypothesis is that AI interrupted courses perhaps could enhance response of residual resistant cells (Colleoni and Maibach, 2007). This area is still in need for more researches. It could be the occasion to cite another example in another cancer i.e. prostate cancer, with different hypothesis. In a phase III randomized trial comparing intermittent androgen suppression IAS versus continuous androgen suppression for patients with PSA progression after radical radiotherapy. IAS was delivered for 8 months in each cycle with restart when PSA reached >10 ng/ml off treatment. Overall survival (OS) was not inferior in the arm of IAS, with improvement of quality of life (QoL), reduced hot flahes. Time to hormone refractory state (HR) was statistically significantly improved on the IAS arm (Klotz et al., 2011).

3.2 Essential drug, relatively cheaper and conventional systemic cancer drugs

Fortunately, the pharmaceutical arsenal of "essential and conventional systemic anticancer drugs" still constitutes the basis of systemic treatment of cancer. In addition, these conventional drugs are relatively inexpensive. For breast cancer the list would include CMF (Cyclophosphamide, Methotrexate and 5 Fluorouracil), FAC (5 Fluorouracil, Doxorubicin and Cyclophosphamide), Tamoxifen and Ovarian ablation. Innovative strategic thinking and approaches should be encouraged to improve the availability and accessibility of first-line systemic anticancer treatments as part of the comprehensive breast cancer control plan for underserved regions (Elzawawy, 2009).

3.2.1 Is anthracycline-based chemotherapy standard as adjuvant breast cancer treatment?

Six cycles of anthracycline-based chemotherapy was considered a standard in adjuvant treatment of breast cancer. However, there is data to suggest that not all patients will benefit from anthracyclines. In a recent study, patients who were Her2 negative did not gain any added benefit from addition of anthracylines as compared to regimens employing CMF (Cyclophosphamide, Methotrexate, and 5 Flourouracil) (Paik, 2008).

3.2.2 Chemotherapy versus ovarian ablation as adjuvant breast cancer treatment

Randomized studies over the past decade have demonstrated that ovarian ablation/suppression equivalence is at least equivalent to CMF regimens in receptor-positive premenopausal patients (Munshi, 2009). In a recent randomized study that included patients with large tumor sizes and nodal positivity, nine cycles of CMF were equivalent to RT-induced ovarian ablation. The study included 762 women who were premenopausal, were hormonal receptor positive, and were at high risk of relapse (defined as metastasis to at least one lymph node or tumor > 5 cm). The patients were randomized to receive either ovarian ablation by RT or chemotherapy with nine cycles of intravenous CMF. A total of 358 first events were observed: 182 in the ovarian ablation group and 176 in the CMF group. The unadjusted hazard ratio for disease-free survival in the ovarian ablation group compared with the CMF group was 0.99 (95% CI: 0.81 to 1.22; $P = 0.95$ by the log rank test). Median disease-free survival time was 130 months in the ovarian ablation group compared with 122 months in the CMF group. After a median follow-up of 10.5 years, the overall survival was similar in the two groups, with a hazard ratio of 1.11 (95% CI: 0.88 to 1.42) for the ovarian ablation group compared with the CMF group. No significant correlation was demonstrated between treatment modality and hormone receptor content, age, or any of the well-known prognostic factors. This strategy may be considered in a low-risk, young, premenopausal woman, whose compliance for chemotherapy is doubtful, and who has a strongly hormone-sensitive tumor. The readily apparent gains from this approach are that repeated visits for chemotherapy can be avoided, as also the toxicity of chemotherapy; there is also considerable savings in cost for the patient or the Medicare. (Ejlertsen, 2006). The ovarian ablation by radiotherapy could be done by simple technique, in 4-5 fractions, during or after the course of post mastectomy or lumpectomy radiotherapy to breast/chest wall. Also, it could be done by surgical ablation.

3.3 The oral route for administration of chemotherapy

The oral forms of chemotherapy could lower the cost of patient transportation, administration, hospitalizations, the subsequent costs of adverse effects of hospitalizations and it may improve the quality of life (Elzawawy, 2008 and Elzawawy, 2009). In fact, this point could be applied to old and new cancer drugs. More pharmacological and clinical researches as well as in manufacture of drugs are warranted. Hence, most known cancers could have regimes of treatment that are totally or partially administrated via oral route. The pros and cons of oral route administration of chemotherapy should be carefully studied in each community in a scientific and realistic ways. Questions of cost-effectiveness and best practices relating to oral and self-administered agents are of considerable interest in LMICs where facilities and providers may be particularly scarce. One of the major realistic obstacles is not the compliance, which should not be taken as an absolute and undefeatable problem in some population, but also, the factors related to oncologists and hospitals with less gain from oral therapy. In a win-win initiative all factors and interests of all stakeholders should be tackled in realistic, transparent, scientific and global ways.

3.4 Genomics and cancer treatment

Pharmacogenomics is the study of individual genetic variation in efficacy and adverse effects of a drug. Radiogenomics is reffered to the same science but for radiotherapy. This science offers a partial explanation for the interpatient variability in treatment response commonly observed in oncology. Small variations in patient germline DNA sequence (genotype), including single nucleotide polymorphisms (SNPs), can alter the expression and functional activity of an encoded protein. Often, genetic variants leading to clinically relevant functional changes occur in noncoding (intron) regions of the genome or in exons that code for protein expression (Guttmacher& Collins, 2003). These changes may lead to individual differences in drug distribution, metabolism, activity and toxicity (Connolly& Stearns, 2009, Lash et. al, 2009).

Pharmcogenomic studies were suggested to guide the adjustment the effective use of some drugs like Tamoxifen (Colleoni, 2002 & Lash, et al, 2009). Patients can be classified as poor, intermediate, or extensive metabolizers according to the genetic variation in CYP2D6, a key enzyme in Tamoxifen metabolism. In the poor metabloizers cases, the use of Tamoxifen, would be a waste of costs for 5 years of probably non sense treatment and with unnecessary risks of hazards. In the other hand, a modeling analysis suggested that the benefit of 5 years of adjuvant Tamoxifen therapy in patients who were carriers of the wild-type CYP2D6,the extensive metabolizers, was similar or perhaps superior when compared with the more expensive aromatase inhibitor therapy. Thus, it was suggested that onetime test for CYP2D6 genotype has the potential to make the patient eligible for 5 years of savings by allowing for the use of -the less expensive- Tamoxifen (Punglia et al., 2007). However, more prospective studies about CYP2D6 and this topic are warranted, as recently there are controversies regarding the significance and value of the adoption of routine CYP2D6 testing in the clinic (Lash et al., 2009). Science is searching for the truth. The road for facts is endless and enjoyable. In fact, once again, not every exciting scientific finding could be translated into the same expected clinical value in the short and the long term clinical researches and trials (Elzawawy, 2010 & 2011).

Besides probable different variations in human host and tumor biology, real local socioeconomic conditions and priorities of problem, cost effectiveness, cost utilty, available services including supportive treatment different, Pharmcogenomics and Radiogenomics are among the possible causes of that protocols and guidelines of treatment shouldn't be copied in different communities without adaptation and without considering these factors in scientific and realistic ways.

3.5 Generic equivalents for off-patent drugs

The World Health Organization (WHO) proposed essential drugs required for cancer therapy (WHO, March 2010). Many drugs included in the 'Essential Drugs for Cancer Therapy' list have generic equivalents that offer the possibility of less expensive treatment. However, we stress on not taking the proposal of using generics off patent cancer drugs as a magic stick and automatically as an ideal solution for more cost effective treatment, without assuring the flow of production and the affordability of generics drugs of good quality. Particularly in developing countries, the quality and bioequivalence of generics drugs should be assured by regulations or developing a transparent system for international testing. A generic of good quality or an "original" essential drug would be more cost effective than generics of less quality, even if the later is of fewer prices. Also, the use of first line treatment of tested good quality drugs could reduce the needs for second and third lines treatment that are usually more expensive. Besides, the risk on patients, results of clinical trials and researches in LMICs would be doubtful if they are done with drugs with questionable quality. We suggested an international body or experts or programs that would assure the quality and bioequivalence of generics delivered to LMCIs. To overcome difficulties in achieving large scale feasibility in quality control, we suggested small scale groups level to test random samples or pilot settings upon invitation from the local

authorities in some developing countries. Hence, it wouldn't be to police, but to advise and it would react only upon request from the locals (Elzawawy, 2008 & 2009).
Contrary to belief, the availability of essential and generics off-patent cancer drugs is very critical issue to rich and developed countries and not only for developing countries. In November, 2010, the American Society of Clinical Oncology (ASCO) announced that across the United States, there is severe and worsening shortage of a big group of these drugs that are placing cancer patients in the US at risk, including -and not limited to- doxorubicin, carboplatin, cisplatin, etoposide, leucovorin, nitrogen mustard, vincristine and morphine. Michael Link, MD, president-elect of ASCO, for the term 2011-2012, said in a statement "Shortages of critical cancer drugs are causing delays in treatment, which can impact survival and the ongoing clinical trials. Additionally, administration of alternative therapies, if they are available, can lead to less optimal treatment, as well as increased costs, for patients and increased administrative burdens for oncology practices". Bona Benjamin, from the American Society of Health System Pharmacists (ASHP) stated "For hospital pharmacists, the shortage of injectable cancer drugs products — many of which have no therapeutic alternatives — is approaching a national crisis in the US. There is no single reason or solution for the shortages. Most of the cancer drugs that are in short supply are generic products and are manufactured by a few companies. There is no financial incentive to manufacture cheaper generic drugs. In a free market, there is nothing to compel manufacturers to make drugs that don't make them money; there is no hammer". (Chustecka, 2010). One of the values of having global scientific approaches for the problems of availability and affordability of cancer is that we could explore and tackle proposals that could help -with variations- in developing and developed countries. The Win-Win initiative concentrates on scientific approaches that could lead finally to the benefit of all stakeholders.

3.6 Old cancer drugs, new uses, news profits

By scientific approaches, old cancer drugs could have new indications, and subsequently offering less expensive treatment to cancer. This implies exploring new indications or innovative combinations or different schedules of administration of older (and relatively cheaper) previously approved cancer. For example, the relatively old like cisplatin has been shown to be useful in the treatment of triple negative (-ve estrogen and progesterone receptors, HER2/neu 0, 1) breast cancer (Gronwald et al., 2009). The metronomic use of prolonged, low oral doses of the cheap drugs cyclophosphamide and methotrexate are used as palliative breast cancer treatment (Colleoni, 2002). In a recent phase II trial, the low dose (6 mg/d) oral estradiol was effective (around 30%) as conventional high dose (30 mg/d) with less adverse events in postmenopausal women with advanced, aromatase inhibitor-resistant, hormone receptor-positive breast cancer (Ellis, 2009).

3.7 Old non cancer drug, new uses in cancer, potential new profits

An example is inexpensive drug called metformin. It's widely used by type 2 diabetics who overproduce insulin. But new researches suggest that it could be useful in breast cancer prevention and treatment. It was found that metformin can also act on lung cancer tumour growth in mice that have been exposed to a common carcinogen in cigarettes. Moreover, new studies suggest that it could be tested for colon cancer too. It's thought the drug works by targeting a cancer tumor's stem cells which, if not killed off, can allow various cancer cell types to regenerate. Hence, have an old molecule, an old drug, a safe drug that may have an unexpected use in cancer prevention and cancer treatment. More studies are currently planned. Each tablet costs 21 cents and must be taken twice daily. Despite the low price, the cost to run such a clinical trial, which involves collecting blood samples, is expected to run at least $15-million. The trial is expected to include 3,582 patients in Canada and the United States who are undergoing standard cancer treatment plus metformin or placebo for up to five years. Until the results are in, patients should not use it unless it is prescribed for diabetes or they are on the clinical trial, where they can be properly monitored (Dowling, 2011).

3.8 New uses for cancer chemotherapy drugs in non malignant indications

An example is the recent researches that revealed that fluorouracil could be used as a skin cream to help repair of sun damage and skin wrinkles on the faces. Topical fluorouracil causes epidermal injury, which stimulates wound healing and dermal remodeling resulting in improved appearance. The mechanism of topical fluorouracil in photoaged skin follows a predictable wound healing pattern of events reminiscent of that seen with laser treatment of photoaging (Sachs et al., 2009)

4. Does evidence-based medicine really reduce costs?

The question is paused by many from time to time. In a wonderful recent article the issue is discussed (Kolodzie, 2011). Till recently the issue was a theory and a hypothesis. It pass now to the phase of having proof. The adoption of pathways based on evidence-based medicine (EBM) in patients with non–small-cell lung cancer (NSCLC) revealed that evidence-based care resulted in an average cost-savings of 35% over 12 months and equivalent outcomes (Neubauer et al., 2010). It is important to note that not all pathways are created equal. Most programs use minimum criteria to develop their pathways; these typically include assessment of efficacy and toxicity. A few pathway programs go beyond these minimum criteria and consider costs as well. These types of programs delineate treatment options based on maximum survival benefits, minimal toxicity, and cost-saving advantages.

4.1 Reduction in expensive supportive care drugs

When two or more therapies are equally effective against a disease, regimens lower in toxicity are typically chosen to be on-pathway. This leads those physicians who adhere to pathways to be less likely to prescribe expensive anti-emetics, growth factors, and other supportive care drugs absent strong evidence to validate their use.

4.2 Fewer hospital visits

One of the most common reasons patients require hospitalization during treatment is adverse effects and complications caused by the agents. The less toxic on-pathway regimens can result in fewer or less severe adverse reactions, therefore reducing the number of unplanned hospital visits.

4.3 Reduction in therapy overall

Treatment guidelines, backed by evidentiary support, lead physicians to confidently recommend the most effective therapy as the first-line treatment with standard order sets that define dosing strengths and number of cycles. For many cancers, especially solid tumors in adults, each successive line of treatment is less efficacious than the preceding line. When patients with late-stage disease face difficult decisions, some will wish to continue a line of treatment no matter what. Others express the desire to improve their quality of life, with many stating that they prefer to die at home rather than in the hospital. (Wennberg et al., 2008). Third and fourth lines of treatments rarely change the course of the disease and can cause incapacitating adverse effects. More often than not, if a patient's cancer has not responded to or has progressed after the first or second line of treatment, the best course for that patient may be to transition into end-of-life or palliative care. A study analyzing Medstat 2007 data in the US, revealed that out of those chemotherapy patients with 10 major cancer diagnoses who were identified as dying in an inpatient setting, 24% received chemotherapy within 14 days of death and 51% received chemotherapy within 30 days of death (Fitch & Pyenson, 2010). While we cannot always predict when death will occur, pathways can help guide physicians in making decisions and treatment recommendations pertaining to whether to offer additional cycles of a treatment or move to second, third, and further lines of treatment. They can also provide practical guidance that can be helpful in end-of-life care discussions. This includes demonstrating that transitioning to hospice care can improve the patient's and the family's quality of life and can reduce the costs borne by the family and payers by avoiding unnecessary and ineffective chemotherapy administered within a few weeks of death (Kolodzie, 2011).

4.4 Use of less expensive drugs

Oncology drug costs are exorbitant, making this line item an obvious target for payers as they search for ways to reduce costs. One way in which EBM can help reduce the costs of cancer care is by optimizing the appropriate use of less expensive drugs. When pathways are developed, it will often be found that evidence supports the use of less expensive therapies, without compromising outcomes or increasing toxicity. For example, if treatment pathways point to two potential therapies that are largely equivalent in efficacy and toxicity, yet these two drugs vary enormously in cost, pathways programs that consider cost a factor would ultimately point to the less expensive drug. Obviously, there are some cases in which cost cannot be a determining factor in deciding which drug to use to treat a patient. Where one therapy is far more effective than others, it is the clear choice and will be indicated as the first choice for that setting. Take trastuzumab as an example. Trastuzumab is unquestionably an expensive drug, but evidence for its efficacy in certain situations is indisputable. As pathways are developed, efficacy is given the highest priority, with cost being considered only when outcomes are equivalent. In the case of trastuzumab, the efficacy of the drug and the lack of available substitutes make it the correct choice- when it is used in appropriate indications- regardless of its price.

5. Control of utilization of a drug as a primary strategy of Medicare, USA

The primary strategy Medicare uses to hold down utilization of a drug (or another health care good or service) is to limit coverage of payment for it. The program does so by actively determining in which settings the drug is or is not "reasonable and necessary" through either a single national or one or more local coverage decisions. When these coverage decisions result in restricted guidelines for the use of the drug, the result is decreased utilization. For instance, in 2007, Medicare narrowed the coverage of erythropoiesis-stimulating agents

(ESAs) for cancer treatment. Medicare limited not only the types of patients who could receive ESAs but also the clinical scenarios in which they could be used (Centers for Medicare & Medicaid Services, 2007). One of the biggest companies who sale ESAs in the USA, reported to their investors in August 2007 that changes in coverage for ESAs by the Centers for Medicare and Medicaid Services (CMS) would reduce annual sales of the company's ESA from approximately $1 billion to $200 million among Medicare patients. In our view, the lesson here, is that if the strategy of control utilization is indicated in a rich country like the USA, then, it would be mandatory in less affluent countries. In a win-win scenarios, our objective is not at all against the sales of drugs per se, but this strategy of controlling utilization of drugs, by whatever the mechanism in each country, would assure more reasonable and justified utilization of drugs (or services). Otherwise, the chaos in its utilizations in some less affluent countries, opens wide doors for the use of these drugs when it is not necessary while omitting patients who are in real big need for these drugs, for more local corruptions and exhausting resources in non cost effective ways without marked improvement of outcome and in non cost effective ways, and finally it could lead to collapse of markets in those of countries in front of new products of companies. Hence, transparent scientifically based measures are encouraged by the win-win initiative for the benefit of all stakeholders.

6. Economic analyses and outcomes assessment

Economic analyses are most valuable to health policy analysis and health care managers who must allocate resources and established health care management. An economic health care analysis tries to directly relate the incremental cost of an intervention to its potential benefit. (Hayman et al., 1996). Clinical Oncologists shouldn't be away from knowing basic information and various terms of such issues. That is why –at least the definitions- are included in many cancer treatment textbooks or in chapters dealing with availability, accessibility and affordability of cancer treatment. Not surprisingly, high costs can be financially devastating to American patients and their families, with some 62% of all bankruptcies estimated to result from medical expenses (Himmelstein et al, 2009). The American Society of Clinical Oncology (ASCO) has issued a Guidance Statement affirming "the critical role of oncologists in addressing cost of care" and stating that "ASCO believes that communication with patients about the cost of care is a key component of high-quality care (Meropol et al.,2009). However, many oncologists feel ill-prepared to discuss the costs of therapy with patients, (Schrag &Hange, 2007) and little is known about how patients factor cost into their decision-making when facing a life-threatening crisis of a cancer diagnosis (Mileshkin, 2009).

6.1 Definitions of various terms used in economic analysis

6.1.1 Cost minimization

It relates to lower cost of an alternative treatment without regard to the efficacy. It is measured in dollars. The major drawback of only using this approach to evaluate cancer treatment is the fact that complex-oncology therapies almost never result in truly identical outcomes.

6.1.2 Cost benefit

It relates to the additional cost of treatment in dollars to its incremental benefit in dollars, as compared to the most reasonable alternative treatment. Results of cost benefit analyses also can be reported as a ratio, where the additional cost of treatment is divided by its added benefit, again compared to the most reasonable alternative.

6.1.3 Cost effectiveness

It relates the additional costs of an intervention to its incremental impact on any clinically relevant measure of benefit. Because one of the primary uses of economic analysis is the allocation of limited resources among different choices, benefit often is measured in units that are universally applicable to all intervention. Years of life saved are the most commonly used measure. For example, the cost-effectiveness of combination chemotherapy, compared with single-agent therapy, for a given disease could be assessed by calculating the additional costs (in dollars or the monetary units) per additional patient reaching the 5-year disease-free survival mark or more frequently, per years of life saved.
The Incremental cost-effectiveness ratio (ICER) or The intervention's cost-effectiveness ratio is calculated by dividing its incremental cost by its incremental impact on survival, as compared to the most reasonable alternative treatment. The intervention's cost-effectiveness ratio, expressed in units of dollars per unit of effect compared to the standard intervention. Years of life saved are the most frequently used measure. Cost-Effectiveness ratios are, therefore, usually expressed in terms of dollars per year of life saved.

6.1.4 The QALY and the DALY

Medical interventions affect not only length of life but also quality of life (QoL). Cancer cure may be brought at the expense of substantial treatment-related morbidity. Conversely, palliative therapy may bring marked relief of symptoms; even it does not lengthen life dramatically. A nonmonetary unit for evaluation is the quality - adjusted life year (QALY). QALY measure the "usefulness "or "utility" of a health state and the length of life lived under those conditions. One attempts to obtain values or utility measures by expert opinion, by using values derived in previous studies, and by surveys of patients. These surveys can be difficult to construct and may involve asking patients to make a "time tradeoff" or engage in a "rating scale "of various conditions or to assign a preference weight on a scale of 0 to 1 to a condition. The DALY is the disability-adjusted life year. WHO has suggested that a health intervention can be considered cost effective if it yields savings of one disability-adjusted life year for less than three-times a country's gross domestic product (GDP) (Torres Edejer et al., 2003).

6.1.5 Cost utility

It relates the additional cost of treatment to its impact on both survival and quality of life, as well as productivity of the patient following treatment. The length of time spent in each outcome is multiplied by the outcome's weighting factor and the product is summed. A cost-utility analysis may be considered as special form of a cost-effective analysis. In the cost-utility analysis, the health outcome of the denominator is valued in term of utility or quality of life. The monetary units of evaluation include the QALY. It is common to express cost-utility analysis as total net cost per unit of utility or measure of quality - for example, a number of dollars or saving per QALY gained. A cost-utility ratio can be calculated by dividing its additional cost by its incremental change in QALYs, compared to a reasonable alternative. Hence, the units of the cost-utility ratio is Dollars/QALY.
We can conclude that over the past decade it has become increasingly clear that, in addition to quantity of life, the impact of treatment on quality of life must be incorporated into measures of benefit. (Hayman et al., 1996 & Weeks, 2003).

It worthwhile to note that the "no treatment" strategy does not necessarily mean it is a "no cost "strategy. Hence, in our view, contrary to belief, the affordability of well-tailored scientifically based treatment or appropriate palliation could -in many cases- reduce variable costs and burden of "no treatment". We hope that this message finds its way to local leaders of health policies decisions makers, leaders of global health departments in the world and in the United Nations Non Communicable Diseases (NCDs) meetings.

7. Health technology assessment (HTA) programs

HTA programs evaluate the value of new therapies and technologies to patients by considering the following (Hutton et al, 2006): Is the new treatment effective? Although surrogate end points such as response rate may be sufficient evidence of efficacy for regulatory agencies (eg, rise in hemoglobin after administration of erythropoietin stimulating agent), HTAs generally demand more direct evidence of benefit (eg, improved quality of life measured by a validated instrument, or improved survival). Which patients benefit? If the clinical trial population excluded particular patient populations, are they likely to have the same benefit as the patients included in the study? How does it compare to other available treatments? At what cost?

Many countries now incorporate HTAs into their decision-making process before deciding to cover new therapies within their publicly funded health care systems. The United Kingdom was the first country to adopt HTA explicitly by creating the National Institute for Clinical Effectiveness in 1999. Since then, many other countries, including Australia, Belgium, Canada, Denmark, Finland, German, Hungary, the Netherlands, Norway, Portugal, and Sweden, have developed processes for HTA to be used in coverage decisions. Although to date the information does not appear to have had much impact on formulary decisions, US private health plans are increasingly requesting pharmaceutical manufacturers to submit evidence dossiers that adhere to the Academy of Managed Care Pharmacy guidelines and include information on clinical and cost effectiveness (Sullivan et al., 2009)

8. Finally, we emphasize on these points

To enhance researches and scientific studies that result in decreasing the total cost of treatment and to increase –or at least not to compromise- effectiveness and quality of life. It is preferred to design -as most as possible- protocols of treatment that require less or no hospitalizations-except in some cases, less costs of auxiliary cares and expensive supportive drugs that could be not available in the community or it could produce high additional financial burden.

To develop more scientific researches that go with the notion of "Resource-level-appropriate use of costly agents" and that necessarily involves inclusion of how to mobilize the locally-available resources and the establishment of viable partnerships with different sectors in the community. Hence, LMICs shouldn't count on financial donations from far, as they would be never enough. The real lasting help to these communities is in assisting of local capacity building, for cooperative scientific researches, training, assistance in reporting and publications and appropriate technology transfer.

To test innovative combinations or different schedules of administration of older (and relatively cheaper) drugs that might lead to improve therapeutic index or newer applications in different societies. Such investigations usually are not supported by pharmaceuticals companies and international conferences, although they might be of benefit to science and cancer patients in LMICs and affluent countries. Conducting such researches in LMICs would be a sort of capacity building for researches and clinical trials that could be used for conducting trials with appropriate ethical guidelines - and subsequent access - for newer drugs in these communities and it could pave the ways for justified use and sales of newer drugs in more cost effective ways in markets that risk to shrink in the upcoming years. Such approach would assist companies in streamlining the development of new drugs and technologies.

To disseminate the concept of global and balanced cancer control including earlier diagnosis and supportive and palliative care. Earlier diagnosis of less advanced cases could decrease the total costs of treatment and increase quality of life. But, screening and efforts for early detection without having affordable treatments that respect what we call "The economic and social dignity of patients and their families" would be fruitless and it would be frustrating for both patients and health professionals. (Elzawawy et al., 2008). Incidence of a particular cancer, total per-capita health spending (WHO, 2010), country's gross domestic product (GDP) should be considered in estimation cost-effectiveness of some screening programs like mammographic screening for breast cancer. Resources in LMCs might be better used to raise awareness and encourage more women with palpable breast lumps to seek and receive treatment in a timely manner and to assure patient navigator services in LMCs, which aim to help women access their health-care system and receive better care once in the system, could be more cost effective than attempts to screen the asymptomatic masses (Harford, 2011). Palliative care is an essential component of comprehensive cancer care (Becker et al., 2011). The availability of supportive and palliative care integrated oncology could improve outcome, reduce overall costs, lessen burden on patients and families and improve qualities of life and death.

Thinking is never enough. We have two preliminary proposals and we cite them here as questions for wider discussion. We suggest the term: "The Relevant Clinical Oncology". It considers the variability in biologic and pharmacologic factors among the human hosts and the nature of tumors, cost effectiveness and cost utility as well as the real socioeconomic conditions. It respects the expectations and priorities of the human beings of each community (A. Elzawawy, 2011). Moreover, we see that the term "personalized" or "customized" cancer treatment is usually concentrated on hitting one or more biological targets that could varied from a tumor to another. We proposed to extend this term to include more aspects of the human host like variability in pharmcogenomics, pharmcodynamics and pharmacokinetics for different drugs, and other personal variations in human beings like socio-economic aspects. Hence, we hope that in the future, the term personalized treatment would pass from "The mechanics" of hitting one target in the tumor by a drug, to the more broader concept and vision of medicine to consider biological tumor factors, human factors and medical wisdom without compromising the overall outcome and via evidence based researches and trials. It is a real challenge. (Elzawawy,2011).

There is a question raised recently in the USA "We have a choice: do we use science to help us reach consensus on what we are willing to pay for new therapies and innovation, or do we leave individual patients to wrestle with the skyrocketing costs of cancer care and treatment determined by their ability to pay?"(Malin, 2010). And globally, we raise the question, are we going to see innovation in cancer treatment and drugs as a of complicating problems of its affordability or we will use science to lessen this rising problem as it facilitates many things in our daily life?.

9. Conclusion

There are no indications that the costs of the novel cancer drugs and radiotherapy of cancer and the incidence and prevalence of cancer will stop increasing in the next decade. Hence, there would be more difficulties and challenges for patients, families, governments, physicians, manufacturers of cancer drugs and radiotherapy equipment, particularly in Low and Middle Income Countries (LMICs). However, there are also increasing concerns in affluent countries and the USA about the increasing costs of cancer therapy. Starting from December 2007, with communications, publications and working meetings, the win-win initiative was proposed by ICEDOC's Experts in Cancer without Borders (ICEDOC: is the International Campaign for Establishment and Development of Oncology Centers www.icedoc.org). The win-win initiative stress on the scientific approaches and in considering stakeholders in win-win scenarios in which no one would lose. Our concerns is to lower the total costs (not necessarily the price of a drug or an equipment), to flourish the system and save it from risk of collapse. In this chapter, we reviewed examples of the recently published scientific works that could lead to lower the overall costs of breast cancer radiotherapy and systemic chemotherapy and hormonal treatment without compromising patients' outcomes. It is presented as a model, to be expanded to other cancers. The cited approaches, with our views, are not presented as wholly inclusive or definitive solutions but are offered as effective examples and as stimuli to hopefully inspire the development of more evidence based management approaches that provide cost effective and more affordable cancer treatment. We recommend to adopt win-win scenarios and to create what Franklin D Roosevelt described as "A Brain Trust" opened for innovative scientific thoughts, ideas and strategies, to foster relevant scientific researches and collaboration that would aim at achieving cost-effective and accessible cancer treatment for more millions of patients with cancers in the world. The win-win initiative is an open movement and it is inspired from the works and publications of many scientists. We don't claim patency. The key leaders of international oncology community and organizations are sharing in the development of the initiative and its working meetings. Hence, it is a concept and an approach that we call all for cooperation for its wide dissemination, to be adopted and to be owned by all who are concerned in the upcoming years. We emphasize on the importance of considering the broad sense for the term science and not to be taken as just to copy the imported protocols or guidelines of treatment. Hence, scientific cooperation, exchange of experiences, customized clinical trials and treatment that respect the realistic biological, human, social and economic conditions, cost -effectiveness, quality of life cost -utility and adapted to each community are recommended. Despite that, the motivation of this initiative is largely humanitarian, but it is based on scientifically derived evidence and reflects 'win-win' scenarios for global cancer management.

10. Acknowledgement

I thank all the international oncology personalities who participated by their thoughtful discussion before, during and after the win-win initiative working meetings. As the list is long, I advise to visit www.icedoc.org/winwin.htm. I particularly thank Prof. David Kerr, President of ESMO (European Society of Medical Oncology), Prof. E. Cazap, President of the UICC (International Union against Cancer) & President of SLACOM (The Society of Latin America and Caribbean of Medical Oncology), Prof. G. Hortobagyi, former President of

ASCO, Prof. M. Piccart, President Elect of ESMO, Dr. Joe Harford, NCI, USA, Dr. Anne Reeler, Paris (Axios and coordinator of CanTreat), Dr. J. Saba, Paris (Axios & CanTreat), Dr. P. Anhoury, Senior Vice President, Kantar Health, Prof. H. Zwierzina, Austria and co-founder of ICEDOC, Prof. H. Mellstedt, Sweden (ESMO DCTF), Prof. P. Parikh, India (ICON Trust), Dr. G. Bhattacharyya, India (ICON Trust), Prof. B. Anderson, Director of BHGI, USA, Prof. B. Koczwara, Australia (ESMO DCTF), Dr. C. Hunter, USA (Vice President of AORTIC for North America, African Organization for Research and Training in Cancer), Mr. Doug Pyle, USA (Director of ASCO International Affairs), Dr. *E. Rosenblatt,* Section Head, ARBR, IAEA,Vienna, Mr. M. Samiei, Head of PACT, IAEA, Prof. M. Hussein, Vice President, Celgene, USA. My deepest appreciation to My wife Dr. Mona Abdulla, Port Said, Egypt, Dr. Pamela Haylock, Secretary General of ICEDOC, Texas, USA, Dr. Atef Badran, ICEDOC & SEMCO and Mr. Dan Rutz, (ICEDOC & Centers for Disease Control and Prevention (CDC), Atlanta, Georgia, USA for their precious advice during preparing the text of the win-win initiative.

11. References

Anderson, B.O.; Shyyan, R.; Eniu, A.; Smith, R.A.; Yip, C.H.; Bese, N.S.; Chow, L.W.; Masood, S.; Ramsey, S.D. & Carlson, R.W. (2006). Breast cancer in limited resource countries: an overview of the Breast Health Global Initiative 2005 guidelines. *Breast J,* Vol. 12, Jan-Feb 2006, Suppl. 1, pp. S3-15

Anderson, B.O. & Cazap E. (2009). Breast Health Global Initiative (BHGI) outline for program development in Latin America. *Salud Publica Mex,* Vol. 51, Suppl. 2, pp. 309-315, ISSN 0036-3634

Bach, P.B. (2007). Costs of cancer care: a view from the centers for Medicare and Medicaid Services. *J Clin Oncol,* Vol. 25, pp. 187-190

Becker,G.; Hatami,I.; Xander, C.; Dworschak-Flach,B; Olschewski, M; Momm, F; Deibert,P.; Higginson, I.J. & Blum,H.E. (2011). Palliative cancer care: an epidemiologic study. *J Clinc Oncol,* Vol. 29, No. 6, pp. 646-50

Bese, N. S.; Munshi, A.; Budrukkar, A.; Elzawawy, A. & Perez C.A. (2008). Guidelines for International Breast Health and Cancer Control–Implementation. Breast Radiation Therapy Guideline Implementation in Low- and Middle-Income Countries. *Cancer,* Vol. 113, No. 8 Suppl., pp. 2306-13

Bhadrasain, V. (2005). Radiation therapy for the developing countries. *J Can Res Ther,* Vol. 1, pp. 7-8

Centers for Medicare & Medicaid Services. (2007). Proposed decision memo for erythropoiesis stimulating agents (ESAs) for non-renal disease indications (CAG-00383N). Available from: <http://www.cms.gov/medicare-coverage-database/details/nca-decision-memo.aspx?NCAId=203&ver=12&NcaName=Erythropoiesis+Stimulating+Agents+&bc=BEAAAAAAEAAA&>

Chadha, M.; Woode, R.; Sillanpaa, J.; Feldman, S.; Boolbol, S.; Furhang, E.; *et al.* (2007). Three-week Accelerated Radiation Therapy (ART) schedule with a concomitant in-field boost as treatment for early stage breast cancer. *Int J Radiat Oncol Biol Phys,* Vol. 69, pp. S137

Chow, E.; Wu, J.; Hoskin, P., *et al.* (2002). International consensus on palliative radiotherapy endpoints for future clinical trials in bone metastases. *Radiother Oncol,* Vol. 64; pp. 275-280

Chow, E., Harris, K.; Fan, G.; *et al.* (2007). Palliative radiotherapy trials for bone metastases: a systemic review. *J Clin Oncol,* Vol. 25, pp. 1423-1436

Colleoni, M.; Rocca, A.; Sandri, M.T.; Zorzino, L.; Masci, G.; Nole, F.; Peruzzotti, G.; Robertson, C.; Orlando, L.; Cinieri, S.; Viale, G. & Goldhirsch, A. (2002). Low-dose oral methotrexate and cyclophosphamide in metastatic breast cancer: antitumor activity and correlation with vascular endothelial growth factor levels. *Ann Oncol,* Vol. 13, pp. 73–80

Colleoni, M.& Maibach, R. (2007). Breast international group newsletter. 9:,pp 22.

Connolly, R. & Stearns, V. (2009). The role of pharmacogenetics in selection of breast cancer treatment. *Current Breast Cancer Reports,* Vol. 1, pp. 190–197.

Chustecka, Z. (2011). Early Warning System for Prescription Drug Shortages. Available from Medscape Medical News, Oncology:
<http://www.medscape.com/viewarticle/737038>

Datta, N. & Rajasekar, D. (2004). Improvement of radiotherapy facilities in developing countries: a three-tier system with a teleradiotherapy network. *Lancet Oncol,* Vol. 5, pp. 695–98

De Souza, J.A. & Bines, J. (2009). The global breast cancer disparity: Strategies for bridging the gap. *JAMA,* Vol. 302, No. 23, pp. 2589-2590

Dowling, R.J.; Goodwin, P.J. & Stambolic, V. (2011). Understanding the benefit of metformin use in cancer treatment. *BMC Med,* Vol. 9, No. 1, 6 April 2011, pp. 33

Drummond, M. & Mason, A. (2009). Rationing new medicines in the UK. *BMJ,* Vol. 338, (22 January 2009), pp. a3182

Early Breast Cancer Trialists' Collaborative Group. (2000). Favourable and unfavourable effects on long-term survival of radiotherapy for early breast cancer: An overview of the randomised trials. *Lancet,* Vol. 355, pp. 1757-70

Ejlertsen, B.; Mouridsen, H.T.; Jensen, M.B.; Bengtsson, N.O.; Bergh, J.; Cold, S.; *et al.* (2006). Similar efficacy for ovarian ablation compared with cyclophosphamide, methotrexate, and fluorouracil: From a randomized comparison of premenopausal patients with node-positive, hormone receptor-positive breast cancer. *J Clin Oncol,* Vol. 24, pp. 4956-62

Ellis, M.J.; Gao, F.; Dehdashti, F.; Jeffe, D.B.; Marcom, P.K.; Carey, L.A.; Dickler, M.N.; Silverman, P.; Fleming, G.F.; Kommareddy, A.; Jamalabadi-Majidi, S.; Crowder, R.& Siegel, B.A. (2009). Lower-dose vs high-dose oral estradiol therapy of hormone receptor–positive, aromatase inhibitor–resistant advanced breast cancer: A phase 2 randomized study. *JAMA,* Vol. 302, No. 7, pp. 774-780

Elzawawy, A.M.; Elbahaie, A.M.; Dawood, S.M.; Elbahaie, H.M.& Badran, A. (2008). Delay in seeking medical advice and late presentation of female breast cancer patients in most of the world. Could we make changes? The experience of 23 years in Port Said, Egypt. *Breast Care,* Vol.3, pp. 37–41

Elzawawy, A.M. (2008). Breast Cancer Systemic Therapy: The Need for More Economically Sustainable Scientific Strategies in the World. *Breast Care,* Vol. 3, pp. 434–438

Elzawawy, A.M. (2009). The "Win-Win" initiative: a global, scientifically based approach to resource sparing treatment for systemic breast cancer therapy. *World Journal of Surgical Oncology*, Vol. 7, pp. 44

Elzawawy, A.M. (2010). Minutes of The 2nd meeting of the Win-Win Initiative, 6th June, 2010, ASCO 2010 Conference, Chicago, IL, USA. Available from <www.icedoc.org/winwin.htm>

Elzawawy, A.M. (2011). Clinical researches and increasing affordability of cancer treatment in middle-income countries: breast cancer as a research model. ASCO International Clinical Trials Workshop, 6th SEMCO-ASCO conference, Cairo, Egypt, January 27-28, 2011. Available from <www.semco-oncology.info/files/15.1.Interactive%20Discussin-Clin%20res_%20increasing%20affordability%20Ca%20tret_Elzawawy.pdf>

Faden, R.R.; Chalkidou, K.; Appleby, J.; *et al.* (2009). Expensive cancer drugs: A comparison between the United States and the United Kingdom. *Milbank Q*, Vol. 87, pp. 789–819

Fairchild, A. & Stephen, L. (2011). Palliative radiotherapy for bone metastases, In: *Decisions Making in Radiotherapy*, Lu, J.J. & Brady, L.W., pp. 25-42, Springer-Verlag, ISBN: 978-3-642-12462

Ferlay, J.; Shin, H.; Bray, F.; Forman, D.; Mathers, C.& Parkin, D. (2010). GLOBOCAN 2008, Cancer incidence and mortality worldwide: IARC CancerBase No 10. Lyon, France: International Agency for Research on Cancer, 2010. Available from: <http://globocan.iarc.fr>

Fitch, K. & Pyenson, B. (2010). *Cancer patients receiving chemotherapy: Opportunities for better management.* Milliman Inc., New York, USA

Foro, P.; Fontanals, A.; Galceran, J.; *et al.* (2008). Randomized clinical trial with two palliative radiotherapy regimens in painful bone metastases: 30 Gy in 10 Fractions compared with 8 Gy in single fraction. *Radiother Oncol*, Vol. 89, pp. 150-155

Gronwald, J.; Byrski,T.& Huzarski, T. (2009). Neoadjuvant therapy with cisplatin in *BRCA1*-positive breast cancer patients. *J Clin Oncol,* Vol. 27, No.15S, pp. 502

Guttmacher, A.E.& Collins, F.S. (2003). Welcome to the genomic era. *N Engl J Med*, Vol. 349, pp. 996–998

Harford, J.B. (2011). Breast-cancer early detection in low-income and middle-income countries: do what you can versus one size fits all. *Lancet Oncol,* Vol. 12, pp. 306–12

Hayman, J.; Weeks, J. & Mauch, P. (1996). Economic Analyses in health care: An introduction to the methodology with an emphasis to radiation therapy. *Int J Radiat Oncol Biol Phys*, Vol. 35, pp.827-841

Himmelstein, D.U.; Thorne, D.; Warren, E.; *et al.* (2009). Medical bankruptcy in the United States, 2007: Results of a national study. *Am J Med*, Vol. 122, pp. 741–746

Hutton, J.; McGrath, C.; Frybourg, J.; *et al.* (2006). Framework for describing and classifying decision-making systems using technology assessment to determine the reimbursement of health technologies (fourth hurdle systems). *Int J Technol Assess Health Care,* Vol. 22, pp. 10–18

Jagsi, R.; Abrahamse, P.; Morrow, M.; Hawley, S.T.; Griggs, J.J.; Graff, J.J.; Hamilton, A.S.& Katz, S.J. (2010). Patterns and Correlates of Adjuvant Radiotherapy Receipt After Lumpectomy and After Mastectomy for Breast Cancer. *J Clin Oncol*, Vol. 28, No. 14, pp. 2396-2403

Jalali, R.; Singh, S.& Budrukkar, A. (2007). Techniques of tumour bed boost irradiation in breast conserving therapy: Current evidence and suggested guidelines. *Acta Oncol* Vol. 46, pp. 879-92

Janjan, N.; Lutz, S.; Bedwinek, J.; *et al.* (2009). Therapeutic guidelines for the treatment of bone metastasis: A report from the American College of Radiology Appropriateness Criteria Expert Panel on Radiation Oncology. *J Palliat Med,* Vol. 12, pp. 417-423

Joensuu, H.; Bono, P.; Kataja, V.; Alanko, T.; Kokko, R.; Asola, R.; Utriainen, T.; Turpeenniemi-Hujanen, T.; Jyrkkiö, S.; Möykkynen, K.; Helle, L.; Ingalsuo, S.; Pajunen, M.; Huusko, M.; Salminen, T.; Auvinen, P.; Leinonen, H.; Leinonen, M.; Isola, J. & Kellokumpu-Lehtinen, P.L. (2009). Fluorouracil, epirubicin, and cyclophosphamide with either docetaxel or vinorelbine, with or without trastuzumab, as adjuvant treatments of breast cancer: final results of the FinHer Trial. *J Clin Oncol*, Vol. 27, No. 34, pp. 5685-92

Kaasa, S.; Brenne, E.; Lund, J.-A.; *et al.* (2006). Prospective randomized multicentre trial on single fraction radiotherapy (8 Gy x 1) versus multiple fractions (3 Gy x 10) in the treatment of painful bone metastases. *Radiol Oncol,* Vol. 79, pp.278-284

Khaled, H.; Emara, M.E.; Gaafar, R.M.; Mansour, O.; Abdel Warith, A.; Zaghloul, M.S.; El Malt, O. (2008). Primary chemotherapy with low-dose prolonged infusion gemcitabine and cisplatin in patients with bladder cancer: A Phase II trial. *Urol Oncol*, Vol. 26, No. 2, pp. 133–6

Klotz,L; O'Callaghan,C.J; Ding, K;, D; Dearnaley P; C. S. Higano, C.S; E. M. Horwitz, E.M;

Malone, S;. Goldenberg,S.L;, M. K. Gospodarowicz, M.K; Crook,J.M. (2011). A phase III randomized trial comparing intermittent versus continuous androgen suppression for patients with PSA progression after radical therapy *J Clin Oncol; 29* suppl 7, abstr 3

Kolodziej, M.A. (2011). Does Evidence-Based Medicine Really Reduce Costs? *Oncology*, Vol. 25, No. 3, Available from <http://www.cancernetwork.com/practice/content/article/10165/1821731?GUID=FB148439-5EF7-471B-8A2A-46E108E67287&rememberme=1&source=NL>

Lash, T.L.; Lien, E.A.; Sorensen, H.T. & Hamilton-Dutoit, S. (2009). Genotype-guided tamoxifen therapy: time to pause for reflection? *Lancet Oncol*, Vol. 10, pp. 825–833

Malin, J.L. (2010). Wrestling with the high price of cancer care: should control costs by individuals 'ability to pay or society wildlings to pay? *J Clin Oncol*, Vol. 28, pp. 3212-3214

Meropol, N.J. & Schulman, K.A. (2007). Cost of cancer care: issues and implications. *J Clin Oncol*, Vol. 25, pp. 180-186

Meropol, N.J.; Schrag, D.; Smith, T.J.; *et al.* (2009). American Society of Clinical Oncology guidance statement: The cost of cancer care. *J Clin Oncol*, Vol. 27, pp. 3868–3874

Mileshkin, L.; Schofield, P.E.; Jefford M.; *et al.* (2009). To tell or not to tell: The community wants to know about expensive anticancer drugs as a potential treatment option. *J Clin Oncol.* Vol. 27, pp. 5830–5837

Mitsumori, M. & Hiraoka, M. (2008). Current status of accelerated partial breast irradiation. *Breast Cancer,* Vol. 15, No. 1, pp. 101-7

Munshi, A. (2007). Breast cancer radiotherapy and cardiac risk: The 15-year paradox. *J Cancer Res Ther*, Vol. 3, pp. 190-2

Munshi, A. (2009). Resource-sparing and cost-effective strategies in current management of breast cancer. *J Can Res Ther*, Vol. 5, pp. 116-20

Neubauer, M.A.; Hoverman, J.R.; Kolodziej, M.; *et al.* (2010). Cost effectiveness of evidence-based treatment guidelines for the treatment of non–small-cell lung cancer in the community setting. *J Oncol Pract,* Vol. 6, pp. 12-18

Overgaard, J.; Mohanti, B.; Bhasker, S.; Begum, N.; Ali, R., Agarwal, J.; Kuddu, M.; Baeza, M.; Vikram, B. & Grau, C. (2006). Accelerated versus conventional fractionated radiotherapy in squamous cell carcinoma of head and neck. A randomized international multicentere trial with 908 patients conducted by the IAEA-ACC study group. *Int J Radiat Oncol Biol Phys.*, Vol. 66, No. 3, Suppl., pp. S13

Paik, S.; Taniyama, Y. & Geyer C.E. Jr. (2008). Anthracyclines in the treatment of HER2-negative breast cancer. *J Natl Cancer Inst*, Vol. 100, pp. 2-4

Phillips, K.A.; Marshall, D.A.; Haas, J.S.; *et al.* (2009). Clinical practice patterns and cost effectiveness of human epidermal growth receptor 2 testing strategies in breast cancer patients. *Cancer,* Vol. 115, No. 22, pp. 5166-5174

Porter, A.; Aref, A.; Chodounsky, Z.; Elzawawy, A.; Manatrakul, N.; Ngoma, T.; Orton, C.; Van't Hooft, E.& Sikora, K. (1999). A global strategy for radiotherapy: A WHO consultation. *Clin Oncol (R Coll Radiol)*, Vol. 9, No. 11, pp. 368–370.

Punglia, R.S.; Winer, E.P.; Weeks, J.C. & Burstein, H.J. (2007). Could treatment with tamoxifen be superior to aromatase inhibitors in early-stage breast cancer after pharmacogenomic testing? A modeling analysis. *J Clin Oncol*, Vol. 25, pp. 502

Ratain, M.J. & Cohen, E.E. (2007). The value meal: how to save $1,700 per month or more on lapatinib. *J Clin Oncol,* Vol. 25, pp. 3397–3398.

Sachs, D.L.; Kang, S.; Hammerberg, C.; Helfrich, Y.; Karimipour, D.; Orringer, J.; Johnson, T.; Hamilton, T.A.; Fisher, G.& Voorhees, J. (2009). Topical Fluorouracil for Actinic Keratoses and Photoaging. A Clinical and Molecular Analysis. *Arch Dermatol,* Vol. 45, No. 6, pp. 659-666.

Sarin, R. (2005). Partial-breast treatment for early breast cancer: emergence of a new paradigm. *Nat Clin Pract Oncol*, Vol. 2, No. 1, pp. 40-7

Sarrazin, D.; Le, M.; Arriagada, R.; Contesso, G.; Fontaine, F.; Spielman, M.; Rochar, F.; Le Chevalier, T.H. & La Cour, J. (1989). Ten Year results of randomized trial comparing a conservative treatment to mastectomy in early breast cancer. *Radiother Oncolol*, Vol. 14, pp. 177

Schrag, D. & Hanger, M. (2007). Medical oncologists' views on communicating with patients about chemotherapy costs: A pilot survey. *J Clin Oncol*, Vol. 25, pp.233–237

Schrag, D. (2004). The price tag on progress -- chemotherapy for colorectal cancer. *N Engl J Med*, Vol. 351, pp. 317-319

Stewart, B.W. & Kleihues, P. (2003). World Cancer Report. IARC Press, Lyon, France

Sullivan, S.D.; Watkins, J.; Sweet, B.; *et al.* (2009). Health technology assessment in health-care decisions in the United States. *Val Health*, Vol. 12, Suppl. 2, pp. S39–S44

The START Trialists' Group. (2008). The UK Standardisation of Breast Radiotherapy (START) Trial B of radiotherapy hypofractionation for treatment of early breast cancer: a randomised trial. *Lancet*, Vol. 29, No. 371, pp. 1098–1107

Torres Edejer, T.T.; Baltussen, R.; Adam, T.; *et al.* (2003). Making choices in health: WHO guide to cost-effectiveness analysis. World Health Organization, Geneva, Switzerland

Truong, P.T.; Olivotto, I.A.; Whelan, T.J.& Levine, M. (2004). Clinical practice guidelines for the care and treatment of breast cancer: 16. Locoregional post-mastectomy radiotherapy. *CMAJ*, Vol. 170, No. 8, pp. 1261–1273

Van den Hout,W.B.;Van der Linden, Y.M.; Steenland, E.;Wiggenraad, R.G.; Kievit, J.; de Haes, H. & Leer, J.W. (2003). Single-Versus Multiple-Fraction Radiotherapy in Patients with Painful Bone Metastases: Cost-Utility Analysis Based on a Randomized Trial. *Journal of the National Cancer Institute*, Vol. 95, No. 3, pp. 222–29.

Weeks, J. C. (2003). Outcomes Assessment, In: *Cancer Medicine*, Kuff, D.W., Pollok, R.E., Weichselbaum, R.R., Bast, R.C., Gansler, T.S., Holland, J.F., Frei, E, pp. 479 -502, BC Decker Inc., ISBN 1-55009-213-8, Hamilton-London.

Wennberg, J.E.; Fisher, E.S.; Goodman, D.C. & Skinner, J.S. (2008). Tracking the care of patients with severe chronic illness. In: Dartmouth Institute for Health Policy and Clinical Practice. The Dartmouth atlas of health care 2008. Available from <http://www.dartmouthatlas.org/downloads/atlases/2008_Chronic_Care_Atlas.pdf>

WHO, World Health Statistics 2010. France: World Health Organization, Department of Health Statistics and Informatics of the Information, Evidence and Research Cluster, 2010.

Yarney, J.; Vanderpuye, V.& Clegg Lamptey, J.N. (2008). Hormone receptor and HER-2 expression in breast cancers among Sub-Saharan African women. *Breast J*, Vol. 14, pp. 510–511

Yip, C.H.; Cazap, E.; Anderson, B.O.; Bright, K.L.; Caleffi, M.; Cardoso, F.; Elzawawy, A.M.; Harford, J.B.; Krygier, G.D.; Masood, S.; Murillo, R.; Muse, I.M.; Otero, I.V.; Passman, L.J.; Santini, L.A.; da Silva, R.C.; Thomas, D.B.; Torres, S.; Zheng, Y.& Khaled, H.M. (2011).Breast cancer management in middle-resource countries (MRCs): consensus statement from the Breast Health Global Initiative. *Breast*, Suppl 2, pp. S12-9.

Zwitter, M.; Kovac, V.; Smrdel, U.; Kocijancic, I.; Segedin, B. & Vrankar, M. (2005). Phase I–II trial of low-dose gemcitabine in prolonged infusion and cisplatin for advanced non-small cell lung cancer. *Anticancer Drugs*, Vol. 16, pp. 1129–1134.